FOURTH EDITION

Maximize Your Body Potential

Lifetime Skills for Healthy Weight and Lifestyle

Joyce D. Nash, Ph.D.

Bull Publishing Company
Boulder, Colorado

Bull Publishing Company
P.O. Box 1377
Boulder, CO USA 80306
www.bullpub.com

Library of Congress Cataloging-in-Publication Data

Names: Nash, Joyce D., author. | Nash, Joyce D. New maximize your body potential.

Title: Maximize your body potential : lifetime skills for healthy weight and lifestyle / Joyce D. Nash, Ph.D.

Description: Fourth Edition. | Boulder : Bull Publishing Company, 2021. | Revised edition of the author's Maximize your body potential, c2003. | Summary: "Here in one book are all of the tools that anyone can use to develop ways to be successful in managing body weight. Using self-tests, checklists, and fill-in forms, Maximize Your Body Potential shows the reader how to make a commitment, how to set realistic goals, and how to design an individualized exercise and eating program"-- Provided by publisher.

Identifiers: LCCN 2021006769 (print) | LCCN 2021006770 (ebook) | ISBN 9781933503202 (paperback) | ISBN 9781945188510 (epub)

Subjects: LCSH: Weight loss. | Weight loss--Psychological aspects.

Classification: LCC RM222.2 .N3718 2021 (print) | LCC RM222.2 (ebook) | DDC 613.2/5--dc23

LC record available at https://lccn.loc.gov/2021006769

LC ebook record available at https://lccn.loc.gov/2021006770

Printed in the U.S.A.

26 25 24 23 22 21   10 9 8 7 6 5 4 3 2 1

Interior design and production by Dovetail Publishing Services

Cover design and production by Shannon Bodie, Bookwise Design

For Morgan,
who has stood by me in all my pursuits.

Also by this Author

Contents

List of Figures, Self-Tests, and Tables

Figures

Self-Tests

Tables

About the Author

Joyce D. Nash, PhD, is a clinical psychologist with specialties in eating disorders and behavioral medicine. She holds two doctorates—one in clinical psychology from Palo Alto University and one in communication from Stanford University, where she also did postdoctoral work in nutrition at the Stanford University School of Medicine. Dr. Nash has authored nine books on cognitive-behavioral medicine and most recently authored her first fiction book entitled *Curveballs*. Dr. Nash lives with her husband in Reno, Nevada.

Introduction

Maximize Your Body Potential, Fourth Edition, is not a diet book. No doubt you've heard that diets don't work! That's true. At least they don't work in the long run. Some experts have offered lots of reasons for this: they aren't sustainable (you can't follow their rules for life), they are a form of starvation and the body reacts negatively to that, diets cause binge eating, diets cause you to obsess over food, diets increase cravings, diets mess up your hunger cues, diets cause your metabolism to slow down, any weight loss you experience on a diet is only temporary—you regain it back and often more in due time, diets make some foods or food groups off limits, diets cause stress, which activates cortisol, the stress hormone, and dieting takes the joy and pleasure out of eating. And there are lots more reasons offered for why diets don't work, many of which are true, if not comprehensive.

But have you ever heard *the real reason why* they don't work? The fact is, obesity is a progressive disease. That means that obesity begets obesity—just being fat causes you to gain more fat! The fact is that temporary or fad diets, cleanses, fasting, and crash dieting cause changes in the body that make it hard to lose weight, and even if weight is lost, it is harder to keep it off. That's because dieting makes the body "think" it's starving. To save energy, the body starts to conserve. The usual amount of fat needed for doing low-grade activities such as walking, cleaning the house, fixing dinner, or working on the computer is reduced. And dieting increases the capacity of the body to store even more fat. These changes lead to a progressive increase in fat accumulation even if the individual is not overeating.

So, what happens when you gain weight? A number of hormonal, metabolic, and molecular changes happen in the body, which increase the risk for even greater fat accumulation. Such obesity-associated biological changes reduce the body's ability to burn fuel for energy, increase the conversion of blood glucose to fat, and increase the body's capacity to store more fat in adipose tissues. This means that more of the calories consumed will be stored as fat. To make matters worse, obesity affects certain regulators of appetite and hunger in a manner that favors further weight gain. Dieting increases the appetite and feelings of hunger. And this is true for both those who are overweight and those who are obese.

Yes, it's unfair, but there is a solution: make gradual basic changes in your lifestyle that lead you to adopt a healthy eating pattern and engage in the right kind of exercise. And, of course, you need to find better ways of coping with stress. The switch you need to make with your health goals is moving from short-term, one-size-fits-all thinking and, instead, learn to make choices you can realistically sustain for years. Shift to gradually building up your changes and new habits over time as if you are building a house—lay a solid foundation of changes and gradually building upon them with more gradual changes. This means taking your wellness vision and breaking it down into tiny action steps. Take one habit or behavior at a time as a target for change. It does not mean waking up tomorrow and trying to do everything at once. Take one behavior at a time and really work through it until it's easy and fully integrated into your life. Then onto the next habit.

Maximize Your Body Potential, Fourth Edition, provides the guide for making lifestyle changes that last. It is based on the most up-to-date nutritional and dietary information available—the "2015–2020 Dietary Guidelines for Americans." These guidelines reflect the evidence that healthy eating patterns and regular exercise are needed to achieve and maintain good health and reduce the risk of chronic disease throughout all stages of your life. The current dietary guidelines provide five specific guidelines and a number of key recommendations to help Americans ages 2 years and older and their families make the lifestyle changes needed for better health.

Maximize Your Body Potential, Fourth Edition, promotes cognitive-behavioral principles such as goal setting, self-monitoring, environmental management, portion control, positive self-talk, and problem solving. It details three healthy eating patterns including the US-style eating pattern, the Mediterranean-style eating pattern, and the Vegetarian-style eating pattern. The dietary guidelines include recommendations for physical activity as well. In addition, recommendations for adequate physical activity from the American College of Sports Medicine are included.

Chapter 1 discusses obesity as a chronic and complex disease. It answers the question: "Is it possible to be healthy at any weight?" It also takes to task the notion that all that counts is doing exercise to be physically fit without having to consider eating habits or body fat.

Chapter 2 defines the terms *overweight* and *obesity*. Body mass index, or BMI, is the common way of assessing these conditions, although there are several other means of doing so. Adults are not the only ones to carry too much weight and body fat. More than 60 percent of Americans are either overweight or obese, and children and teens are gaining weight. Help for younger folks is included here. Does fat sit there in the body and just hang out? No. This chapter provides information on the dynamics of body fat.

Chapter 3 presents important information on the chronic diseases that put a heavier person at risk for poor health. This chapter considers the effect of excess weight on both physical and mental health. It provides information on how to get professional help for both, as well as suggests ways you can cope now.

Chapter 4 gives detailed information on the causes of overweight and obesity. This chapter discusses genes and heredity, hormones, culture, and other outside influences, as well as personal indulgences.

Chapter 5 helps the reader differentiate between "good" and "bad" cholesterol. Most importantly, it details the danger of *metabolic syndrome*, also known as *insulin resistance syndrome*. One means of assessing this syndrome is through measuring waist circumference. Finally, medical treatment of obesity is considered.

Motivation for changing behavior is always a problem. Chapter 6 discusses the roles of goal setting and values on habit and how to get motivated to adopt a new healthy eating pattern. Social support can be a source of motivation, and this chapter focuses on the role of a social support person and how to choose that person to help you.

Chapter 7 addresses the all-important need for behavior change and how to achieve it The basics of changing cues and using rewards are given. Cognition refers to all forms of knowing and awareness, such as perceiving, conceiving, believing, remembering, reasoning, judging, imagining, and envisioning problem solving. In short, thinking. Cognition and feelings affect behavior, and one way to understand them is as a series of cues and rewards. Subconscious thinking and cognitive distortions are discussed in this chapter. How to undertake new responses to challenging situations is examined. Help for overcoming cravings is also provided. The chapter outlines the need for mindfulness to change behavior.

The "2015–2020 Dietary Guidelines" put out by the government outline three healthy eating patterns—a US-style eating pattern, a Mediterranean-style eating pattern, and a Vegetarian-style eating pattern. Chapter 8 discusses shifts needed to achieve any of these eating patterns. The dietary guidelines also provide key recommendations, which are included in this chapter.

Chapter 9 provides basic nutrition and weight management information. It also discusses whether food addictions or sugar sensitivity can be problems for the person who wants to adopt healthier eating. To help the reader accomplish healthy eating without sugar issues, the chapter gives information on the glycemic index and glycemic load and summarizes the food exchange system for choosing foods. Reading food labels and meal planning are covered as important ways of adopting healthy eating.

Chapter 10 focuses on exercise and health. Physical activity guidelines for ages through 65 and older ages are provided. Information on how to begin an exercise program or how to work toward greater exercise fitness are included. Guidance for choosing a gym or hiring a personal trainer is covered in this chapter. Most important, instructions are given for walking for health and weight loss. Learn how to increase activities of daily living to improve health.

Chapter 11 introduces important aspects of thinking and altering self-talk to promote behavior change. This chapter covers cognitive distortions that interfere with thinking and behavior, and it describes the kind of helping and hindering self-talk that can undermine motivation. Attention is given to core beliefs, the stories we tell ourselves, and how these affect behaviors.

Chapter 12 extends the focus of chapter 11 on thinking and behavior. Behavior is affected by automatic thoughts and "inner voices." Some of the types of inner voices include the "Internal Critic," the "Victim," and others. Identifying inner voices and fostering a supportive voice helps change behaviors. Creating counterbalancing statements or thoughts is one way of coping with inner voices.

Managing stress is the mandate of chapter 13. Assessing the cause of stress and available coping skills is the first step toward reducing stress. Problem-focused coping and emotion-focused coping are discussed here. This chapter highlights the need to fight back against the "inner bully." Additional topics in this chapter include mindfulness for managing stress, assertiveness, coping with interpersonal conflict, and managing emotions.

Chapter 14 takes aim at stopping the binge-eating cycle and binge-eating disorder (BED). The first step is to analyze and understand the binge cycle. Types of binges are discussed and the need for forgiveness—of self and others—is described. To interrupt and change binge eating, the eating pattern needs to be "normalized."

It is also necessary to "binge proof" the house and cope more effectively with "danger" foods.

Backsliding is a big problem for most people trying to change habits. Chapter 15 analyzes the causes of lapses and gives tips for handling high-risk situations. Triggers for backsliding are provided here, and suggestions for translating intentions into action are described.

1

Health and Lifestyle

Nita was considerably overweight. Her young daughter, Gaby, was too. Nita worked two jobs trying to make ends meet. Often it was easier to pick up dinner at the local McDonald's than try to cook at home. Nita disliked the taste of diet drinks and preferred drinking Classic Coke. Gaby went to a nearby grade school, which provided lunches—typical choices included corn dogs, chicken nuggets, chips, cookies, apples, and sweet drink options. Nita worried that Gaby had to walk back and forth to school, even though it was only a few blocks, because the neighborhood was known to be unsafe. She insisted that Gaby stay inside to play or do her homework. Gaby didn't have many friends at school anyway; she was teased about her weight and her mother's weight. The doctor told Nita that her blood pressure was high, as was her cholesterol, and she needed to lose weight. Nita had tried diets before, but none worked.

Perhaps you have heard of mumps, measles, smallpox, malaria, polio, and other "old" diseases that were the scourge of your grandparents and great-grandparents. These were often the cause of death during their lifetimes. At the turn of the century, in the early 1900s, the average life expectancy was 50. By 2020, it had increased to 79. Now society has medicines, injections, vaccines, and other means that have virtually eliminated these earlier diseases. With advances in medicine, people are living longer, but now there are health conditions that our ancestors mostly didn't have to deal with—heart disease, type 2 diabetes, hypertension, stroke, musculoskeletal disease, cancer, obesity, Alzheimer's, and the like. To meet these and newer challenges to health and longevity requires making lifestyle changes.

Ask any doctor or nurse. They will say that most of today's diseases are influenced to a large degree by a poor-quality diet, lack of adequate exercise, and difficulty dealing with stress. When it comes to eating a healthy diet, many people understand they should avoid saturated fats, eat a varied diet, and keep sodium and alcohol to a minimum. Most people know that too many calories consumed combined with not enough of the right kind of exercise leads to weight gain. Even though gyms and fitness centers have proliferated, most people don't take advantage of them. Carbohydrates, in general, have gotten a bad reputation for causing weight gain, and dietary supplements claiming to reduce cravings and promote weight loss, increase mental sharpness, or promote energy are doing a booming business.

When it comes to improving health, many people say, "I know what to do. I just don't do it." And there's the rub. Some people think they know what to do to achieve good health, but many have been duped by misinformation and bad health claims. Perhaps their knowledge is simply out-of-date. Even if they are well-informed, some people can't find the motivation to change.

Obesity Is a Disease

Obesity is a complex chronic disease that should be properly assessed and treated seriously. It is second only to smoking tobacco as the leading cause of preventable death in the United States. According to the Centers for Disease Control and Prevention (CDC), the prevalence of obesity (defined as a body mass index [BMI] between 30 to 39.9) in the United States was 42.4 percent between 2017 and 2018. Between 1999 and 2000, and between 2017 and 2018, the prevalence of severe obesity (>40 BMI) increased from 4.7 to 9.2 percent.

Taking overweight as well as obesity into account, more than 70 percent of US adults are overweight or obese according to the 2013–2014 National Health and Nutrition Examination Survey (NHANES) data. Men are more overweight or obese than most women (73.7 percent versus 66.9 percent respectively). Only at a BMI of 30 or greater do women surpass men in having obesity.

Body mass index is the tool commonly used to estimate and screen for overweight and obesity in adults and children. BMI is defined as weight in kilograms divided by height in meters squared. For most people, BMI is a good estimate of the amount of body fat in their bodies, which can raise the risk of many health problems. Obesity-related conditions include heart disease, stroke, type 2 diabetes,

Table 1.1 BMI Categories

	All (Men and Women)	Men	Women
Overweight or Obese	70.2	73.7	66.9
Overweight (BMI 25 to 29.9)	32.5	38.7	26.5
Obesity (BMI 30 to 40)	37.7	35	40.4
Extreme Obesity (BMI >40)	7.7	5.5	9.9

and certain types of cancer, all of which are leading causes of pre-ventable, premature death.

Of course, weight is just one measure of health. People who are slimmer but don't exercise or eat nutritious foods aren't necessarily healthy just because they don't appear to be overweight. Excess body fat can be a killer for both those who are obese as well as for some who fall in the healthy weight range of a BMI table.

What Is a Healthy Weight?

A healthy weight is the weight your body naturally settles into when you consistently eat a varied and nutritious diet of moderate caloric intake appropriate to your age, gender, and body type, and when you are physically active on a regular basis so that calories in and calories out are balanced. A body mass index chart is used by many people to determine a healthy weight range. A BMI chart is shown in chapter 2 on page 17.

Recommended BMI ranges work for most people, although it is not a good measure for a few elite athletes, such as football players, who may be "overweight" according to the chart when, in fact, they simply have a lot of muscle, which weighs more than fat. Similarly, a marathon runner, bicycle racer, or ice skater may register at the lower end of the BMI scale because they have long, lean muscles and a high proportion of lean body mass. Thus, the BMI scale is not a good approximation of body fat in the case of many highly trained athletes. Similarly, a BMI chart is not considered a good single mea-sure of healthy weight for children, pregnant women, or the sick or elderly, the latter of whom have, in most cases, lost muscle mass as well as bone density.

At the same time, persons who are in the upper regions of the "healthy" weight range on the BMI chart may need to consider los-ing some weight if they have two or more factors indicating risk for heart disease (for example, a person with high levels of low-density lipoprotein cholesterol or LDL—one type of lipid or fat that circu-lates in the blood—who also has high blood pressure or other risk factors). And people who have other diseases associated with a high weight, such as coronary artery disease, type 2 diabetes, or sleep apnea may be advised to lose weight even if their BMI is within the healthy range.

Despite the existence of different methods for measuring levels of body fat in individuals, there is general agreement that excess weight can be a health risk. But it is safe to say that a truly healthy weight is one that minimizes risk of weight-related diseases (like metabolic syndrome, defined in a later chapter), is realistic for your body and heredity, and is one that can be comfortably maintained with healthy choices and habits, including regular exercise. Even those whose jobs require a lot of activity and who don't appear over-weight may have risk factors for disease that are undiagnosed.

Other factors such as inactivity and smoking must be considered when assessing what is a healthy weight. Smoking contributes to lower weight but increases the risk of disease and premature dying. BMI alone should not be used to determine a healthy body weight, but it is a good guide for beginning to assess disease risk. Other body measures that correlate with health are waist circumference and waist-to-hip ratio. Both of these have been shown to be related to higher risk of coronary heart disease. Experts agree that BMI together with waist girth and waist-to-hip ratio are important initial screen-ings for unhealthy body weight.

Is It Possible to Be Healthy at Any Weight?

Healthy obesity refers to excess body fat without the presence of metabolic syndrome, which is discussed more in chapter 5.

People who are overweight but healthy typically have some lev-els of fat in the abdomen and lower cardiovascular risk compared to people within the healthy weight range and those with more severe obesity as indicated on a BMI chart. However, studies have found that at least half of those without metabolic syndrome ultimately convert to metabolically unhealthy obesity with increased risk of cardiovascular disease. In the Nurses' Health Study, 84 percent of women who had healthy obesity—that is, no metabolic syndrome factors—converted to unhealthy after twenty years of follow-up. The Multi-Ethnic Study of Atherosclerosis (MESA) study reported that 48 percent of those with healthy obesity developed metabolic syndrome and an increased risk of cardiovascular disease during a median of twelve years of follow-up.

Apparently positive reports of people who are metabolically healthy but are obese are highly dependent on how *healthy* is defined. According to one health expert with more strict definitions, it is hard to find obese but healthy individuals. So, the answer to the question of is it possible to be obese and healthy is: "*Yes—as long as the person does not have metabolic syndrome.*" Over time, however, it is unlikely one can sustain good health and be obese. In the long run, it is healthier to focus on weight management and leading a healthy lifestyle.

Some obese people have been led to believe that it is more important to "just be fit" and have added 10 to 15 minutes of walking to their daily routine or have purchased a Fitbit wrist device to track their physical activity. Of course, such efforts are to be applauded. But for many obese people, the message that physical activity is more important than managing weight is not only unhelpful but also not true. When it comes to health and wellness, fatness can matter more than fitness. Focusing on healthy eating is just as important. Furthermore, for most people, excess weight can make exercise much harder.

> **Metabolic syndrome** is a cluster of conditions that occur together, increasing your risk of heart disease, stroke, and type 2 diabetes. These conditions include increased blood pressure, high blood sugar, excess body fat around the waist, and abnormal cholesterol or triglyceride levels.

Happy Weight Versus Healthy Weight

Odds are you weigh more now than you did twenty years ago. Most of us do. And not only has your waistline grown, but your idea of an "ideal" weight may have changed. In a recent Gallup poll,

60 percent of respondents described their present weight as "just about right." That's just about the percent of people who are identified in research as overweight or obese. It may be that the respondents to the poll were not entirely truthful. Or, hopefully, they aren't experiencing body dissatisfaction or worry about their weight. In essence, they are saying that they are at their happy weight.

In 2013, a study came out that claimed people who were up to 30 pounds overweight were less likely to die earlier than people who were in a healthy weight range as defined by body mass index. In fact, this study had major flaws, and its conclusion, while hopeful, was wrong.

Decades of research has demonstrated that obesity leads to many serious health problems as well as increased mortality. Extra pounds make you more likely to develop coronary heart disease, type 2 diabetes, high blood pressure, stroke, some types of cancer, and even dementia. The key to reducing your risk of these diseases and others is to evaluate your situation and your lifestyle. You'll need to identify your body mass index and, if it is unhealthy, consider what lifestyle changes you need to make to bring your weight more in line with the healthy range. Measure your waist size for a start. Your waist size can give you a better picture of your health than your bathroom scale. Simply take a tape measure and put it around your waist right above your belly button. If your waist size is over 35 inches if you are a woman, or if it is over 40 inches if you are a man, it's time to take some action.

Don't get caught up in tables of "ideal" weights. Some health professionals don't even like to talk about ideal weight. The fact is, even small amounts of weight loss can help reduce risks of chronic diseases. Instead of focusing on an ideal weight, focus on making changes in your lifestyle that will bring about improvement. A 7 to 10 percent weight loss makes a huge impact on your metabolism. Small changes are more likely to become permanent, and one small change often leads to another. Remember: it's never too late to make healthy changes in your lifestyle.

Defining Overweight and Obesity

Hideko weighed herself at home and checked her weight against an online BMI table. She was pleased to learn she was in the "healthy weight" range. All of Hideko's friends told her she looked great. Hideko tried to make healthy food choices, but she didn't get any exercise. She was surprised when her doctor told her that her cholesterol was high. He prescribed a medication that would help lower her cholesterol. When she got home, she did an internet search to find out more about cholesterol. She learned that there was more she could do to get healthy.

Overweight and *obesity* are both labels for ranges of weight that are greater than what is generally considered healthy or that have been shown to correlate with the risk of certain diseases and other health problems. Body mass index, or BMI, is the ratio of body weight to height and is highly correlated with body fat. Although there are some exceptions, for most adults BMI is a reliable indicator of body fatness and is one measure commonly used to assess whether one's body weight is healthy.

Body Mass Index

Body mass index, which is a statistical measure of the relationship between a person's weight and height, is useful when generalizing about groups of people. Healthcare professionals use BMI to classify people as underweight, healthy weight, overweight, or obese. Although BMI correlates well with the amount of body fat, it does not directly measure body fat. As a result, it is no more than one possible indicator and is not necessarily accurate when applied to all individuals. In addition to body fat, race, gender, and age also must be considered. For example, compared to whites, Asians tend to have lower BMIs but higher percentages of body fat. Women have more fat under the skin than men, who have a greater muscle mass than women of the same weight. Elder adults tend to weigh less than middle-aged adults because they have lost muscle mass.

There are various formulae for determining body mass index, but the easiest way is to look up BMI in a table that gives weight ranges correlating to BMI. To check your BMI, refer to table 2.1.

Although the cutoff points for weight ranges of BMI can vary, for adults, a healthy weight is generally defined as a BMI in the 18.5 to 24.9 range. Overweight is defined as a BMI of 25.0 to 29.9, and obesity as having a BMI of 30.0 or more. Those with a BMI of 40.0 to 49.9 are designated as morbidly obese (i.e., having serious health risk) or severely obese, while those with a BMI equal to or greater than 50.0 are termed *super obese*. People with a BMI less than 18.4 points are termed *underweight*, and a BMI of 17.5 or less is one criterion used to diagnose anorexia nervosa. Younger people should be closer to the lower end of the healthy weight range while middle-aged adults may be in the upper ranges of healthy BMI weights.

Assessing Body Composition

While BMI is easy to use and is a far better method for assessing healthy weight than weighing on a scale, there are a number of other methods for estimating body composition. These include skinfold thickness measurement, hydrodensitometry (underwater weighing),

Table 2.1 BMI

Height	Underweight			Healthy Weight								Overweight						Obese		
BMI	17	17.5	18	18.5	19	20	21	22	23	24	24.9	25	26	27	28	29	29.9	30	35	40
4'10"	81	84	86	89	91	96	101	105	110	115	119	120	124	129	134	139	143	144	168	192
4'11"	84	87	89	92	94	99	104	109	114	119	123	124	129	134	139	144	148	149	173	198
5'	87	90	92	95	97	102	108	113	118	123	128	128	133	138	143	149	153	154	179	205
5'1"	90	93	95	98	101	106	111	117	122	127	132	132	138	143	148	154	158	159	185	212
5'2"	93	96	98	101	104	109	115	120	126	131	136	137	142	148	153	159	164	164	191	219
5'3"	96	99	102	105	107	113	119	124	130	136	141	141	147	153	158	164	169	169	198	226
5'4"	99	102	105	108	111	117	122	128	134	140	145	146	152	157	163	169	174	175	204	233
5'5"	102	105	108	111	114	120	126	132	138	144	150	150	156	162	168	174	180	180	210	241
5'6"	105	108	112	115	118	124	130	136	143	149	154	155	161	167	174	180	185	186	217	248
5'7"	109	112	115	118	121	128	134	141	147	153	159	160	166	173	179	185	191	192	224	256
5'8"	112	115	118	122	125	132	138	145	151	158	164	165	171	178	184	191	197	197	230	263
5'9"	115	119	122	125	129	136	142	149	156	163	169	169	176	183	190	197	203	203	237	271
5'10"	119	122	126	129	133	139	146	153	160	167	174	174	181	188	195	202	209	209	244	279
5'11"	122	126	129	133	136	143	151	158	165	172	179	179	187	194	201	208	215	215	251	287
6'	125	129	133	137	140	148	155	162	170	177	184	184	192	199	207	214	221	221	258	295
6'1"	129	133	137	140	144	152	159	167	174	182	189	190	197	205	212	220	227	228	265	303
6'2"	132	136	140	144	148	156	164	171	179	187	194	195	203	210	218	226	223	234	273	312
6'3"	136	140	144	148	152	160	168	176	184	192	199	200	208	216	224	232	239	240	280	320
6'4"	140	144	148	152	156	164	173	181	189	197	205	206	214	222	230	238	246	247	288	329

bioelectrical impedance analysis (BIA), dual-energy X-ray absorptiometry (DXA), and a number of other methods. Each of these procedures has advantages and disadvantages and all have some margin of error. Regardless of the method used, 10 to 25 percent body fat is generally considered healthy in an adult man and 18 to 32 percent in an adult woman. Fat percentages above these levels are deemed unhealthy.

Skinfold Thickness

For skinfold thickness measurements, an instrument called a caliper is used to measure the thickness of fat at one or more sites on the body. This is one of the most common ways to assess body fat. However, it is more prone to error than other methods, in part because it requires skill on the part of the person measuring and it depends on the number and location of sites measured. If the calipers are not accurate, the readings will be false. If fewer locations are measured, there is a greater chance for error. Furthermore, skinfold thickness does not measure interstitial body fat (fat within and between muscles and organs). Skinfold thickness measurement assumes that the subcutaneous adipose layer (that is., the layer of fat just under the skin) reflects total body fat, but this association varies with age, gender, and race.

Underwater Weighing

Underwater weighing, also called hydrodensitometry, is based on the principle that fat tissue is less dense than muscle and bone. The process involves a specially constructed water tank in which the individual is submerged while exhaling the air from his or her lungs. Until recently, this method has been considered the reference standard for body composition studies and the most accurate method for measuring body composition. However, measurements are often difficult to obtain because the process requires special equipment, and many people have difficulty exhaling all their breath underwater.

Bioelectrical Impedance Analysis

Bioelectrical impedance analysis (BIA) is done by passing a small, harmless electrical current through the body and measuring electrical resistance. The underlying principle is that lean body mass conducts electricity better than body fat. Taken together with height and weight, the resistance measurement yields an estimate of the percent of body fat.

Results can vary based on how much water is in the body and where the electrodes are placed. To obtain the most precise reading, the person being tested should fast for four hours and lie down for several minutes prior to testing. (This is why most bathroom scales that presume to measure body fat are not very accurate even though they use a small current passing through the feet to assess body fat.) BIA may not be accurate in very obese individuals, and it is not useful for tracking short-term changes in body fat brought about by calorie reduction or exercise.

Dual Energy X-ray Absorptiometry

Dual energy X-ray absorptiometry (DXA) is emerging as the new reference standard for body composition studies, replacing underwater weighing. However, like BIA, this method can be affected by how much water is contained in body tissues at the time of measurement. (Dehydration will affect its accuracy.) It is also unclear how this method can be used for assessing body composition except for repeated measurements that would show changes. For now, DXA remains a method used more by scientists and medical professionals than for common assessment of body composition.

Health Measurements

The beer belly (also called the "Buddha belly") is a visible manifestation of abdominal fat and has been recognized as the type of fat most associated with the highest health risks (as compared with fat located elsewhere in the body). The primary reason abdominal fat is unhealthy is that it is metabolically active, producing hormones and chemicals that harm the cardiovascular and other body systems. When waist size shrinks, levels of interleukin-6 (an inflammatory chemical produced by fat and certain other tissues) also decrease. Even if you aren't a lot overweight but you carry excess weight in your trunk, and you have other weight-related factors such as high blood pressure or high cholesterol, it is best to reduce your abdominal fat in order to decrease your risk of coronary heart disease and diabetes.

The purpose of determining waist and hip girth is to gain a measure of the amount of abdominal fat (also known as visceral fat). A flexible tape measure is all that is needed to assess waist circumference and hip circumference or girth. The waist measurement is taken at the narrowest waist level, or if this is not apparent, at the midpoint between the lowest rib and the top of the hip bone. The tape should not be pulled too tight or left too loose. The hip girth measurement is taken over minimal clothing at the level of the greatest protrusion of the buttocks muscles. When such measurements are taken, the gluteal muscles should be relaxed and not tensed. A person should stand with feet slightly apart when the hips are measured.

Waist Girth Measurement

The National Institutes of Health contends that risk for developing diseases increases greatly for women with a waist girth measurement of 35 inches or more and for men at 40 inches or more. Table 2.2 gives risk levels for waist or abdominal girth. Those in the High or Very High risk levels should consider undertaking a serious weight-loss endeavor.

Waist-to-Hip Ratio

The ratio of waist circumference to the hip circumference is related to the risk of coronary heart disease. To assess waist-to-hip ratio, simply divide the waist measurement by the hip girth. Table 2.3 shows levels of waist-to-hip ratios for men and women. Men with a

Table 2.2

Waist or Abdominal Girth in Inches by Risk Level

Risk Level	Men	Women*
Very High	>47	>43.5
High	39.5–47	35.5–43
Low	31.5–39	28.5–35
Very Low	<31.5	<28.5

Table 2.3

Levels of Risk for Waist-to-Hip Ratio

Risk Level	Men	Women*
Extreme	>1.00	>.90
High	.95–1.00	.85–.90
Average	.90–.95	.80–.85

*ACSM. (2005). *ACSM Guidelines for exercise testing and prescription*, 7th ed. New York: Lippincott, Williams, and Wilkins, 61.

waist-to-hip ratio of greater than .95 or women above .85 have unacceptable levels of risk.

Children, Teens, and Weight

Adults aren't the only ones getting fatter. Overweight is a serious health concern for children and adolescents.

In 2020, obesity was estimated in 18.5 percent of children and adolescents ages 2 to 19 years old and affected about 13.7 million children and adolescents. What's more, overweight and obesity are increasing in our young. Among 2- to 5-year-olds, obesity affected 13.9 percent of this cohort. For those 6 to 11 years old, 18.4 percent were deemed obese. And of those 12 to 19 years old, 20.6 percent were obese. Furthermore, obesity is more prevalent in certain populations of children. More than 25 percent of Hispanic children are obese, while 22 percent of non-Hispanic Blacks are obese. Non-Hispanic Asians had lower obesity prevalence than Hispanics or non-Hispanic Blacks.

In the United States, body mass index is the measure used to determine overweight and obesity in children and adolescents. Overweight is defined as having a BMI at or above the 85th percentile for age and sex. Obesity is having a BMI at or above the 95th percentile.

Adolescents who are overweight or obese are at a higher risk of low self-esteem, distorted body image, depression, anxiety, discrimination, and strained peer relationships. Girls are at greater risk of this than boys, but they too suffer.

Obese boys and girls are starting to develop illnesses that used to be associated only with adults in their 40s and beyond—diabetes, heart disease, gallstones, and liver disease. Overweight and obese children and teens are increasingly being diagnosed with type 2 diabetes (originally termed *adult-onset diabetes*) as well as hypertension. Overweight and obese kids are also at greater risk for heart attacks and stroke. These diseases were unheard of among young people just a few decades ago. Overall, 90 percent of overweight kids have at least one avoidable risk factor for heart disease. What's more, large kids are more likely to be teased and bullied by peers and to suffer social stigma and ostracism, and are at greater risk for depression.

A chart of body mass index adjusted for children and adolescents is recommended by the CDC and the American Association of Pediatrics (AAP) for initial screening for overweight or underweight in children beginning at the age of 2. BMI helps identify children at risk for health problems such as type 2 diabetes and high blood pressure, but it is only a rough measure and not the only measure recommended for use. Other assessments such as skinfold thickness and evaluations of diet, physical activity level, and family history are also considered in assessing health risk.

Dynamics of Body Fat

To understand the damage that obesity can do, it is helpful to understand the dynamics of fat, but keep in mind that experts do not completely understand everything about fat. Past accepted wisdom was that people are all born with a fixed number of fat cells, and gaining or losing weight is simply a matter of filling or emptying those cells. But things appear to be more complicated than that. As weight increases beyond "normal," the number of fat cells also increases. Presumably fat cells, including these additional ones, can never be lost, and the more fat cells a person has, the harder it is to lose weight.

And fat cells don't just sit there and do nothing—at least not the ones deep inside the body. While fat stores just under the skin are relatively benign, deeper visceral fat inside the body can surround and even suffuse vital organs such as the liver. Visceral fat cells (those in the belly) also secrete hormones and cytokines (proteins that affect the immune system), which regulate the way cellular fuel is maintained and managed in the body. As food calories are absorbed, the pancreas secretes insulin, which prompts the liver to convert sugars into fat. Fat cells then release leptin, a hormone that tells the body it has received enough calories. (Hormones are chemical messengers that regulate body processes.) In essence, leptin puts the brakes on eating by making you feel full. Eating too many calories keeps insulin levels high and eventually leads to insulin resistance and, in due time, to type 2 diabetes. In the meantime, the disruption in these feedback mechanisms causes the brain and body to feel constantly hungry.

Additionally alarming to doctors is the impact of excess weight on the liver. This organ orchestrates the breakdown and distribution of fats and sugars from the diet. When too many calories from fat or sugar are consumed, the liver starts to keep some of the excess for itself, causing the development of a liver streaked with fat—that is, a fatty liver. Many overweight children already show abnormal levels of liver enzymes, and one-third suffer from liver damage. The remedy for these children is to get active and keep calorie input in line with what's burned off in activity. For children, as with adults, the bottom line is to eat moderately and get plenty of exercise.

Should I Have a Goal Weight in Mind?

Many people have in mind how much they want to lose to achieve a goal weight. Sometimes they pick this number from a BMI table. More often, they want to return to a weight they were when they were younger, or to some number they think they can accomplish. Or the number may be fanciful. Maybe a doctor told them how much they needed to lose. The problem is that these "goals" are putting the cart before the horse.

If you make gradual changes as you switch over to one of the healthy eating patterns that are described in *Maximize Your Body Potential* and you get adequate exercise, your weight will settle naturally to the "right" weight for your body. No more dieting. No more getting on the scale and feeling bad, or temporarily feeling good if you lose a pound. In fact, if you do weigh yourself, don't do it daily. Weigh only once a week, or once a month, at the same time of day and wearing the same clothes each time (or weigh yourself naked). The "goal" or "goals" you need to focus on are the small changes you can make that will take you closer to a healthy lifestyle. Diets make you crazy. Maintaining small changes over the long haul is the best goal.

Chronic Disease and Weight

At age 42, Lou knew he wasn't in the best of shape. He had a beer belly and going up stairs caused him to stop at the top to catch his breath. His father had died of a heart attack when he was Lou's current age, so Lou was a little worried. Lou didn't get much exercise. After work he liked coming home, getting in his easy chair in front of the TV, and having a cold beer. His wife, Milly, was a good cook, and she enjoyed making nice dinners for Lou. Milly was 40 pounds overweight too, but she and Lou had settled into a comfortable routine with their two young children. When Lou's doctor told him he should lose weight because his blood pressure was high, Lou asked Milly to try to cook differently. He bought her a new cookbook, which they went over together, picking out recipes that sounded good.

About 97 million adults in the United States are overweight or obese. Obesity and overweight contribute to increased risk of poor health, including heart disease, high blood pressure, high cholesterol, type 2 diabetes, insulin resistance, stroke, gallbladder disease, osteoarthritis, sleep apnea, as well as endometrial, breast, prostate, and colon cancers, and other diseases. Obese women are at risk for pregnancy complications and obese people have a higher incidence of arthritis and joint problems.

Cardiovascular Diseases

According to the World Health Organization, cardiovascular diseases (CVDs) are defined as disorders of the heart and blood vessels and are the number one cause of death globally. Multiple risk factors contribute to CVDs. Such risk factors can often be reduced with proper diet, adequate exercise, and weight reduction.

Coronary Heart Disease

Based on the National Health and Nutrition Examination Survey (NHANES) 2007–2010 survey, 15.4 million Americans above 20 years of age have coronary heart disease (CHD). In 2009, CHD accounted for 49 percent of cardiovascular deaths. Coronary heart disease refers to ailments of the heart caused by a narrowing of the coronary arteries (*atherosclerosis*), which reduces the blood supply to the heart. In people with CHD, fatty substances—primarily cholesterol—and fibrous tissue accumulate on artery walls, forming raised tissue patches called *plaques*. An accumulation of plaques reduces the supply of oxygen to the heart muscles causing pain (*angina*). If a plaque breaks loose and shuts off or reduces blood flow in an artery, the heart muscle is deprived of oxygen and nutrients, and a heart attack or stroke occurs.

Research has found that those who had heart attacks and who were overweight but not obese typically had heart attacks up to four to six years earlier than people in the healthy weight range. Obese people had heart attacks nearly a decade earlier than their healthy weight counterparts. In a study by the Mayo Clinic that adjusted for other health conditions, such as high blood pressure, high cholesterol, and diabetes, excess weight was still directly related to earlier heart attacks. Overweight patients had heart attacks an average of

3.6 years earlier than healthy weight people, and obese people had heart attacks an average of 8.2 years earlier. What's more, there is only a one in two chance of surviving a heart attack. Higher body weights are also associated with increases in premature death from other causes as well.

A diet low in saturated fats and high in fiber, fruits, whole grains, and vegetables reduces cardiovascular risk. Likewise, regular exercise and avoiding smoking are necessary to protect your heart. Blood pressure tends to rise with age, so you may want to purchase a blood pressure cuff from a drugstore to check your blood pressure at home as you get older. Your physician should monitor your blood pressure and prescribe medications as necessary to manage hypertension. A diet low in salt is also considered a good idea by many healthcare professionals.

Lou and Milly took his doctor's advice to change his diet seriously. They also decided they should get some exercise, so they started taking walks together right after dinner. Lou helped Milly with the dishes so they could get out and walk. When winter set in and they couldn't go for walks, they joined a gym. Lou went to the gym first thing in the morning before he went to work. He took his work clothes with him, showered at the gym after working out, and then dressed for work. Milly had to get the children off to school, so she decided it was easier to go to the gym once the kids were off.

Stroke

Each year, 795,000 people experience a stroke, and for most of them it is their first. On average, a stroke occurs in the United States every 40 seconds. According to the NHANES 2007–2010 survey, 6.8 million Americans above the age of 20 years of age have had a stroke. A stroke occurs when there is a lack of oxygen delivery to the brain. During this time, brain cells begin to die.

There are two main types of stroke. Ischemic stroke is the most common, accounting for 87 percent of all strokes. Hemorrhagic strokes, which account for 13 percent of all strokes, occur when a blood vessel in the brain leaks or ruptures. Stroke is caused by disruption to the flow of oxygenated blood to the brain. This disruption can be due to plaques or blood clots that have formed in the blood vessels.

Risk factors for stroke include hypertension, atrial fibrillation, obstructive sleep apnea, diabetes, physical inactivity, and high blood cholesterol. Obesity is the common link among these risk factors.

Heart Failure

As body weight increases, the total blood volume and the amount of blood pushed by the heart through the body also increases, resulting in increased cardiac output. The increase in the body's total blood volume also increases the volume of blood that flows into and out of the heart muscle. This causes dilation and enlargement of the ventricles of the heart. Throughout time, the muscle wall thickens, which leads to heart failure. The heart cannot pump blood to the lungs for oxygenation, which the brain and body require. A BMI greater than 25 is associated with risk of heart failure. For every unit of BMI increase, the risk of heart failure increases 5 and 7 percent in men and women, respectively.

Type 2 Diabetes

Type 2 diabetes affects nearly 24 million Americans. Three of every five people with type 2 diabetes have at least one complication of the disease, according to the American Association of Clinical Endocrinologists. Complications include cardiovascular disease, vision loss, kidney disease, or loss of limbs. Officially, diabetes is the seventh deadliest disease in the United States and is known to be an underreported contributing factor in deaths.

Diabetes is a disease in which the body does not produce or properly use insulin. Insulin helps your body convert sugar, starches, and other food into the energy needed for daily life. Type 2 diabetes, the type associated with obesity, primarily involves insulin insensitivity rather than lack of insulin production, as in type 1 diabetes. When insulin resistance occurs together with hypertension, high LDL and low HDL cholesterol, and certain other abnormalities, it is called *metabolic syndrome* or *syndrome X*. People classified as having this syndrome have a greater risk of premature death than those without it.

One out of four Americans ages 60 or older now has type 2 diabetes. Another 40 percent of those ages 40 to 70 are prediabetic—that is, their blood sugar levels are higher than normal but not quite high enough to be diabetic—and many do not know they are prediabetic. The link between weight and type 2 diabetes is clear: more than 80 percent of people with diabetes are overweight or obese. Scientists now know that fat cells—especially in the deeper, visceral fat around the belly—send out signals to other cells in the body, which result in the cells functioning abnormally. Some of these signals produce low levels of chronic inflammation and interfere with the insulin receptors on cells. In the process, these fat cells raise the risk of heart disease and other illnesses, such as cancer and stroke.

Trans fats in the diet are especially bad for diabetics, but a diet high in refined carbohydrates—sugar, corn syrup, white flour, white rice, white bread, some cereals, and even some supposedly whole wheat breads—also increases risk. Sugar itself does not cause diabetes, but sweetened foods, especially liquid calories from sweetened beverages, are a major contributor to obesity and subsequently to type 2 diabetes. The bottom line? It is best to stay away from sugary soft drinks, fruit juices (which are high in sugar), white bread, potatoes, white pasta, and sweets. Avoiding these products can help with weight loss and reduce the risk of developing type 2 diabetes. The good news is that risk can be reduced without a lot of weight loss. Of course, exercise is also necessary to lose weight and improve the health of diabetics.

If you already have diabetes, you know you need to be careful about what and when you eat, and you need to monitor your blood glucose. People with diabetes need to eat a low-glycemic diet, avoiding refined carbohydrates and choosing foods that have a low impact on blood sugar levels. A later chapter on nutrition provides more information on glycemic diets and advice on keeping a food record, measuring portions, tracking calories, and, of course, choosing foods wisely. Losing weight and keeping it off is the best way to make the most of living with diabetes.

Cancer

Evidence is now in that fat cells produce hormones that contribute to the development of certain cancers, especially those of the breast, endometrium (uterine lining), prostate, and colon. As discussed in the section on hormones in the next chapter, the fat cells of over-weight people are sometimes less sensitive to insulin, a hormone that regulates blood sugar. When fat cells are less sensitive to insu-lin, the body has to produce more insulin in order to remove sugar from the bloodstream. Extra insulin spurs cells to divide faster than they would otherwise, thereby increasing the chances of random mutations or glitches in a cell's life cycle. This can ultimately lead to the runaway cell growth seen in cancer.

Colon cancer is a particular risk, since colon cells divide much more rapidly than other body cells and are thought to be especially sensitive to insulin. With weight gain, existing fat cells expand and additional ones are added to accommodate more stored energy. More or bigger fat cells work even harder to make the hormones that put the overweight or obese person at high health risk. One-third of cancer deaths each year are attributed to nutrition factors, including obesity. Eating more plant-based foods and less saturated fats and trans fats can reduce the risk of cancer.

Dementia

Obesity is also associated with dementia. A meta-analysis study of research (a summary or overview of research outcomes that assesses the degree of effect of those outcomes in many studies) from 1995 to 2005 found that obesity and high cholesterol increased the risk of dementia and associated illnesses such as Alzheimer's-type demen-tia. This review suggested that obesity increased the risk of dementia in general by 42 percent, Alzheimer's by 80 percent, and vascular dementia by 73 percent. Alzheimer's is the eighth leading cause of death in the United States. The researchers found no elevated risk of dementia in people who were in the healthy or overweight BMI weight ranges. Prevention or early treatment of obesity can decrease risk by 20 percent, which is important because it is expected that 50 percent of all people who reach age 85 will develop symptoms of Alzheimer's disease.

Sleep Apnea

Many people who are obese suffer from *obstructive sleep apnea* (OSA)—disrupted breathing during sleep, technically defined as "repetitive interruption of ventilation during sleep caused by collapse of the pharyngeal airway." An estimated 15 million adults in the United States, Europe, Australia, and Asia suffer from OSA. One in five adults have mild OSA, whereas one in fifteen have moderate to severe OSA. Most of those with clinically significant and treatable OSA have never been diagnosed or treated. According to a large study conducted by the Wisconsin Sleep Cohort, obesity is a confounding factor in obstructive sleep apnea. That is, obesity raises the risk of premature death due to OSA, primarily when the degree of visceral obesity—that is, fat in the abdomen—is high. Visceral fat is associated with metabolic syndrome, and the higher the volume of visceral fat—often seen most obviously in the "beer belly" or potbelly appearance—the greater the risk of cardiovascular disease, regardless of BMI. Men, in particular, are at greater risk of death from OSA. In other words, men who have OSA and a beer belly but are not fat elsewhere are at increased risk of dying from heart disease. Additional factors associated with OSA include hypertension, type 2 diabetes, and cardiovascular disease. Untreated OSA is associated with an increased rate of cardiac events and cardiovascular mortality. Not only is it important to lose weight if you are obese, especially if you have a beer belly, it is necessary to see your doctor to treat excessive snoring and other symptoms of OSA, such as daytime sleepiness.

Osteoarthritis

The impact of obesity is especially felt in osteoarthritis of the hip and knee joints. Every pound of body weight puts four to six pounds of pressure on each knee joint. Individuals with obesity are twenty times more likely to need a knee replacement than those who are not overweight. From 2002 to 2009, the number of total knee arthroplasty procedures performed on patients with obesity doubled. The detrimental effects of obesity on surgical outcome results and complication rates are well documented in medical literature. These effects include higher rates of infection and prosthesis failure—loosening of the implant—when compared to patients of normal weight. Obesity contributes to arthritis and other musculoskeletal health issues. In combination with other conditions, such as heart disease and diabetes, obesity can adversely affect orthopedic surgical outcomes. Pre- and postoperative complications may include difficult wound healing, infections, blood clots, blood loss, and dislocation of the replacement joint, especially in the hip.

Excess Weight and COVID-19

Being obese puts people at risk for many serious chronic diseases and increases their risk of severe respiratory illness from COVID-19. Twelve states had adult obesity rates at or above 35 percent, according to the CDC 2019 Behavioral Risk Factor Surveillance System, up from only nine states in 2018 and zero in 2012. A majority of those states were in the South, with Mississippi seeing the highest rate of obesity in 2019 at 40.8 percent. Colorado, on the other hand, saw the lowest rate of obesity at 23.8 percent, according to the report. Residents of these states are likely to be at high risk for COVID-19. A high-risk state is one in which the seven-day moving average of daily new COVID-19 cases is ten or more per 100,000 persons.

Obese adults, and possibly overweight adults, in all states are at risk for developing COVID-19. Obesity may triple the risk of hospitalization due to a COVID-19 infection. Obesity is also linked to impaired immune function. Because of decreased lung capacity and reserve, obesity can make ventilation more difficult. As BMI increases, the risk of death from COVID-19 increases. Studies have demonstrated that obesity may be linked to lower vaccine responses for numerous diseases, such as influenza, hepatitis B, and tetanus.

Obesity disproportionately negatively impacts certain racial and ethnic minority groups. CDC data from 2017 to 2019 highlight the following notable racial and ethnic disparities:

- Black adults had the highest prevalence of self-reported obesity (39.8 percent), followed by Hispanic adults (33.8 percent), and white adults (29.9 percent).

- Six states had an obesity prevalence of 35 percent or higher among white adults.

- Fifteen states had an obesity prevalence of 35 percent or higher among Hispanic adults.

- Thirty-four states and the District of Columbia (DC) had an obesity prevalence of 35 percent or higher among Black adults.

- Hispanic and Black adults have a higher prevalence of obesity and are more likely to suffer worse outcomes from COVID-19. Racial and ethnic minority groups have historically not had broad opportunities for economic, physical, and emotional health, and these inequities have increased the risk of these groups getting sick and dying from COVID-19. Many of these same factors are contributing to the higher level of obesity in some racial and ethnic minority groups.

At this writing, the CDC recommends wearing face masks, staying at least six feet from the nearest person, avoiding gatherings, and washing hands to decrease the risk of contracting the virus. Other steps to take include eating a healthy diet, being active, getting enough sleep, and coping better with stress.

Excess Mortality from Obesity

Despite much controversy, some research evidence demonstrates that obesity—defined as a BMI equal to or greater than 30—is strongly associated with increased mortality and impaired quality of life in men and women of all racial and ethnic groups. Some people argue that this conclusion does not apply to those who fall into the overweight category (based on some evidence that a few extra pounds do not pose a threat). However, a study published in 2006 in the *New England Journal of Medicine* that followed over 60 thousand participants over ten years found that significant excess body weight during midlife (over age 50) is associated with an increased risk of early death. In further analysis, after controlling for health status and smoking, a higher risk for death was still associated with being overweight, as well as being obese. The results suggested that men and women in midlife (ages 50 to 55 years) who had never smoked but were overweight or obese had a 20 to 40 percent increased risk for premature death. Another study published in the *Journal of the American Medical Association* provided some good news: the older an overweight person is—that is, the longer they have already survived—the less his or her risk of premature death due to overweight. If overweight and obesity doesn't get you by the time you are a senior, it becomes less of a threat of dying prematurely later in life. Some people do survive excess weight.

Excess Weight and Mental Health

Overweight and obesity are associated with psychological problems as well as social difficulties. Studies of children's preferences have found that a child who is overweight is less acceptable to other children than a child who has a perceived physical defect such as a cleft lip or large ears. Healthy weight children are considered more attractive and are preferred by parents, teachers, and peers and are rated as possessing more positive traits of every kind than overweight children. Discrimination based on appearance is a fact of life for both children and adults, and obese individuals are often the most blatantly ostracized. Social rejection contributes to low self-esteem and even self-hatred.

Body Dissatisfaction

Body dissatisfaction is pervasive among those who are obese. Even those who are overweight and not obese are often extremely self-critical and obsessed about their size and weight. Increasingly, this applies to men as well as women. Even though some obese people subscribe to the healthy-at-any-weight concept of size acceptance, most obese people would prefer to be thinner. Remember, it is possible to be healthy at a higher weight, defined as being in the healthy weight range, if you do not have risk factors such as hypertension, diabetes, have metabolic syndrome, are a smoker, and you are eating a well-balanced diet, getting enough exercise, keeping calories in and calories out equally balanced.

Not surprisingly, overweight and obesity are likely to contribute to depression and anxiety. The diagnosis of an eating disorder is often appropriate for those who are obsessed with food, eating, and weight; who binge eat; who suffer guilt, shame, or self-criticism about eating or weight; or who detest their appearance.

Depression

Depression often accompanies overweight and obesity. One type of depression is characterized by an increased appetite and a need to sleep a lot, as well as low self-esteem and other symptoms. Alternatively, depression may be characterized by loss of appetite, loss of weight, and difficulty sleeping. Both types can be symptoms of a major depressive disorder. Another kind of depression is a chronic and persistent feeling that life just isn't very good. A study of 200,000 adults in thirty-eight states found that respondents who were currently depressed or had a previous diagnosis of depression were 60 percent more likely to be obese and twice as likely to smoke as those who were not depressed.

Feeling depressed can cause some people to seek food as a relief. Eating is often used as a salve for painful emotions, as well as boredom, loneliness, and anger. Food is also used to provide entertainment and pleasure to counteract down feelings. Although exercise has been shown to help mild depression equally as well as antidepressant medication, most obese people don't engage in regular exercise of adequate intensity to alleviate depression. Those who succeed in losing weight with the more invasive type of bariatric surgery—for example, the Roux-en-Y procedure—find that their depression lifts as they begin to lose weight. For others, dieting without success can itself contribute to depression. It is not known whether depression causes obesity or the reverse. However, eating is often a means of coping with depression, whatever its source. When symptoms of depression are evident, the help of a therapist or physician is indicated.

Anxiety

Anxiety is a common ailment that brings people into therapy. Anxiety can interfere with sleep and makes daily life exceedingly uncomfortable. People who are overweight or obese typically use food and eating to assuage anxiety. They may even become anxious at the thought of not having enough food in the house in case they need to eat.

Many who are obese suffer from social anxiety—anxiety about being around strangers or authority figures or having to perform at work or in public. Those with social anxiety tend to isolate and avoid social contacts whenever possible. If they isolate themselves, and thus avoid the anxiety of being around others who they fear will judge them, they are more vulnerable to eating out of boredom or loneliness. Some people also use alcohol to escape anxiety, which can lead to weight gain and more problems.

Seeking Professional Help

Depression and anxiety are best treated by seeing a professional such as a psychiatrist (MD), a psychologist (PhD, PsyD), or another type of counselor such as a Marriage and Family Therapist (MFT) or

Licensed Clinical Social Worker (LCSW). Only psychiatrists or other physicians can prescribe medication and some psychiatrists also provide therapy. Some people avoid or delay seeking help because of a perceived stigma about "going into therapy." Most people who suffer depression do not seek treatment. The best course is to seek professional help.

Ask for a referral or recommendation from a doctor or a trusted friend or check out the website of one of the organizations that provide referrals to therapists. Once you have names of potential therapists, contact them and ask how they would work with you and your issues. That first contact should tell you a lot about that therapist. If he or she spends some time on the phone asking about your situation and explaining how they work, make an appointment. If necessary, see several therapists before making the decision about whom to continue seeing. Allow yourself a few sessions with a therapist before deciding if he or she is right for you. You should feel that the therapist understands you, and you should feel safe talking to the therapist.

Medications for Treating Obesity

Eating less and moving more are the basics of successful weight management. For some people, however, prescription weight-loss medications may help. Only a doctor can decide if prescribing a medication to treat obesity is indicated. He or she needs to know in advance your medical history, including allergies or other conditions you have. Provide the doctor with a list of medicines or supplements (even if they are herbal or natural) that you are taking. Advise the doctor if you are pregnant, breastfeeding, or planning to get pregnant soon.

Several prescription medications are available to treat obesity (BMI >30) for those who have an increased medical risk because of their weight. However, these drugs are not a cure-all, and they are most often useful in producing a rapid initial weight loss. In general, these medications are modestly effective, leading to an average weight loss of 5 to 22 pounds above that expected with nondrug obesity treatments. People respond differently to such medications, and some people lose more weight than others while some lose little weight. Maximum weight loss usually occurs within four to six months of starting medication, after which weight tends to level off or increase during the remainder of treatments. Research studies conducted in people with obesity all show that people who eat less, increase physical activity, and take medication lose considerably more weight than people who use medication without lifestyle changes. Medication is not a substitute for exercise and cutting calories.

Most weight-loss medications are approved for only a few weeks or months of use, although some of the newer medications may be used for longer periods. The possible benefit of these drugs in the short term includes weight loss, which may lower obesity-related health problems. Whether these drugs actually improve a person's health over the long term is not known. All medications have side effects that should be discussed with a doctor.

Currently Available Weight-Loss Medications

Currently, most available weight-loss medications approved by the US Food and Drug Administration (FDA) are for short-term use. These include Xenical (orlisat), Contrave (naltrexone HCl/bupropion HCl), Saxenda (liraglutide) and Qsymia (phentermine and topiramate). Available over the counter without a prescription is Alli, which has half the dose of the same active ingredient as Xenical.

Xenical is a fat-absorption inhibitor that works by preventing the body from breaking down and absorbing about 30 percent of dietary fat eaten with meals. The undigested fat is then eliminated in bowel movements, thus lowering calories absorbed. The undigested fat causes increased frequency and number of bowel movements, which are likely to be oily in consistency. Side effects include oily spotting, gas with discharge, and an urgent need to go to the bathroom. Patients who take Xenical must adhere to a reduced-calorie diet that contains no more than 30 percent fat, otherwise the effect on bowel movements will be more pronounced. The medication will also block digestion of the fat-soluble vitamins A, D, E, and K, so a supplement with these ingredients should be taken.

Contrave doesn't work in the abdominal system like Xenical and Alli. It works in the hypothalamus, the brain's central thermostat that controls appetite, temperature, and how the body burns energy. Contrave combines two drugs already on the market—bupropion (an antidepressant) and naltrexone (an antiaddiction drug). Contrave's side effects are constipation, headache, possible vomiting, dizziness, insomnia, and dry mouth. It has been associated with suicidal thoughts and may cause seizures or increase blood pressure and heart rate.

Saxenda is a higher dose of the type 2 diabetes drug Victoza. It mimics an intestinal hormone that tells the brain your stomach is full. (It is unlikely to work for emotional eating.) Side effects include nausea, vomiting, diarrhea, constipation, low blood pressure, and increased appetite.

Qsymia curbs appetite. It can work in several ways, including helping you feel full, making foods taste less appealing, and burning more calories. The most common side effects are tingling hands and feet, dizziness, altered sense of taste, insomnia, constipation, and dry mouth.

Some antidepressant medications have been studied as appetite-suppressant medications. While these medications are FDA approved for the treatment of depression, their use in weight loss is "off-label." (*Off-label* refers to the practice of prescribing drugs for a condition for which they have not been officially approved by the FDA.) Studies of these medications generally have found that patients lost modest amounts of weight for up to six months. However, most studies found that patients who lost weight while taking antidepressant medications tended to regain it while they are still on the drug treatment unless they made concurrent lifestyle changes.

4

Causes of Overweight and Obesity

A 29-year-old middle-class woman, Delia was worried about her weight. Both her mother and father were obese. Her BMI was 32, and she went on any "new" diet promoted on TV or in the media to drop excess pounds. At times, she lost weight but then regained it back in a month or two. Delia knew that snacking was a bad idea, but when she was feeling down, she bought cheese to snack on before her evening meal. That, together with some wine, usually made her less hungry for dinner, so she often skipped it altogether. Delia reported to her therapist that when she was a child, she had been sexually abused by an uncle.

Many factors play a role in the development and maintenance of weight problems, including genes and heredity, hormones, peptides in the brain, culture, gender, age, differences in metabolism, a history of abuse, emotional eating, and lack of exercise.

Genes and Heredity

Genes play a part in how your body balances calories and energy. Children whose parents are obese are at greater risk of becoming overweight or obese also. A family history of obesity increases the chances of becoming obese between 25 and 30 percent. A child who is obese in childhood is all but certain to become an obese adult. Where weight is carried—in the hips or abdomen—is also a matter of heredity. But heredity alone does not doom a person to becoming overweight or obese; genes merely create a susceptibility to gaining weight. Behavior and other factors combine to make that vulnerability a reality.

A person can influence the amount of body fat he or she has with a good diet and regular exercise. It is not possible to change genetic makeup by willpower any more than it is possible to make yourself taller or shorter by wishing it so, but people can and do achieve a healthy weight even with a family history of obesity. A person with a family that is overweight or obese must commit to a lifestyle that includes regular exercise and healthier eating.

Hormones and Peptides

The endocrine system is made up of glands that secrete hormones into the bloodstream. (Recall that hormones are chemicals that regulate body processes.) The endocrine system works with the nervous system and the immune system to help the body cope with different events and stresses. Excesses or deficits of hormones can lead to obesity. Several hormones are involved in obesity. Some of the important ones include leptin, estrogen, ghrelin, and insulin. Neuropeptide Y has been associated with a higher intake of carbohydrates.

Leptin, the Fat Hormone

The hormone leptin is produced by fat cells and is secreted into the bloodstream from body fat stores called adipose tissue. In healthy bodies, leptin reduces appetite by acting on specific centers of the brain to lessen the urge to eat. It also seems to control how the body manages its store of body fat. Since leptin is produced by body fat, leptin levels tend to be higher in obese people than in people in the healthy weight range. A key issue currently being researched is why obese people are obese in spite of having higher than usual levels of this appetite-reducing hormone. In other words, why do heavier people have higher than average levels of leptin, yet still eat more than they should? One theory is that obese people are not as sensitive to the effects of leptin. Thus, leptin is not effectively controlling appetite for them.

This theory has arisen from various studies that have shown that blood leptin levels drop after people undertake low calorie diets. Dramatically reduced leptin levels that result from strict low-calorie diets are believed to upset the balance in the body and, in fact, increase, rather than decrease, appetite and slow metabolism. This may be one factor in explaining why crash dieters usually regain their lost weight, and it is another argument in favor of combining exercise with calorie control to reach a healthy weight. It argues for slow, steady weight loss from making lifestyle changes instead of engaging in dieting that restricts many calories.

Estrogen, the Female Hormone

As noted earlier, body fat distribution plays an important role in the development of obesity-related conditions such as heart disease, high blood pressure, stroke, type 2 diabetes, gallbladder disease, breathing problems, certain cancers, and some forms of arthritis. Abdominal fat poses a greater risk factor for disease than fat stored in the buttocks, hips, and thighs. Estrogen, one of the female reproductive hormones (made by the ovaries and responsible for prompting ovulation every menstrual cycle) helps determine body fat distribution. Women of childbearing age tend to store fat in the lower body and have a "pear shape," while men and postmenopausal women tend to store fat around the abdomen and upper back and are "apple shaped." Postmenopausal women with reduced estrogen often tend to store excess weight in the breasts as well as the abdomen, contributing further to the apple shape. Postmenopausal women on estrogen supplements don't accumulate fat around the abdomen but are more likely to add fat around the thighs and hips. In terms of health, pear shapes are preferable to apple shapes.

Ghrelin, the Hunger Hormone

Ghrelin is a growth hormone found in the stomach lining as well as other places in the body. It is responsible for stimulating the appetite before eating. In laboratory tests, humans who are injected with ghrelin report an increase in hunger. In addition, research demonstrates that ghrelin suppresses the utilization of fat in adipose tissue. (Adipose tissue is where the body stores fat.) In essence, ghrelin appears to be at least partially responsible for letting the body know when it is hungry and for keeping the brain and body informed about the energy balance in the body. Those who are obese may be acutely sensitive to ghrelin and, thus, experience more hunger than people who are not overweight. Interestingly, those who undergo certain types of weight-loss surgery may experience a drop in ghrelin production and feel less hungry.

Insulin, the Metabolism Hormone

Insulin is a key hormone in metabolism; its levels rise as levels of body fat increase. Obese people often have chronically high insulin levels and as a result they are resistant or insensitive to the hormone. This puts them at risk for developing type 2 diabetes. It is well established that tissue such as muscle and fat can become insulin resistant. Research provides evidence that insulin receptors in the brain help control food intake and body weight. It is possible that insulin resistance and leptin resistance act together to increase hunger and thus contribute to obesity and type 2 diabetes.

Neuropeptide Y, the Appetite-Regulating Peptide

One of the most potent peptides found in the brain is neuropeptide Y or NPY. It not only increases total food intake but also seems to be associated with increased ingestion of carbohydrates—especially snacks high in fat and sweets favored by many who struggle with their weight. As such, it is one of the most potent appetite-regulating substances in the body and causes the deposit of body fat. NPY is associated with insulin resistance too. Fasting or seriously reducing calories appears to magnify the effect of NPY. Research is currently underway to see if a drug can be found to alter the function of NPY.

Other Factors That Influence Body Weight

Many factors besides hormones influence body weight. Admittedly, obese people have hormone levels that encourage the accumulation of body fat. But they also engage in behaviors such as snacking, overeating, and not exercising that, over time, "reset" the processes which regulate appetite and body fat distribution. Thus, those who are obese are physiologically more inclined to gain weight or to maintain a higher weight. The body is always trying to maintain balance, so it resists any short-term disruptions such as crash dieting and seriously restricting calories. However, there is evidence to suggest that long-term behavior changes, such as healthy eating and regular exercise, can retrain the body to shed excess body fat and keep it off. This is accomplished by making gradual changes in eating and exercising.

Culture

Hunger is not always the cause of unhealthy eating. Numerous cultural factors influence the choices you make about when and how much you eat. You learn to cook and to eat the way you were brought up. Food preferences and choices are learned early in life. Social events and family rituals are often centered on meals that are large as well as high in fat and calories. In today's high-stress and high-achieving culture, it is often perceived to be easier to go to a restaurant or buy take-out or processed foods, rather than cook a healthy meal at home from scratch. Even though many people have gotten the message to reduce fat in their diets, many Americans believe they can eat as much as they want if only the food is labeled low fat or nonfat. As a result, they still take in too many calories to maintain a healthy weight. Children are still rewarded with sweets for behaving well, and adults treat themselves with food using almost any excuse to do so.

Gender

Muscle uses more energy than does body fat. Men have more muscle than women and they are heavier to begin with. As a result, at rest men burn 10 to 20 percent more calories than women. For this reason, a woman who eats about the same number of calories as the average man is more likely to become overweight or obese than is a man. What's more, men often have an easier time losing weight. A good analogy is a car with a big engine versus one with a four- or six-cylinder engine. The bigger the engine, the more gas a car consumes. Men have bigger engines than women, so they can consume more calories without gaining weight.

Age

Remember the way your body morphed at puberty? One day a girl is a beanpole and the next day an hourglass. Or in the case of a young man, his shoulders and chest seem to grow broader almost overnight. Well, once she hits about 40, a woman's shape starts shifting again. Although premenopausal women tend to gain fat in the lower body to nourish children, women whose reproductive years are drawing to a close gain fat in their upper bodies. The results can be larger breasts, the emergence of fat on the back, and little fat pouches near the armpits that hang over the bra. To make matters worse, fat can also accumulate around the hips.

As a person gets older, the amount of muscle in the body tends to decrease without exercise, and body fat accounts for a greater percentage of weight. (This decline is worse in people who haven't been doing muscle-building exercise.) This lower muscle mass leads to a decrease in metabolism and results in slower calorie burning. In this way, changes in muscle mass and metabolism reduce caloric needs as time goes on. If food intake is not decreased and exercise increased, weight is gained over time and with age. On the other hand, muscle-building exercise such as weightlifting can preserve or increase muscle mass despite aging. The message is: exercise your body to hedge your bets against accelerated aging.

Metabolism

The body gets the energy it needs from food through metabolism—the chemical processes in the body's cells that convert the fuel from food into the energy needed to do everything from growing to thinking to moving. Some people have a fast metabolism and burn calories easily; others have a slow metabolism (actually, a more efficient system for extracting and storing calories) and may struggle with gaining weight and trying to lose it. Restricting calories slows down metabolism (i.e., makes the body's metabolism more efficient) making it harder to lose weight. This is because the body is naturally "wired" to resist significant changes in weight, especially over short periods of time.

Losing weight is difficult and requires sustained effort, especially for those who are obese. The failure to lose weight quickly can make you think your body has a metabolic problem. In fact, less than 2 percent of all obesity is the result of metabolic problems such as thyroid or endocrine problems. Your doctor is the only one who can assess if a metabolic problem is contributing to your weight. In the meantime, the best way to boost metabolism is through exercise. Metabolic benefits from exercise can last up to twenty-four hours after exercising.

History of Abuse

Research has found that those who suffered childhood abuse are far more likely to become obese adults. This research showed that early trauma is so damaging that it can disrupt a person's entire psychology and metabolism. One analysis of 57,000 women found that those who experienced physical or sexual abuse as children were twice as likely to become addicted to food as a coping mechanism. Many obese women said they felt more physically imposing when they were bigger. They felt their size helped ward off sexual advances from men.

Emotional Eating

Food is often a source of solace or celebration. Painful emotions often lead to problem eating. If you feel blue, sad, lonely, or bored, you may turn to food. Some people refer to food as their "best friend" because it is easily available, and it pushes troubles to the background. Obesity, for some, is a solution for feeling vulnerable. But even pleasant feelings can produce overeating. Most people celebrate social events with food, and feeling happy can lead to eating more than you'd like.

Many people use food to escape the pain and dissatisfaction inherent in everyday life. No one feels happy all the time, but some people feel unhappy or "blah" most of the time. The former is the normal state of things, but the latter state is likely to be a kind of chronic, low-level depression that some people come to accept as "normal." Accepting that life has its disappointments—an unsatisfactory job, ungrateful children, an emotionally detached partner, demanding parents, or whatever—and working with or around them is necessary for creating a satisfactory life. This means changing what can be changed and accepting what can't. We need to do what we can to influence a difficult situation, but if, in the end, little in the situation changes, then we must either learn to accept what is and make the best of it or leave the situation. Too many people resort to food to salve emotions instead of acting according to their core values—for example, making healthy choices, contributing appropriately to a happier family life, working toward financial stability, and being guided by other overarching life values.

Emotional eating behaviors can have roots in childhood. When a parent has issues with a child's eating or weight, that parent may set limits on eating or criticize the child's behavior. This often leads to sneaking food and lying about eating or weight. This problem can carry into adulthood, especially when weight continues to be an issue. Wanting to avoid criticism or even any discussion of weight, the now-adult child is likely to continue to lie or to get angry with or resent parents or other adults who disapprove.

Experience with one or more parents playing "food police" can set up an unhealthy psychological situation from which emotional eating often results. Many people in this situation talk of having an internal "rebel" that rejects any attempts to set limits on their eating, even self-imposed limits. In such cases, the emotional connection between past humiliation and the need for more adaptive behavior in the present is the challenge to be met.

Alternatively, people who are sensitive about their weight may become "people pleasers" in the hope of winning the approval and love of others who, they hope, won't notice their weight. They care for others and put their needs before their own and thereby gain the satisfaction in life they crave. When they feel lonely or bored, they eat, and when they feel unappreciated, they resort to food to fill the void. Likewise, being raised in a dysfunctional family can contribute to unhealthy eating.

Some people who have experienced an eating disorder, such as anorexia or bulimia, in their youth may find themselves struggling with overeating later in life. Likely, their original issues with food and body image were never adequately resolved even if their original disorder temporarily abated. When stress or a crisis in their current life occurs, they either fall back into old habits (for example, restricting, bingeing and purging), or they follow the opposite path and overeat. In either case, food is being used to avoid the pains and unpleasantness that life presents.

Or someone who was an athlete earlier in life may find themselves later in life with a weight problem. What worked in the past to maintain weight no longer works in the present. While the athlete probably never had to think much about managing weight, or just did more exercise or cut back on calories when they needed to "make weight," the person now finds it harder to stay at a healthy weight.

If they engage in compulsive eating, they further defeat finding a solution. It is necessary for such people to redefine their relationship with food and exercise, that is, "This is what I usually eat," "This is what I rarely eat," "This is what I do in terms of physical activity."

Other psychological factors that can produce emotional eating include how a person thinks about food and eating. A person may make excuses and rationalizations to give themselves permission to eat in unhealthy ways. "This has been such a stressful day. I deserve a treat," or "Well, I've blown it, so why not keep eating?" If you have difficulties being assertive, you may resort to food to stuff down painful feelings. Thinking of yourself as someone who can't resist food or who has a sweet tooth makes it harder to incorporate changes in lifestyle that are necessary for weight management success. "I'm a chocoholic" is a self-definition sure to make it harder to resist temptation. To overcome emotional eating and succeed in making a lifestyle change that leads to a healthy weight, you must redefine who you are and how you act in relation to food and exercise.

Lack of Adequate Exercise

Overweight or obese people are usually less physically active overall than those in the healthy weight range. And when people with weight problems do exercise, the frequency and length is often inconsistent. (Those who are obese but do exercise regularly are few and far between, and they still maintain a higher weight probably because they eat too many calories despite their high activity level.) Obese people often have difficulty moving around to get exercise. Additional weight can cause pain in the feet, ankles, and knees. It can also cause shortness of breath and bring on fatigue easily. In addition, self-consciousness may keep an obese person from going to the gym or exercising in other public places.

In general, opportunities for exercising, as well as motivation to do so, can be hard to come by. Adults as well as children spend more time in front of the TV, playing video games, or using the computer, and less time getting out and moving. Exercising is not often a high priority for overweight people, especially if they have busy schedules, despite promising research showing that regular exercise can significantly improve the quality of life of inactive, overweight, older men and women. Just exercising three to four times a week for at least six months provides these benefits, and the more exercise, the better the benefits.

High-Fat and High-Calorie Foods

What we eat is important. Different kinds of food provide our bodies with different types of nutrients and different amounts of energy. Ounce for ounce, fat has more calories than carbohydrates (nine versus four, respectively). Foods high in sugar are often high in fat as well. Vegetables are complex carbohydrates that are high in fiber and they cause the body to burn more calories to digest them than do foods high in fat. These are the "good" carbohydrates. That is, they help to lower overall cholesterol in the blood. (Cholesterol is a blood lipid, or fat. In the right kind and the right amount—as in high density or HDL cholesterol—it is needed by the body, but too much of the wrong type of cholesterol—low density or LDL cholesterol—can have negative health effects.) The "bad" carbohydrates are the "white" ones—that is, white bread, white rice, white pastas, foods made from white flour (even if it is "enriched"), and foods made from white sugar (in any of its forms), such as sugary soft drinks, juice drinks, and sweets. Bad carbohydrates contribute to weight gain. Increased consumption of sugary sodas and fast foods account for a large part of the additional calories consumed by most Americans. For many people, alcohol is a source of excess calories as well.

Trans fats are man-made fats created by adding hydrogen to vegetable oil to make a more solid substance that extends shelf life and preserves taste. When you see the words *partially hydrogenated* or *shortening* on the label, these terms refer to trans fats. Saturated fats (found in animal products like red meat and butter) and trans fats actually raise the level of low density (LDL) cholesterol, the "bad" cholesterol, in your blood, and they decrease the level of high density

(HDL) cholesterol, the "good" cholesterol. Foods in which saturated and trans fats are typically found include crackers, candies, cookies, snack foods, baked goods, fried foods, and processed foods.

And, of course, it is not just what you eat but how much you eat that affects your weight. Many people focus so much on avoiding "fat" calories, they forget to monitor total calories. Portion size is always important, even if a food is designated as low fat or low calorie. Restaurants serve large portions to attract customers even though the "serving" provided is equal to multiple servings.

Why do we keep eating once our basic energy needs are met? Science has uncovered some important instigators of overeating. Three food components in various combinations tantalize taste buds: fat, salt, and sugar. Think about a typical American chain-restaurant meal. Start with tortilla chips—lots of fat and salt. (Try putting some chips on a paper napkin or in a paper bag and see what happens; the grease quickly seeps into the paper.) Add cheese dip for the chips; the ingredients are heavy cream (fat), and cheese (fat), plus some onion or spices. How about a bacon cheeseburger for your entree? Ground beef has a high-fat content, bacon is fat and salt, cheese adds more fat, and finally the sauce is mostly fat and salt. And to drink? What about one of those flavored coffee drinks? A flavored frozen cappuccino drink is made up of coffee and a mix that might include sugar, whipped cream (fat and sugar), chocolate chips (fat and sugar), and chocolate drizzle (sugar). Why do these foods win over our appetites rather than healthy and weight-reducing vegetables? Because they are mouth entertainment!

Humans typically eat in part for stimulation. The environment gives us lots of cues to eat. Plus, food is entertainment. Food should be enjoyed. The three ingredients just mentioned that drive consumption—fat, salt, and sugar—also stimulate the neurotransmitter dopamine—the "feel good" chemical—in the brain making us want to eat. Any combination of these "big three" produces a roller coaster sensation of taste in the mouth that is very satisfying. The sight of food that has texture, color, temperature, and mouth feel can trigger appetite when you are not really hungry. Just an attractive photograph or ad for food can do this alone, and the smell of fatty food cooking is very compelling even to people without overeating problems.

What to do about this? First, you need to develop a new way of eating that conforms to your own definition of healthy (and happy) that keeps the three taste teasers (fat, sugar, and salt) in check. That means you should eat foods that contain these ingredients in moderation. What satisfies is personal, but a good strategy is to focus your eating on foods that occur in nature, like whole grains, beans, vegetables, and fruit, combined with lean protein and an appropriate amount of "good" fats—that is, monounsaturated fats such as canola oil, avocado oil, and olive oil. It is best to avoid prepared foods as much as possible. It is also necessary to plan ahead to deal with temptations and to be on the alert for emotions that might make you more vulnerable to inappropriate eating and the use of food as a means of self-soothing.

CHAPTER

Cholesterol, Metabolic Syndrome, and Weight

Stella is 56 years old and has a BMI of 36. She also has high blood pressure, which is under control with medication. Her doctor recently told her that her high cholesterol put her at risk for developing metabolic syndrome. Stella replied that she walked every day and tried to stay fit that way. "Isn't being fit a good way to be healthy?" she asked.

Heart Disease

The leading cause of death in the Western world is heart disease, a chronic disease affected by diet. Cholesterol is an important factor in the high incidence of heart disease. *Cholesterol* is a waxy, fatlike substance that is found in all cells in the body. The body needs some cholesterol to make hormones, vitamin D, and substances that help in the digestion of foods. But the body makes all the cholesterol it needs. Some foods claim to be cholesterol free and the implication is that makes them better to eat. While eating foods that do not contain cholesterol is important, not eating foods with saturated fat is more important.

Foods that are touted as cholesterol free are misleading. Part of the confusion comes from the fact that cholesterol in food isn't the same thing as the cholesterol that clogs arteries. To be sure, foods high in cholesterol can cause blood levels of cholesterol to rise, but only about one in three people seems to be especially susceptible to the effects of cholesterol in food.

"Dietary cholesterol isn't the biggest worry when it comes to heart disease," says Kathy McManus, MS, RD, director of nutrition at Brigham and Women's Hospital in Boston. "Studies show it's only about half as important as saturated fat and *trans fat* in raising serum cholesterol levels."

Heart disease includes *coronary heart disease* (CHD), also known as *coronary artery disease.* CHD is the most common type of heart disease and happens when plaque sticks to the walls of the coronary arteries forming a clot that limits the blood flow to the heart's muscle by narrowing or even blocking the arteries. This buildup of plaque is known as *atherosclerosis.* The narrowed or blocked blood vessels can lead to a heart attack, chest pain (angina), or stroke.

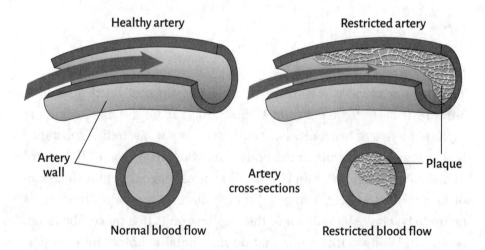

Figure 5.1 **The Effects of Atherosclerosis**

What Is the Difference Between "Good" and "Bad" Cholesterol?

What Is HDL, LDL, and VLDL?
HDL (or high-density lipoprotein), LDL (or low-density lipoprotein), and VLDL (or very low–density lipoprotein) are all *lipoproteins*. These are a combination of fat (lipid) and protein. Lipids need to be attached to proteins so they can move through the blood.

High-density lipoprotein cholesterol, or HDL, is sometimes called the "good" cholesterol because it acts like a scavenger and carries LDL cholesterol from the inner walls (*endothelium*) of blood vessels back to the liver. There, HDL reduces, reuses, and recycles the LDL cholesterol.

Low-density lipoprotein cholesterol, or LDL, is sometimes called the "bad" cholesterol because a high LDL level leads to the buildup of plaque in arteries. As the blood vessels build up plaque over time, the inside of the vessels narrow, blocking flow to the heart and other organs. When blood flow to the heart is blocked, it can cause *angina* or a heart attack.

Very low–density lipoprotein cholesterol, or VLDL, is also a "bad" cholesterol, because it too contributes to the buildup of plaque in arteries and blood vessels. VLDL and LDL are different; VLDL mainly carries triglycerides and LDL mainly carries cholesterol. *Total cholesterol* is the total amount of cholesterol in the blood. This includes all sources of cholesterol in the blood, including triglycerides. A total cholesterol of 180 to 200 mg/dL or less is considered best for health.

What Affects Cholesterol Levels in the Blood?

A diet high in the "bad" fats—particularly those from saturated fats as found in some meats, dairy products, chocolate, baked goods, and deep-fried and processed foods—can raise blood cholesterol. Being overweight and sedentary are also contributors to high cholesterol. Lack of physical activity is a risk factor for heart disease. Regular physical activity can help lower bad LDL and raise good HDL. The goal is to be physically active for thirty minutes on most, if not all, days.

Smoking lowers good HDL, the type that helps remove bad cholesterol from arteries. Smoking causes chemical changes in the body that raises levels of LDL, the bad cholesterol, and raises triglycerides in the blood. Smokers who kick the habit may improve their levels of good HDL cholesterol within one year.

Lower "good" HDL accompanies a higher level of "bad" cholesterol, and this is more prominent when a person is stressed or economically depressed. There is compelling evidence that high stress can indirectly cause an increase in bad cholesterol. For example, one study found that stress was positively linked to having less healthy dietary habits, a higher body weight, and a less healthy diet, all of which are known risk factors for high levels of bad cholesterol.

Those who are economically depressed fall prey to fast foods because fast-food restaurants are disproportionally located in poor neighborhoods, and the food is cheaper than buying fresh fruits and vegetables.

Metabolic Syndrome (Insulin Resistance Syndrome)

High plasma cholesterol is associated with *metabolic syndrome*, also called *insulin resistance syndrome*, which is not a disease but a group of characteristics that include obesity, high blood pressure, elevated blood sugar levels, and high triglycerides (fatlike substances in the blood). These factors increase the risk of developing type 2 diabetes, which is also a significant cause of death and disability.

Metabolic syndrome is characterized by a high plasma insulin concentration that fails to suppress plasma glucose (blood sugar) normally. It involves glucose intolerance, diabetes, and risk of heart disease. The components of metabolic syndrome include reduced HDL cholesterol (the good cholesterol), raised triglycerides, high blood pressure, and high fasting plasma glucose (blood sugar).

Diet and physical activity are key modifiable risk factors that play a significant role in the development, progression, and reversal of

Triglycerides

Triglycerides are a type of fat (lipid) found in the blood. When food is eaten, the body converts any calories it doesn't need right away into triglycerides that are stored in fat cells. Later, hormones release triglycerides for energy between meals. A normal triglyceride level is below 150 mg/dL. Higher levels may require treatment. Recent evidence suggests that persons with higher than normal levels should work to reduce triglycerides, especially if they have heart disease or other risk factors such as diabetes, high blood pressure, or are smokers.

insulin resistance and fat accumulation. Not only is caloric intake an issue, but so is the quality of the diet. Depending on the diet, the macronutrients in the diet may affect insulin sensitivity. Obese and overweight individuals with more severe insulin resistance have a decreased ability to switch from carbohydrate to fat oxidation.

Prevalence of Metabolic Syndrome

Between 10 and 30 percent of people have metabolic syndrome, the prevalence of which increases sharply in most European countries and the United States, especially in older age groups. By the age of 70, the prevalence of metabolic syndrome has been estimated at 42 percent among American men and women. Rising trends in obesity, especially in young people, are predicted to give rise to more cases of metabolic syndrome and greater risk of heart disease.

What Is the Test for Diabetes?

The fasting plasma glucose test is performed after a person has fasted for at least eight hours. A sample of blood is taken from a vein in the arm. If the blood glucose level is greater than or equal to 126 mg/dL, the person is retested and, if the results are consistent, the person is diagnosed with diabetes.

The Development of Metabolic Syndrome

Adults who gain weight and accumulate body fat are at risk for developing metabolic syndrome. Some people have a predisposition to accumulate fat in intra-abdominal sites (that is, in the belly). Excess belly fat may lead to ectopic fat deposition. *Ectopic fat* is the storage of triglycerides in tissues such as the liver, skeletal muscle, heart, and pancreas. Notably, a vicious circle exists between insulin resistance, or metabolic syndrome, and ectopic fat storage, and together they increase the risk for heart disease. Large waist circumference is a good indicator of excess belly fat and elevated risk.

Large Waist Circumference as a Risk Factor for CHD

As noted in chapter 2, belly fat is an active organ that has a direct role in the development of metabolic syndrome. Men who have a waist measurement between 37 and 40 inches are at high risk for heart disease and should lose 5 to 10 percent of body weight and prevent further weight gain. Women who have a waist measurement between 31 and 35 inches are at high risk and should lose 5 to 10 percent of body weight and prevent further weight gain. Men with a waist measurement above 40 inches and women who are above 35 inches are at high risk for heart disease. They need to lose more than 10 percent of body weight through effective weight-loss treatment.

What Is Insulin Resistance?

When *blood glucose* (blood sugar) remains elevated despite normal or high levels of insulin, this is called *insulin resistance*. One of insulin's jobs is to help move glucose from the blood into the cells for energy. Nutrition is a key determining factor for both insulin resistance and ectopic fat deposition. To reduce the risk of insulin resistance, one's diet should be low in fat. A healthy Mediterranean diet, which is discussed in chapter 8, can help lower weight, blood pressure, and lipids, and improve insulin resistance. Likewise, a healthy Vegetarian diet, also discussed in chapter 8, can do this. Becoming more active is also an important factor in lowering insulin resistance.

Genetic Factors That Play a Role in Insulin Resistance

Insulin resistance represents a physical state in which the action of the hormone insulin is impaired. As a result, the body is not effectively able to adapt to its metabolic or energy demands.

Sex, age, lifestyle, and other factors may play a role in fat accumulation. In general, women accumulate more fat in their glutes and hips than in their abdominal area, whereas men tend to store fat in their bellies. Notably, abdominal fat is associated with increased risk of developing type 2 diabetes and cardiovascular diseases. Abdominal fat has also been linked to higher levels of inflammation and insulin resistance.

Lifestyle factors, such as an unhealthy diet and lack of physical activity, are key factors in the accumulation of body fat and insulin resistance. Exercise's different modalities—such as resistance training, endurance training, and other physical activities—bring improvements not only in cardiovascular fitness but also in fat reduction and in better insulin sensitivity.

Individual macronutrients in the diet—specifically fats, carbohydrates, and proteins—seem to determine metabolic adaptations that are related to body fat and insulin resistance. Dietary fat quality (the type of fat consumed) has significant effects on ectopic fat and insulin sensitivity. Diets high in saturated fat promote heart disease. Simple carbohydrates, such as candies, cakes, cookies, and plain sugar in the sugar bowl have been linked to metabolic disorders. Consuming protein helps improve insulin sensitivity.

Generally, a Mediterranean or high-fiber diet is recommended for reducing risk of metabolic syndrome, but because people may respond differently to the same dietary intervention, a more personalized approach may be needed. This might require the assistance of a registered dietitian.

Metabolism and Metabolic Disorder

Metabolism is the process by which the body gets or makes energy from food. A *metabolic disorder* occurs when the body disrupts the process of getting or making energy from the food eaten. Food is made up of proteins, carbohydrates, and fats. Chemicals in the body's digestive system break the food parts down into sugars and acids that end up as the body's fuel. The fuel can be used right away or it can be stored in body tissues, such as the liver, muscles, and body fat. A metabolic disorder occurs when abnormal chemical reactions in the body disrupt this process. When this happens, the body may have too much of some substances or too little of others that are needed to stay healthy.

There are different groups of disorders. Some affect the breakdown of amino acids, carbohydrates, or lipids. Another group, *mitochondrial diseases*, affect the parts of the cells that produce the energy. A person can develop a metabolic disorder when organs, such as the liver or pancreas, become diseased or do not function normally. Diabetes is an example. (See chapter 1, page X, for more information on diabetes.)

New Insights from Recent Research on Weight and Obesity

Genes play an important role in weight and blood lipids. They help regulate appetite and energy expenditure, body mass index (BMI), fat distribution, and metabolic syndrome. Those people carrying ten or more genetic variants have a greater risk of obesity than those carrying only one or two genetic variants. Also, childhood obesity increases the risk of developing massive obesity and a predisposition to carry fat in the abdominal area.

> *Impaired Glucose Tolerance*
> Impaired glucose tolerance is a pre-diabetic state of high blood sugar that is associated with insulin resistance and increased risk of cardiovascular pathology. It may precede the diagnosis of type 2 diabetes by many years and is also a risk factor for mortality.

Signs of Metabolic Syndrome
1. Having a large waistline, also called *abdominal obesity* or "having an apple shape"
2. Having a high triglyceride level
3. Having a low HDL (good) cholesterol level
4. Having high blood pressure
5. Having a high fasting blood sugar, which may be an early sign of diabetes

Management of Metabolic Syndrome Through Changes in Lifestyle Factors

Dietary Changes

To reduce the risk of metabolic syndrome, dietary intake must change. It has been unequivocally shown that levels of total plasma cholesterol can be substantially altered by dietary changes involving reduction of saturated fats. Calories from saturated fat are associated with high levels of total plasma cholesterol.

Daily intake of five portions of fruit and vegetable is recommended. Because excess alcohol intake is a factor in the development of metabolic syndrome, it is important to reduce or eliminate regular alcohol consumption. Likewise, reducing weight is needed. Individual differences, however, may determine the response to a particular diet. Implementation of more personalized nutrition can be complex, and the help of a registered dietitian may be required. More research on this is warranted.

Weight Management

Evidence-based weight management with a cognitive-behavioral approach should be undertaken. Weight loss of 5 to 10 percent has been shown to substantially benefit metabolic factors in overweight individuals. Research finds no difference in metabolic syndrome from weight loss with low-carb compared to higher-carb diets after twelve weeks. Similar findings were for low-carb and low-fat diets. Reducing calories is the key to successful weight management.

Physical Activity

Inactivity promotes the risk of heart disease. It is recommended that a person restrict television viewing and computer use, avoid motor transport for short journeys and walk or use a bicycle instead, and increase moderate daily activities. Engaging in regular swimming, climbing stairs, brisk walking, dancing, and household activities can be helpful. If using an internet app to monitor step counts, set weekly targets, aiming to reach an average of 10,000 to 15,000 steps per day.

6

Getting and Staying Motivated

Olivia wanted to lose weight for her daughter's upcoming wedding. One possible obstacle to her success was that Olivia and her husband liked going out to dinner and socializing with friends. She was about 15 pounds overweight, but her husband didn't mind. "I like a woman with meat on her bones," he had been heard to say. Olivia wished she could wear slimmer clothes, even though she was already a well-dressed woman. It was hard for Olivia to get enough motivation to undertake a serious weight-loss effort. She had to examine carefully her reasons for wanting to lose weight and determine whether she really needed to lose weight or if she just needed to make some changes toward a healthier lifestyle. One thing she realized was that she wasn't exercising as much as she could. She asked her sister, who also wanted to lose some pounds, to join her in her effort.

Motivation

Motivation can be elusive. The dictionary defines it as "that which causes a person to do something or act in a certain way." Motivation steers you toward or away from goals. Both *internal factors*—like thoughts, beliefs, and values—and *external factors*—like friends or tangible rewards—stimulate desire and energy to exert effort toward attaining a goal. Expectations about the likely consequences of a behavior affect motivation. If you expect a pleasant reward, you are more likely to be motivated to act. On the other hand, if you think a behavior will lead to something unpleasant, you are likely to avoid that action. If a good friend invites you to walk with her several times a week, you are more likely to do it than if you had to walk alone. If later she stops going for walks, you may stop too. Unless you have internalized the value of getting exercise, your motivation is likely to slip away.

Generally, most people want to do things that feel good and avoid those things that feel bad. Tasting something good motivates you to take another bite. The motivation to keep eating generally continues until you are full or satisfied—or until the food is all gone. Motivation to stop eating is signaled by a *cue*, for example, a feeling of fullness or an empty plate or food container. Eating motivation is governed not only by cues, but also by the rewards expected from the behavior. So how do you get motivated?

Motivation can come from learning without necessarily experiencing. Getting burned by a hot stove motivates you to avoid touching stoves or other heat sources in the future or, at least, generally motivates you to be more careful around them. Fortunately, people don't have to be burned to avoid a hot stove; they can learn by being warned not to touch sources of heat. Being told not to touch something because you will be hurt is usually enough to motivate you to move away from a heat source. Similarly, learning that red meat contains lots of saturated fat might motivate you to limit your red meat consumption. In this case, warnings about the unhealthiness of eating fat motivate you to choose other food options. This book provides lots of information about how to maintain a healthy eating pattern, and this information may motivate you to make changes.

Motivation also comes from thoughts, beliefs, expectations, goals, and personal values without any external cue necessarily being involved. You may feel motivated to take food to a grieving neighbor because you think it will help them and you believe neighbors should help one another in times of need. You do this because you have a personal value of being kind to others in need and because it "feels like the right thing to do." Or you might hear of a new diet that promises easy success and be motivated to try it, hoping this time it will work for you. All too often, eventually your hopes for the diet are dashed, at which point motivation to continue disappears. What's worse is you may blame yourself instead of the fad diet for the failure. Your subsequent expectation may be that "you are one of those people who can't lose weight," which decreases your motivation to try again.

Motivation and Habit

Sometimes, what starts as a motivation to behave in a certain way evolves into a habit. *Habits* are behaviors people engage in without complete conscious control. A habit results from doing the same thing enough times that it becomes more or less mindless. With repetition of a behavior, the initial motivation to seek pleasure or avoid pain caused by a behavior dissipates and is replaced by a habit that involves little, if any, conscious thought. For example, suppose you walk by a coworker's desk and take a handful of M&M candies; if you do it almost every day, it becomes a habit. You do it without thinking. At one time, this behavior was pleasurable, but that pleasure may have been forgotten or diminished and now you act simply out of habit. Taking the elevator when you could take the stairs can also become a habit. This habit is one of avoiding the energy expenditure of walking the stairs; it's just easier to take the elevator. So habits are behaviors that have "gone underground" in our consciousness. Habits are easy to do because they have become automatic.

Motivation and Goal Setting

Change is a big word. It can strike fear into the hearts of many people. To some, it means giving up something they like. To others, it means having to do something they'd like to avoid. Usually, people expect change to mean *big* changes that take time and effort and even money. But the best way to approach change when it is needed for health is to take a gradual approach—set goals that are reasonable but still challenging. Choose to make small changes over time and keep revising your goals until you reach your ultimate goal. For example, if you now drink 2-percent milk and want to get to drinking nonfat milk, first move to 1-percent milk until you are used to it. Later, move to nonfat milk. If you don't currently get much exercise, choose a small goal, such as walking for ten minutes two or three days a week. Once you achieve that, move your goal up to walking fifteen minutes. When you've been able to do that, plan to do this activity three or four days a week. Keep revising your goal upward until you reach your desired end. This is called *shaping behavior*.

Setting appropriate goals is a valid and useful way to increase motivation. To be motivating, goals need to meet certain criteria. To be most effective, they need to be specific, measurable, attainable, sufficiently challenging, and time bound. Clear goals with appropriate feedback are the key to improved performance. Dr. Edwin Locke's pioneering research on goal setting and motivation is relevant. His research showed that there is a relationship between how difficult and specific a goal is and a person's performance of the behavior. *Specific* means that the goals are defined in terms of behavior, are measurable, and have a time frame. For example, saying "I will take at least 6,000 steps (behavior) today (time frame) as measured on my fitness tracker (measurement)" is more motivating than "I'll try to go for a walk later."

Activity Trackers

Usually worn on the wrist, activity trackers, such as the Fitbit, Koretrak, and Apple Watch, can automatically record the distance you walk, run, swim, or cycle, as well as the number of calories you burn and consume. Some also monitor your heart rate and sleep quality.

Likewise, a goal's level of *difficulty* is important. Difficulty can range from easy to hard. A goal that is too easy will not be challenging and, therefore, not very motivating. A goal that is too challenging can be less motivating, and you may decide not to even try. So a goal must be reasonably attainable but challenging enough to be worth doing. And the goal must be relevant and desirable to the person setting it. Setting a specific goal such as walking 6,000 steps a day is relevant to the larger goal of managing weight and living a healthy lifestyle.

Specific and sufficiently challenging goals lead to better task performance than vague or easy goals. Achievement is also motivating and important. That first time the scale shows a decrease in body weight is rewarding and stimulates more effort. Likewise, noticing your pants are fitting better is feedback that is motivating. More success boosts enthusiasm and the drive to keep trying. Some research shows that those who lose weight early in a weight-loss effort (within the first four weeks) tend to be more successful in the long run, whereas those who do not tend to drop out early. Even though the bathroom scale is a poor measure of body fat, it is a common source of feedback and motivation—or disappointment.

Feedback and Goals

In addition to setting goals, feedback about progress is important for motivation. Feedback provides opportunities to adjust your goals or efforts. Knowing that you have made progress allows you to measure success along the way, which is particularly important if it's going to lead to a healthier lifestyle.

Feedback can come in a variety of forms. As mentioned, your bathroom scale is but one means of assessing progress, although it isn't a reliable source. Tracking steps or mileage with an activity tracker like a Fitbit is another. Monitoring daily calories and calories consumed over time is yet another type of tracking and gives you feedback relevant to your behavior. Many smartphone apps are available that can be useful for tracking progress with calories, foods, and exercise. Even changes in the way clothes fit, although difficult to measure precisely, can be motivating.

This book provides a variety of ways for getting feedback and determining progress. One is the calendar-and-stickers method, which can be individualized to any smaller type of goal. (See chapter 7, "Changing Behavior," for more about this method.) Keeping track of steps when using a fitness tracker is another. Many internet programs and smartphone applications help chart progress and give feedback. Using these resources can help you keep count of calories consumed throughout the day or calories burned in daily exercise, as well as tracking weight loss and graphing exercise. Of course, keeping a food journal or tracking food eaten and emotions experienced at the time of eating in a personal journal is a powerful, if less technological, means of getting information about progress. Some people prefer to use the old, reliable paper and pencil method of journaling and tracking.

Motivation and Values

Motivation is influenced by values. Your actions are guided by those things you value or act as guiding principles in your life. For example, if you value being an honest person, you generally don't tell lies. Motivation comes when a person embraces and refers to his or her personal values. Maybe you make sure to get exercise every day because you value being healthy and believe that participating in regular exercise is a necessary means of achieving physical well-being. In this case, striving to be physically fit is your value. Likewise, you may choose to reduce portion size to manage your weight.

Getting exercise and making healthy food choices are in alignment with your value of striving for good health.

Values are a key concept in mindfulness- and acceptance-based therapies. Values are global, desired, and chosen life directions. They embody intention and are exhibited in every purposeful act. Usually, values are deliberately chosen combinations of verbs and adverbs. To embrace relating (verb) to others lovingly (adverb) is a value. Paying (verb) your bills on time (adverb) is a value. Maintaining (verb) a healthy lifestyle (adverb) is another value.

A personal value, such as being honest, might motivate you to give back money to the insurance company if you find the lost item you had received a reimbursement on earlier. Of course, having a goal of personal gain might motivate you to forget your value of honesty and tempt you to keep the money, especially if you think you would not be caught. If you generally think of yourself as an honest person, your mind might try to trick you with rationalizations such as, "It's just a big insurance company and they make lots of money anyway." Any value, such as that of being honest, doesn't stop and start depending on circumstances. It guides what you do *consistently*, not just now and then. Of course, many people stray from their values given certain circumstances, but it is important to return to your values as soon as possible. Motivation is influenced by both goals and values.

Goals Versus Values

Humans are endowed with the capacity to conceptualize a future. For example, wanting to become a firefighter or a doctor provides inspiration and motivation to take actions to realize such long-term goals. These goals are in service to the larger value related to career direction. Goals are things you can obtain, like owning a Corvette, for example, or getting a graduate degree. They are concrete events, situations, or objects, and they can be completed, possessed, or finished. Not so values. Values are permanent dispositions.

Over time, and with experience, goals may change, but the personal value system guiding your actions is not as changeable. Values help you define what your life is about. They point you in a direction, but they are not a destination. Values are about having a particular code or philosophy that you live by—like honesty, reliability, integrity, having a sense of humor, treating others respectfully, and so forth. They act as a compass that guides your actions. Most importantly, values are chosen.

Defining Your Values

Identifying your values and associated guiding principles is important for motivation and for choosing healthy behaviors. This may seem like a daunting task. You may never have thought about your values or what principles you want to guide your life choices. You may even conclude you have no values. Answering just one question can start you on the road to having awareness of your values and a way to define them: "What do I want my life to be about?"

It is not uncommon for people to deny that they have any values at all. It can be painful to look at your past actions and inquire what values they express. For example, it may be easier to profess no values than to acknowledge to yourself that snacking indiscriminately suggests a disregard for health or perhaps an easy way to avoid unpleasant feelings. Or that lack of exercise might suggest a disregard for healthy behavior. Such realizations can be painful but can also stimulate new behavior. The good news is that it is never too late to examine and redefine your values.

Most people learn values in the context of their family and culture. If your family put high stakes on doing the "right thing," you probably adopted that value too. You learn your initial values mostly from your family. If you were imbued with the idea that paying your bills on time is important, you will likely do that. If your parents were spendthrifts, you may not have learned budgeting nor to stay within your credit limits. Or you may react to some parental behavior you don't like by adopting the opposite behavior that expresses a different value. All your experiences inform your values. As an adult, with hindsight and the ability to discover what is working and what isn't in your life now, you may adopt new values.

The values you choose to live by define who you are and what your life is about. It helps to think of values in terms of verbs and not as nouns. So instead of saying "honesty" is your value, it might be more usefully expressed as "to be honest without hurting others." Instead of "health," you might say "to make life-enhancing choices." Frame your values so they point to actions. Table 6.1 features a partial list of domains of values framed as actions (verbs and adverbs).

Living consistently with your values and guiding principles may allow you to feel good at times, but not always. Giving back a large sum of money to a faceless insurance company may be painful, at least initially. You may wonder if you really should have done that, especially if friends question your actions. But your value to be honest guides your actions. Getting out and exercising five days a week

Table 6.1 Values Framed as Actions

Value Domain	Value Expressed as a Chosen Life Direction
Health	To make healthy choices
Relationships	To treat others respectfully
Family	To create loving relationships
Friendship	To nurture friendships
Career	To do my job well
Education	To pursue personal development
Recreation/Leisure	To engage in revitalizing activities
Financial	To be financially responsible and secure
Spiritual	To feel connected to something larger than myself
Citizenship	To contribute to society and the community

may not always be what you want to do, but you do it because of the value you place on the benefits of exercise. Note the difference between the *value* of exercising for health and the *goal* of exercising a certain number of days. Values inform a higher level of meaning in your life; goals are changeable. Values may hit bumps in the road, but you persist in the direction they point; goals can be easily discarded. A person who values creating a loving family may, nevertheless, have to go through a divorce. To adhere to the value of creating a loving family during a divorce would mean not allowing children to be used as weapons against an ex-spouse, and it would mean agreeing to a fair division of assets. Even when you have failed to live up to your values, you can take corrective action and bring your life back into alignment with your values.

Values are the overarching guides that give direction to behavior and make life meaningful. Goals are the targets for action that help you live the life you say you want. Behavior is directed toward attaining a goal and should be consistent with personal values. Goals are motivators of action. You need to have plans for putting your intentions or goals into action. How many times have you said, "I'll start tomorrow," but tomorrow never seems to come? You may have an intention but no way to implement it. Good intentions and lofty goals are just not enough to get you where you want to go.

Motivation is helped when you define and stay in touch with what you want for yourself in the long run. Of course, some people have never given much thought to the direction they want their life to take. They may simply follow opportunities as they present themselves. And even those who have thought about what they value in themselves may still struggle with behavior change. A helpful way of understanding this is through the Stages of Change model discussed next, which characterizes different phases of the change process.

The Five Stages of Change

Behavior change is rarely a discrete, single event. Instead, the person who wants to change moves gradually from being uninterested in changing, to considering a change, to deciding and preparing to make a change, and finally to actually changing. The person eventually takes genuine, determined action and, over time, works to maintain the new behavior. Lapses or backsliding are almost inevitable and are not excuses to stop taking action, rather they must simply become part of the process of working toward permanent lifestyle change.

The five stages of change describe how a person can modify a problem behavior or acquire a new and healthier behavior. *Precontemplation* is the stage at which there is little or no acknowledgement of the problem and no intention to change behavior in the foreseeable future. A person in this stage may be unaware of his or her problems or be in denial. He probably has not thought about his or her values. Such a person is unlikely to be motivated to change. In the *Contemplation* stage, a person is aware a problem exists, acknowledges it, and is in the process of seriously thinking about overcoming it, but has not yet made a commitment to take action. The person may not yet be clear about their values. Such a person may or may not make lifestyle changes. *Preparation* is the stage in which a person is intending to take action in the next month or so or has unsuccessfully taken action in the past year. At this stage, the person has more clearly identified and embraced personal values. *Action* is the stage in which a person takes steps to modify behavior or the environment to overcome personal problems. This stage requires a considerable commitment of time and energy to change behavior patterns. Successful action is guided primarily by values. In the *Maintenance* stage, a person works to prevent relapse and consolidates the gains attained during the Action stage. Even when there is a slip, values guide behavior back on track.

These stages are not lockstep, and people may slide to a previous stage or move back and forth between stages. Learning to recover from small slips to prevent total relapse is important, especially at the latter two stages involving taking action. The first two stages of change, Precontemplation and Contemplation, are characterized primarily by thinking and emotions. The third stage, Preparation, involves both taking action and cognition (thinking and feeling). Taking action is the focus of the latter two stages, Action and Maintenance.

Stage 1: Precontemplation

People may be in the Precontemplation stage because they are uninformed or underinformed about the consequences of their behavior, or they simply don't want to acknowledge the negative consequences of their current behavior. They are in denial. Some in the Precontemplation stage may have tried to change their behavior a number of times before and have become demoralized about their inability to change. Both those who are uninformed and those who are discouraged may tend to avoid reading, talking, or thinking about their high-risk behaviors. They may be "resistant" or "unmotivated," but the end result is that they avoid or discount disturbing information about their health.

If you are in the Precontemplation stage, it is important to realize that you are not ready to jump into action of any sort except to give thought to your personal life direction and values. There are important questions for you to answer before you attempt to change. What do you want your life to be about? What do you value? That is, what principles do you want to guide your behavior? What are your goals? Do your current behavior patterns serve your larger goals and values related to leading a healthy and fulfilling life? What would have to happen for you to accept that significant overweight or obesity or lack of exercise is a problem for you? Naturally, the answer to these questions and the decision to change is entirely yours. But before answering these questions, acquaint yourself with the health risks you face if you do not understand and accept the research evidence about what constitutes a healthy lifestyle.

Stage 2: Contemplation Stage

If you are reading this book, you are probably in the Contemplation stage or a later stage. In the Contemplation stage, you are thinking about change but don't yet know if you can or will make changes in your life. You are aware of the pros of changing but are also acutely aware of the cons. In essence, you are sitting on the fence. The balance between the costs and benefits of changing versus not changing can produce profound ambivalence that can keep you stuck in this stage for long periods of time. The prospect of giving up an enjoyed behavior that has helped you cope can cause you to feel an anticipated sense of loss despite the possible gain in changing.

Completing the cost-benefit analysis provided later in this chapter is meant to tip the balance toward the Preparation and Action stages of change. It is intended to help you evaluate the pros and cons of behavior change. During the Contemplation stage, it is important to assess the barriers to change, such as time, expense, hassle, fear, and uncertainty, as well as the benefits of change. At this stage, the potential to change exists and the threat of inertia prevails.

Important questions to answer are: "What are my reasons for changing?" "Why am I thinking about change at this time?" "What would keep me from changing at this time?" "What difficult challenges have I faced and overcome in the past?" "What might help me overcome barriers to change?"

Stage 3: Preparation Stage

The Preparation stage is marked by experimentation. In this stage, you are testing the waters. In all likelihood, you are thinking about what specific changes you would like to make. You may experiment with small changes as your determination increases. All this is in preparation for taking action in the immediate future. Perhaps you have already taken some significant action, such as talking to your physician or checking out a program for changing your lifestyle. You may have other action items in mind, such as joining a gym, calling a therapist, or reading and completing the exercises in this book. Maybe you have already made some changes in what you eat or your exercise. For example, you may have already tried eating smaller portions as a first step toward additional dietary modifications.

Now is the time to identify your plan of action and assess obstacles. Seek social support for your plan to change. Talk to friends, family, or professionals who are likely to be supportive. Contact others who are interested in managing weight and plan to do things with them. Get them involved. Check out websites that offer tools and blogs for social support. Start with small initial steps. Preparing and planning your approach is an important step before swinging into full action.

Step 4: Action Stage

In this stage, you are already undertaking changes in your lifestyle. Within the past six months, you have made positive changes to your eating behavior or you have been working out, perhaps with a trainer or in a gym. You are restructuring your environment to better manage eating cues, or you are using rewards to reinforce new behaviors. You may be using the tools provided by various websites and apps for help with tracking food and exercise. If you have been a binge eater, you are taking care to eat three adequate meals a day plus planned snacks as necessary. You are implementing new ways of managing stress to avoid emotional eating. You have someone who listens when you need to talk. You may have enlisted a "buddy" or joined a social network to support you during your change process. Perhaps you have joined a forum or blog for support.

During this stage, you may have feelings of loss about your old ways of eating or using food, and you need to reiterate to yourself the long-term benefits of managing weight and living a healthy lifestyle. It is helpful to be aware of the causes, consequences, and cures for problematic lifestyle behaviors. At this point, a vigilant response to relapse becomes critical. Relapse or backsliding is common during lifestyle changes and need not spell the end of motivation. A slip is an opportunity to learn something new about yourself and the process of changing behavior. After a slip, deconstruct what happened: What were the triggers? What was the function of the behavior? Knowing what you know now, what would you do differently? Problem solving, not self-blame or giving up, is in order. Evaluating what triggered a slip or lapse and learning from it is important for making forward progress.

You need to learn to recover from small slips before they lead to a total relapse into old habits. If you slip, reassess your motivation and reaffirm your plan to overcome the barriers to permanent change. Learning coping strategies is important. As you become more confident in your ability to sustain change, your awareness of the cons of changing—the difficulties—starts to shift to an awareness of the pros of changing—the rewards. In this stage, you have successfully redefined who you are and what you will do with regard to your life values about health.

Step 5: Maintenance Stage

In the Maintenance stage, the change process is mostly complete, and your new lifestyle has become part of your new self-definition. You must still prevent relapse and recover from lapses, but you are more confident about handling small slips. There is less need for external rewards because you have internalized the rewards of a healthy lifestyle. Your beliefs about how you choose food and what you do for exercise guide your actions. You think of yourself as a person who leads a healthy lifestyle. You have a firm commitment to

Table 6.2

Stage of Change	Motivation
Precontemplation	No motivation. Doesn't know or denies there is a problem. Needs information.
Contemplation	No motivation. Is thinking about changing but needs more information.
Preparation	Some motivation. Gathering information about problem and thinking about changing.
Action	Motivated to take action. Undertaking lifestyle changes.
Maintenance	High motivation. Solidifying lifestyle changes.

sustaining your new lifestyle and have incorporated the new behavior for the "long haul."

Cost/Benefit Analysis for Change

To create and maintain motivation, especially in the Contemplation and Preparation stages, you need to assess the benefits and costs of either undertaking a change effort or not doing so. If weight loss is your goal, the first step is to examine and strengthen your reasons for wanting to lose weight. Your aim is to create clear, concrete goals that will guide your behavior that can be consciously retained over the long term.

Begin by completing the self-test "Why Do You Want to Lose Weight?" Rate yourself on each of the reasons for losing weight according to *how important that reason is in your decision to undertake weight reduction at this time.* (Be careful to avoid the common temptation to rate all or most of the reasons as "extremely important.") After you have rated each reason, go back and choose the top three reasons you rated most important. Use the spaces provided to the left of each statement to rank the first most important reason that made you decide to want to lose weight at this time, the second most important reason, and the third most important reason. Later, you will use this information to help bolster your motivation and to create a clear commitment that will increase your chances of success.

The reasons you cited in Self-Test 6.1 for wanting to lose weight reflect either the benefits you expect to get by succeeding in losing weight or the costs you want to avoid paying if you remain overweight. Benefits include the rewards, pleasure, or satisfaction you perceive for losing weight. Benefits also accrue if you think you can avoid something unpleasant or bad—like avoiding gaining more weight or preventing or overcoming a chronic health condition. Of course, there are also perceived benefits for *not* losing weight—that is, the easiness of not changing, letting yourself avoid effort, and so forth. A benefit of not trying to lose weight might be that of not having to take responsibility for your food choices.

Self-Test 6.1 Why Do You Want to Lose Weight?

Rank	Extremely Important	Somewhat Important	Not at All Important
___ 1. I want to wear slimmer clothes.	1 2 3	4 5 6 7	8 9 10
___ 2. I want to feel better about myself.	1 2 3	4 5 6 7	8 9 10
___ 3. I want praise and approval from others.	1 2 3	4 5 6 7	8 9 10
___ 4. I want to move around more easily.	1 2 3	4 5 6 7	8 9 10
___ 5. The doctor said I need to lose weight.	1 2 3	4 5 6 7	8 9 10
___ 6. Someone I care about isn't happy about my weight.	1 2 3	4 5 6 7	8 9 10
___ 7. I have a health problem and losing weight could help.	1 2 3	4 5 6 7	8 9 10
___ 8. I want to avoid potential health problems from too much weight.	1 2 3	4 5 6 7	8 9 10
___ 9. I'm afraid of getting fatter, so I better start now.	1 2 3	4 5 6 7	8 9 10
___ 10. I don't like the criticism and ridicule I get from others.	1 2 3	4 5 6 7	8 9 10
___ 11. My weight gets in the way of my feeling sexy.	1 2 3	4 5 6 7	8 9 10
___ 12. I want to present a better professional image.	1 2 3	4 5 6 7	8 9 10
___ 13. If I don't lose weight, I may lose my job.	1 2 3	4 5 6 7	8 9 10
___ 14. Other: _____ _____ _____	1 2 3	4 5 6 7	8 9 10

Likewise, costs are associated with changing as well as not changing. The costs are the punishments, pain, or discomfort you experience whether or not you change. Costs of changing include having to impose self-discipline about exercise and food choices, as well as accepting the expenditure of time, money, effort, or the loss of certain personal pleasures in order to succeed at changing. Costs of not changing are likely to involve diminishing health and vitality and increasing social problems.

When you believe that the rewards or benefits from doing a particular thing outweigh the costs involved, you tend to keep doing whatever produces benefits. Conversely, you tend to stop doing whatever produces punishment or displeasure or costs you more time and effort than the resulting benefits are worth. Since both benefits and costs are involved in every behavior pattern—whether it involves eating, exercise, or some other area of life—you make tradeoffs between the two.

For example, exercising may provide the immediate benefits of feeling good and the long-term benefits of improved cardiovascular fitness, but it also takes time that you might prefer to spend differently, and, in the beginning at least, exercise may involve some discomfort. If you like feeling good after exercise and you want to ensure long-term cardiovascular health, you decide to pay the costs involved in exercising, including making time for it and expending the effort.

People who exercise regularly usually have a long list of the benefits they get from it—feeling good, having more energy, being able to eat more than sedentary people, and so forth. If asked what they *don't* like about exercise, they are likely to minimize the costs. They exercise frequently because they perceive greater benefits than costs. It's important to redefine yourself as a person who gets regular exercise, not a person who *tries* to get exercise. On the other hand, people who don't exercise or who used to exercise occasionally but don't at all anymore are more likely to give a long list of the costs of exercise while minimizing the benefits.

Exactly what constitutes a cost or a benefit depends on your point of view. What is rewarding to one person may be punishing to another. The benefits you derive, or the costs you perceive, are what *you* think they are, not what someone else judges them to be. If you get enough benefits from behaving a certain way, your tendency is to ignore the costs that go along with this behavior pattern or ratio-nalize them away. People who smoke, for example, manage to ignore smelling bad, persistent coughing, stained fingers and teeth, and the long-term negative health consequences. By ignoring the costs of smoking and focusing on the pleasure or relief smoking provides, they allow themselves to continue smoking. Human beings are good at distorting or denying the very real health costs of a particular behavior pattern—whether it is smoking, eating inappropriately, or not exercising—in order to keep enjoying the rewarding aspects of unhealthy behavior. Denying the costs of bad habits or rationalizing them is a common reason for procrastination and loss of motivation. It is this kind of denial that leads to putting off losing weight or to periodically starting a weight-reduction effort and losing momen-tum before achieving success.

Immediate Versus Delayed Costs and Benefits

Some of the benefits and costs associated with a behavior are imme-diate. When you eat a hearty meal, you feel satisfied. When you over-eat, you feel uncomfortable. Other benefits and costs are delayed. You can eventually wear a smaller size when you lose weight. If you don't lose weight, your clothes may feel tight and you may someday develop diabetes or another health problem.

The benefits and costs that have the most powerful influence on how you act are those that occur immediately, at the time you are acting. Results that come later have far less influence. When faced with the choice of whether to eat a hot fudge sundae and get plea-sure now, or to pass it up to lose weight so you can wear slimmer clothes later, it is much easier to decide "I'll start tomorrow." When the alarm goes off a half hour earlier than usual to remind you to get out and jog, the immediate pleasure of continuing to snuggle in bed is often more compelling than the idea of the exhilaration that will come an hour from now from exercising or having better health months or years down the road. That's why values are so important—they make long-term rewards more immediate by providing lifestyle guidance. (People who think of themselves as valuing their health may occasionally choose a hot fudge sundae, but they make sure to exercise regularly.)

To be successful in losing and managing weight, you need to keep the delayed benefits you expect from losing weight and the costs you pay for not doing so in the forefront of your thinking at all times. At the same time, you need to minimize and discount the immediate rewards you get from staying the same and ignore or minimize the costs of changing. Unfortunately, as you begin the work of changing your habits, choosing food differently, and increasing your exercise, you may find that your attention shifts to the more immediate benefits of not trying to change as well as to the immediate costs of making such efforts.

It is crucial that you avoid dwelling on the pleasures you used to get before starting weight management, otherwise it is only a matter of time before you revert to old patterns and give up your weight-management efforts once again. You need to constantly bring your focus back to your values and what you expect to get by losing weight and the realistic assessment of the costs you will pay for not losing weight. When you find yourself dwelling on the effort involved in losing weight, you need to refocus your thinking to the motivating aspects of changing. Doing a cost-benefit analysis can help in that.

Doing a Cost-Benefit Analysis

Completing a cost-benefit analysis will help you assess the costs and benefits you expect to experience from undertaking behavior change. In the sample shown in table 6.3, the change is that of losing weight, although you could specify some other behavior change,

Table 6.3 Sample Cost-Benefit Analysis

#1 Benefits of changing	#2 Benefits of *not* changing
What good things do you expect to get, now or later, from losing weight, like better health? ■ *feel better physically* ■ *able to put on panty hose without getting out of breath* ■ *wear smaller-sized clothes* ■ *like myself more*	What enjoyable things do you get to do or have by not trying to lose weight? What unpleasant things do you avoid, like having to exercise? ■ *don't have to deal with men* ■ *don't risk getting hurt* ■ *eat and drink what I want* ■ *control is unnecessary* ■ *don't have to exercise*
#3 Costs of changing	**#4 Costs of *not* changing**
What don't you want to give up in order to lose weight? What do you have to do that you would rather not do? ■ *give up junk food* ■ *cut down on alcohol* ■ *make time for exercise*	What unpleasant or undesirable things are you likely to get now or in the future if you don't lose weight, like lower self-esteem or a chronic disease? ■ *poor health* ■ *feeling fat* ■ *feeling bad about myself* ■ *lack of a relationship*

such as quitting smoking or undertaking exercise. Later, when you feel tempted to return to old habits, review what you have written. Post the form in a place where you can see it easily and be reminded of your reasons for changing. If you are keeping a journal, put your cost-benefit analysis in the book.

First, look at the sample cost-benefit analysis in table 6.3. Then fill out the blank form in table 6.4 or create your own form by drawing a line down the center of a paper and another line across the center forming four quadrants or boxes. Label the one in the upper left-hand corner #1, the one in the upper right-hand corner #2, the one in the lower left-hand corner #3, and the one in the lower right-hand corner #4. Box #1 should also be labeled "Benefits of changing," box #2 is labeled "Benefits of *not* changing," box #3 is labeled "Costs of changing," and box #4 is "Costs of *not* changing." Changing, of course, can relate to losing weight, exercising more, adopting a particular healthy lifestyle behavior, or some other lifestyle change you want to make.

In box #1 on the form, note the benefits you expect to get both now and later from undertaking behavior change. (If this change is to lose weight, as shown in the sample, you can get some help on this topic from the "Why Do You Want to Lose Weight?" checklist in table 6.2 that you completed earlier in this chapter.) Unfortunately, the benefits expected from weight reduction are often not well thought out. You need to develop persuasive but realistic ideas of the benefits you expect to receive by making lifestyle changes. Moreover, these benefits must be important to you regardless of what others think. If the benefits you expect from losing weight are not powerful enough to compete successfully with the benefits of staying the same—that is, not changing—or if they are not powerful enough to overcome the costs involved in losing weight, you must give this question more thought. Your odds of long-term success will not be good unless you have powerful reasons for wanting to lose weight.

In completing this analysis, Olivia from the chapter-opening vignette wrote that the benefits she expected to get from losing weight were to be able to wear a size eight dress and get more compliments. She was asked if she presently got compliments about her appearance from her husband and people she cared about. Olivia replied that she did. She was then asked if her husband and friends particularly cared what size she wore. Olivia conceded that they probably didn't. "Is wearing a size eight dress going to be powerful enough to carry you through the tough times when you don't feel like exercising or do feel like making less healthy food choices?"

Table 6.4 Sample Cost-Benefit Analysis

#1 Benefits of changing	**#2 Benefits of _not_ changing**
What good things do you expect to get, now or later, from losing weight, like better health?	What enjoyable things do you get to do or have by not trying to lose weight? What unpleasant things do you avoid, like having to exercise?
#3 Costs of changing	**#4 Costs of _not_ changing**
What don't you want to give up in order to lose weight? What do you have to do that you would rather not do?	What unpleasant or undesirable things are you likely to get now or in the future if you don't lose weight, like lower self-esteem or a chronic disease?

"I guess not," replied Olivia.

Olivia was given this good advice in response to her reply: "Then you need to rethink your reasons for wanting to lose weight. Try to develop some powerful but realistic ideas about what dressing slimmer will do for you. Maybe there is something else that you seek and losing weight seems like the most readily available solution. Don't start weight reduction efforts until you examine the situation.

Perhaps you should check the BMI chart and, if you are within the healthy range, reconsider whether you need to lose weight at all. If you are not in the healthy range, consider the health benefits of losing some weight. Or even if you are in the healthy weight range, give some thought to losing weight if you have risks of cardiovascular disease such as hypertension or high cholesterol. Perhaps you can benefit from increasing your exercise and just making some small changes in the way you eat, like reducing your intake of red meat."

In box #2, indicate the benefits you expect to get now and later by staying the same—by not changing or not trying to lose weight. Examples might be "not having to exercise" or "continuing to eat whatever I want." These are the sorts of things you get to enjoy right now when you are not trying to lose weight, and these are the things that are most likely to come to mind when you are in the middle of a weight-loss effort.

In box #3, state the costs you expect to pay both now and later by undertaking change or losing weight. In the enthusiasm of a fresh start, you may be tempted to ignore or minimize these costs. Don't. Acknowledge them now so you can make an informed decision to pay the costs. It is important to recognize and acknowledge them in the beginning so that they will not come as a surprise later. When you find yourself thinking about the costs in the future, it will be easier to accept them if you have anticipated them. You will need to discount and minimize the costs then as much as possible and to turn your attention back to what you have noted in boxes #1 and #4.

Finally, in box #4, write the costs you now pay and may pay in the future as a result of not losing weight—of not changing. Some of the reasons you checked earlier on the Self-Test 6.1 "Why Do You Want to Lose Weight?" may give you a clue to your costs for staying the same. For example, one cost could be lower self-esteem. Once your change effort is underway, your natural tendency will be to deny or minimize the costs you pay for not losing weight. By listing them now, it will be harder to dismiss them later. Be honest with yourself here; it will be important later.

At the moment, as you anticipate beginning a change effort, the boxes that tend to exert the most influence on your behavior are boxes #1 and #4—the benefits you get from losing weight and the costs of not losing weight. As a result, you feel motivated to get going. Box #1 is "the carrot" and box #4 is "the motivational stick."

People who focus on boxes #2 and #3—the benefits of not changing and the costs of trying to lose weight—find it hard to start on a change effort or to stay with one. These "demotivating" boxes are shaded on your sample and the blank forms as a reminder that focusing on these concerns is likely to undermine your motivation. If thoughts about these do arise, notice they are there and remind yourself that these are just tricks your mind is playing; you don't have to act on those thoughts. These demotivating thoughts come from that part of you that doesn't like change and wants you to take the easy way out. Simply acknowledge to yourself that they are coming from the part of you that isn't in touch with your values. Refocus your thoughts on the ideas in the unshaded "motivation" boxes—box #1 (the benefits you expect to get from changing) and box #4 (the costs you will pay for not changing). By reminding yourself of these ideas and staying in touch with your values, you can motivate yourself to undertake change and to stick with it.

Periodically, you should go back and review your cost-benefit analysis. As you progress in your change endeavor, you may find new reasons to continue with your effort, or you may need to acknowledge and accept some costs you hadn't recognized previously. If your motivation starts to flag, review your analysis. Use it to keep your commitment clear and your motivation on track.

Social Support and Motivation

Finding other people to support your behavior change or weight-management efforts is important for success and sustaining motivation. Some weight-loss internet programs and smartphone applications provide social support in a variety of ways. They may provide bulletin boards or chat rooms for interaction or other means of social networking with others trying to lose weight or get more exercise. Another way to get social support can be to choose a "buddy" or support person to help you in your change efforts. A buddy or friend is someone with whom you check in on a regular, perhaps daily, basis for praise, encouragement, and a listening ear when necessary. Perhaps they join with you in making lifestyle changes. Having a support person means being accountable to someone else for your actions. When you report on your efforts to someone else, you are more likely to stay on track.

If you are participating in a group or formal weight-loss program, it is a good idea to choose your support person from among this group. In larger groups, the leader may suggest choosing a buddy. Alternatively, there are people who perform the services of a weight-loss coach for a fee. You may be able to find one near you by checking the internet. If you are trying to lose weight on your own, try to find someone who is interested in losing weight with you. It is okay to have more than one support person. Working with a buddy is usually a reciprocal arrangement and, in most cases, you will act as a buddy in return, but be careful you don't make your support person into the "weight police." What you need is someone to talk to and get encouragement from when you slip and who will praise your efforts when you succeed at making even small changes.

Some people in a group program don't like the idea of having a buddy in their weight-management efforts. They think they should be able to succeed without outside help, or they want their weight-management effort to be a private affair. If forced to choose a buddy, they are likely to find someone who shares these sentiments, and the two of them, in effect, enter into a contract to *pretend* to be buddies. In other cases, one person genuinely wants to have and be a buddy, but the other person isn't as committed to the idea. For the buddy system to work, you need to believe that it can benefit you, and you must be willing to make the extra effort to stay in touch with your support person. For the buddy system to pay off, it has to be a mutually cooperative effort.

One of the most important aspects of weight loss is keeping in contact with others who are working on losing weight or making another behavioral change. When there are others who are in tune with your change ups and downs, and are waiting for your responses, you are more likely to lose weight and keep it off. To find a buddy, you could check out the internet for chat rooms of others who are engaged in a weight-loss effort.

The Role of a Support Person

A good support person has an optimistic attitude. There is no place for pessimism or criticism in the buddy system. Support persons not only talk to each other about their progress but may engage in other helpful activities, such as exercising together or sharing healthful recipes. Support persons should:

❖ Maintain a positive, accepting, success-oriented attitude.

❖ Avoid judging or criticizing.

❖ Make regular contact as mutually agreed upon.

❖ Listen with the intent of hearing the other's feelings.

❖ Share progress and positive experiences.

❖ Offer advice or suggestions only when asked or given permission.

❖ Avoid complaining or rejecting suggestions without consideration.

❖ Avoid giving permission to backslide.

Choosing a Support Person

Some people are shy about asking an actual person (as opposed to someone online) to be a buddy or a support person. If they are in a weight-management group, some people simply turn to the person nearest them to get the awkward selection over with. A more productive approach is to get to know a few of the people in the group before choosing a candidate. Take time to find out how a prospective support person feels about having a buddy and what their expectations are. (It also helps to have a second choice in mind.)

If you are not in a group program, consider asking a friend or coworker to be a support person. It is great if the prospective support person is also engaged in a similar change effort, but it is not absolutely necessary if they are understanding and accepting. No matter how you find a support person, it is necessary to exchange information, including email addresses, phone numbers, and the best times to be in contact to talk.

If you decide to find a support person who is not currently involved in a weight-management effort, be sure to explain to them how they can be of help. Explain to the person you choose what you need him or her to do and not do. For example, you do not want your support person to watch over your every move or to comment negatively on what you are eating.

Often a willing spouse or significant other can be a valuable and supportive buddy. Spouses who also keep track of what they eat, who are also striving to improve eating and exercise habits, who praise partners for day-to-day progress and for attaining goals, and who exercise with them are most helpful. If possible, spouses should attend weight-loss program meetings and learn more about weight management. Spouses who are involved together in weight management generally report increased marital satisfaction.

Competitive Buddies

Some people find that engaging in a competition is helpful to their change efforts and helps increase motivation. Often deciding to compete is done informally, such as when one person poses the challenge to another that "whoever loses 20 pounds first wins." The pair may wager some money or another prize to boost their motivation. Such an approach is more likely to work if it is done a little differently. First, instead of issuing a challenge for losing a number of pounds, establish a proportion of body weight to lose, such as

5 or 10 percent of your total weight. In that way, people of different sizes or genders can compete equally. Likewise, set a time limit that allows for the reasonable possibility of losing that percentage of weight, and be specific about the prize. For example, the challenge might be "The first one to lose 10 percent of their body weight by [a set date] (say, four months from now) will be owed $50 by the other." Next, involve a monitor for each competitor. The monitor is present when each competitor weighs in at the beginning and end of the competition and periodically asks about progress. The monitor also makes sure the prize is awarded.

Contests and competitions involving groups of people can also be helpful in promoting motivation and weight loss. Whole organizations sometimes compete against another organization, or departments within one organization might wage a contest with one another. Just as when two individuals compete, it is important that a definite time frame be established with rules and there is an agreed-upon impartial person to monitor the process. When contest participants exercise together, monitor eating, and support one another's efforts, they are more likely to stay motivated and succeed.

7

Changing Behavior

Emma was always going on a diet. She could be "good" for a while, but at some point, usually when stress got to her, she would have a cookie or two, at which point she felt she had crossed some imaginary line. "Well, now I've blown it. I may as well keep on eating." All her resolve went out the window. She felt terrible about herself when she went off a diet, but whenever she heard of a new, "breakthrough" diet, she would try again. She had heard that diets don't work and that adopting a healthy lifestyle including exercise was the key, but she didn't know how to go about it.

Behavior is to people what water is to fish—you don't usually pay much attention to it. But to adopt a healthier lifestyle, you need to understand and learn how to notice behavior so you can make changes. The first model for understanding behavior was *behaviorism*, which was fostered by B. F. Skinner's work. This came to be known as the *first wave* of psychology. Behaviorism focused on observable behavior only—what can be seen and counted. Later work recognized that thinking and emotions are also involved in behaving, and the *cognitive-behavioral model* was proposed. This was called the *second wave* of psychology. More recently, mindfulness has been recognized as an important means of fostering helpful behavior and managing emotions. *Mindfulness* considers personal values and what a person focuses on—what they attend to in their mind. It has come to be known as the *third wave* of psychology. All three of these ways of understanding behavior are important for adopting healthier habits.

The ABCs of Behavior

In the first wave of psychology, early psychologists explained behavior in terms of the ABCs. This approach involved stimulus (the A), behavior (the B), and reward or result (the C or Consequence) to formulate the ABC model of behavior. According to this model, an *Antecedent* (stimulus or cue) prompts a *Behavior* (an action) that is followed by a *Consequence* (what happens next). If the consequence is sufficiently rewarding—you like it—it keeps the behavior happening again and again. So, for example, if you see a cookie (cue), eat the cookie (behavior), and it tastes good (rewarding consequence), you are likely to have another one, and the sequence happens again, perhaps until you have eaten all the cookies.

If the consequence is not rewarding or feels bad, the behavior is abandoned. For example, if you don't like getting up early in the morning to go to the gym (and who does?), you are likely to stop going. Sometimes the consequence involves losing something you want or like, and this too can prevent the behavior from happening again. For example, if the friend you normally walk with every day gets sick or decides to stop walking, you may stop walking, at least until they can join you again.

If the consequence is rewarding, the cycle is likely to repeat. That consequence becomes a new cue for a new cycle. Take note of figure 7.1.

Of course, things are actually a little more complicated than that, but this simple model made it possible to instruct people how to

Figure 7.1

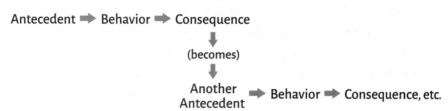

change behavior themselves and start new habits by intervening at one of these points.

From a behavioral perspective, environment sets the stage for behavior and influences the success of any endeavor. It provides the *circumstances* for behavior—the setting that includes the external cues (antecedents) that prompt behavior and indicates the rewards or results (consequences) that are likely to follow. An example of circumstances that can trigger unhealthy eating behavior would be having something inviting—like cookies—sitting out on the counter or table. Just the sight of cookies can make your mouth water. To change behavior, it is important to manage cues in the environment. Based on behaviorism, early suggestions for losing weight included not having tempting food in the house (managing the environment and avoiding cues to eat) or using a smaller plate (creating a cue to eat less). Many such behavioral suggestions are still pertinent.

Cognitive-Behavioral Model

The ABC model was intended for only observable actions. In the second wave of psychology, the ABC model was expanded to include thoughts, beliefs, and feelings as internal actions, which were designated *private events* or *cognitions*.

Psychiatrist Aaron Beck at the University of Pennsylvania and New York psychologist Albert Ellis pioneered the work called *rational thinking*. Thoughts could be cues, behaviors, or consequences. As a result of their work, the influence of thoughts and feelings became a legitimate focus of research. Unlike behaviorism's sole focus on observable behavior, private events were legitimately conceived by the cognitive-behavioral perspective as antecedents, behaviors, or consequences. Thus, thoughts can trigger eating, or eating can trigger self-criticism and feeling bad, for example. Or, feeling bad can trigger a thought about food, which then leads to eating, followed by more thoughts and feelings—often self-criticism and upset. The idea of examining *overt behavior* (observable actions) in conjunction with *covert behavior* (thinking and feeling) came to be known as the *cognitive-behavioral revolution*.

Cognition

The word *cognition* refers to all forms of knowing and awareness, such as perceiving, conceiving, believing, remembering, reasoning, judging, imagining, and envisioning solutions. In short, *thinking*. Thinking can occur silently in the privacy of one's own mind through "talking" to ourselves (sometimes out loud). Thinking can also involve picturing things or places in our heads, imagining something that doesn't yet exist, recalling past memories, or considering what to do about problems. Research has shown that cognition is an important part of how and why behavior happens.

Subconscious Processing

More and more research involves investigating cognitive processes that operate in the background of conscious processing and influence behavior. Such processes are also referred to as the *unconscious* or *subconscious* mind. These might be defined as that part of the mind which gives rise to a collection of mental phenomena that manifest in a person's mind but which the person is not aware of at the time of their occurrence. These phenomena include automatic skills (like driving a car without knowing how you got to your destination), unnoticed perceptions (like attending to nonverbal behaviors in others or subtle physical sensations in your body), or unconscious thinking habits. One example of an unconscious thinking habit is a cognitive distortion, a common error in thinking that many people make. An example would be to think "I'm either perfect or I'm a failure." Many people experience this type of *dichotomous thinking*, also known as *all-or-nothing thinking*.

The Mindfulness Model

The more recent third wave of psychology preserves many of the techniques from behaviorism and cognitive-behaviorism but focuses on *context*—how we see and understand thoughts and feelings so they don't have to determine action—and on learning to hold thoughts lightly (i.e., not believing thoughts and feelings must be acted on). It emphasizes the broad constructs of values and mindfulness, whereas the first- and second-wave models focused mainly on immediate problems and relief of symptoms. For example, a unhealthy might seek to identify and challenge cognitions, but a third-wave therapist might focus on the need to accept thoughts and feelings and understand how they tie into a person's value system. The aim is to change by identifying and referring to values and life goals and ultimately changing that which can be changed or accepting that which cannot be changed. In this new psychology, thoughts and emotions are conceptualized as events of the mind that may conform to or distract from personal values. Recognizing that thoughts can be problematic and bringing behavior back in line with one's values is important for permanent success.

Doing What Works

Managing the external environment, including observable cues and reinforcements, is still an important part of changing behavior, as is paying attention to thinking. It is important to manage thinking and cope with feelings to bring about permanent lifestyle change. The new ingredient to successful change is *mindfulness*, which is the ability to observe thoughts without judging them and without becoming overwhelmed by mind chatter—the stream of thinking that occupies everyone's mind when they aren't focused on one thing. A good way to learn more about mindfulness is to search the internet for "youtube everyday mindfulness."

Cues and Rewards

To change behavior, attention needs to be paid to external cues and consequences. *Cues* are the signals or conditions that elicit or prompt behavior or suggest reward is available. Seeing someone walking down the street with an ice cream cone, or seeing an ice cream store, might cause you to want to buy an ice cream cone. Seeing ice cream is a cue. Putting your running shoes by the door or assembling and putting out your exercise clothes the night before can be a cue to exercise the next morning.

Rewards, or consequences of a behavior, determine whether behavior will be repeated or abandoned. What if healthy behavior is rewarded, say, by an employer like Safeway? In fact, the Safeway grocery chain did once initiate a program whereby employees who stopped smoking or who lost weight were rewarded with a small amount of money. That action got some of them to adopt a new behavior. Is this type of change in behavior lasting? Maybe. But for many people who participate in similar programs, the new behavior lasts only while the reward is in effect. Once the environment reverts—in this example, once Safeway ended the program—old habits often come back. (Notice that Safeway was implementing an *extrinsic* reward system—one that came from outside and not from the people themselves. *Intrinsic* rewards—those motivated from within the person—are more powerful for reinforcing new behavior.) While Safeway's intentions were probably good, the reward offered may not have helped the behavior become firmly held.

Behavior is influenced by many cues happening at the same time and by anticipated rewards. Think of a time when you went out to dinner with friends. Looking forward to being with friends in a social setting may have been a cue to feel pleasant. Being in a nice restaurant was another cue—and probably part of why you were feeling good. Finding appetizing dishes on the menu probably stimulated interest—more cues for the desire to eat. All these cues set the stage for choosing food. Anticipating what would taste good was also a cue. Once you ordered and started dining, your physical sensations hopefully were pleasant and rewarding, which made you keep eating. The fact that you were satisfied with your entrée and wanted to continue feeling good—and, possibly, you were excited by a dessert description on the menu—may have prompted you to order dessert. The rewards of the experience made you want to go out to dinner again, probably with the same people. Of course, if you didn't like the food or the people you were with, you would decline the next invitation. This is how cues and rewards work. But beliefs and mindfulness also influence behavior.

Cognitive-Behavioral Influences

Self-talk is a way of thinking that influences behavior and emotions. Chapters 11 and 12 are devoted to this topic. For now, be aware that negative self-talk—self-criticism, taking things personally, rationalizations to make poor choices, thoughts focusing on unfulfilled expectations or perceived failure, and more—can often undermine goal-directed behavior and lead to discouragement. Becoming aware of such thinking and refocusing on more positive thinking is needed for lifestyle change and success.

Beliefs and Mindfulness

Behavioral changes really only stick if they are internalized as the natural outcome of beliefs and life values. A *value* is a belief or philosophy that is personally meaningful in some way. Whether you are consciously aware of them or not, every individual has a core set of personal values that guide behavior. Values can range from the commonplace, such as a belief in hard work and punctuality, to the more psychological, such as self-reliance, concern for others, and harmony of purpose. Some people have values that are not socially acceptable, such as that of a thief, who only wants personal gain.

Mindfulness is having an open and nonjudgmental attitude in the present moment; mindfulness helps you stay in touch with your values. It involves paying attention to the present and whatever is

happening now. Mindfulness is a state of alert, focused consciousness that involves paying attention to thoughts and sensations without judgment. It is a focus on the present moment without resorting
to thoughts about the future or the past.

Those who value their health and well-being find it easier to
engage in behaviors that reflect their values. To change behavior
permanently, it is necessary to reevaluate personal values. There
must be a basic change in the way a person views themself and their
life and the values by which they want to live. Otherwise, an old
habit returns when previous circumstances are reinstated or values
remain unexamined.

You may be one of those people who, in the past, undertook a serious
effort to lose weight and maybe even succeeded for a while. Perhaps
you were able to take weight off and keep it off for an extended period.
If you eventually regained weight, it was probably because you gradually—or quickly—returned to old behaviors. Old habits encroached
on, and eventually overtook, your success. Having returned to previous behaviors and your prior weight, you were probably left with a
quiet fear that you will never really succeed in maintaining a healthier
weight or lifestyle. And you were also left with a question: How can I
alter my behavior to make changes permanent?

Changing Behavior Patterns

The first step toward changing a behavior is to uncover unhealthy
patterns by keeping a record of the circumstances of the bad habit
or behavior. The behavior pattern in question could be overeating,
not exercising, smoking, gambling, spending, skin picking, and so on.
Remember that thoughts and feelings are also behaviors, albeit mental ones. Recording the cues to behavior, what actions you took, and
the consequences are the circumstances of interest. You might choose
to use a smartphone app to record eating and exercise behavior, or
you might choose to record your actions in a less technical way by
keeping a journal or a spreadsheet. Doing so is called *self-monitoring*.
If you use this latter method, the following is a list of behaviors you

might want to record. Self-monitoring brings behavior to the front of your consciousness and is one of the most powerful ways to change behavior.

Self-Monitoring

Behavior doesn't just happen. It is embedded in a context that includes the events (both private thoughts and feelings and observable events) that elicit, or cue, and reinforce behavior. For eating, these include the time of eating, the location, related thoughts and feelings, the anticipated and real results of the action, and a variety of other influences. You need to uncover the circumstances of the behavior you want to alter to change it. One approach to identifying behavior patterns is with self-monitoring. Self-monitoring involves keeping a daily record of behavior and the circumstances—i.e., cues and consequences that surround the behavior. The following information should be recorded each time you eat, for instance:

❖ **When:** What time of day or night did you eat?

❖ **What:** What did you eat? A brief description of the food should suffice, but some people find it helpful to track calories or nutrients.

❖ **Degree of hunger:** How hungry were you at the time? Rate your hunger from "not at all hungry," to "ready to eat hungry," to "overly hungry."

❖ **Location:** Where were you when you were eating (at the kitchen table, in the car, at your computer, in front of the TV, etc.)?

❖ **Triggers:** What triggered your desire to eat? What were your cues for eating?

❖ **Stressors:** What stressors were involved—people, thoughts, emotions? That is, did something stressful lead you to eat, or did you eat out of boredom or some other emotion?

❖ **Emotions:** How did you feel about eating? What were your feelings before, during, and after?

❖ **Reward:** What were you getting (besides food) from eating (e.g., relief from emotional distress, escape from boredom, pleasure, hunger satisfaction, following a routine, avoiding thinking, etc.)?

❖ **Binge:** If you felt *out of control* with the food when you were eating, you were probably amid a binge; indicate this on your record. You might also want to check out chapter 14, "Stopping the Binge-Eating Cycle." If you simply ate a lot but didn't feel out of control, it wasn't a binge, it was just overeating.

The idea is to identify the cues and rewards of your eating behavior. Observable cues and rewards—what you can see—may be people, places, or things. Also record what your thoughts and feelings are at the time of eating, as well as just beforehand and afterward. Self-monitoring keeps you mindful of what you are eating, what is cueing the eating, the emotions that may be involved in the eating event, and the function of the eating behavior—what the behavior serves to do in the moment. Does it satisfy hunger or relieve an unpleasant feeling like boredom, for example? By self-monitoring, you can determine what changes you need to make.

It is also highly recommended that you keep your self-monitoring record at the ready so information can be recorded *at the time the behavior occurs*. Unfortunately, many people who try to self-monitor do not record as they eat. Instead, they try to recall it and they write down the information at the end of the day—that is, they record what they can remember, which usually results in an inaccurate and unhelpful record. Some wait even longer to record, perhaps the next day, further diminishing the usefulness of self-monitoring as a behavior change strategy.

Keeping a simple paper record on hand is one way to make sure you can record the circumstances each time you eat but, these days, a paper record is not your only option. Many internet programs allow people to input their daily calorie intake and calories expenditure information. None of the online programs currently allows recording of thoughts and feelings except in blogs and on forums. Some people prefer to create and update their self-monitoring record on a personal computer, although this may require data entry sometime after the behavior occurs. Some people may keep track of their food consumption and the context of eating on a spreadsheet. Smartphones have many applications for counting calories and nutrients by recording food eaten that also allow you to keep track of your exercise. In some cases, these records can be printed out to show your therapist, dietitian, or support person.

Research has shown that about a quarter of weight-control success is attributable to consistent self-monitoring. No matter how it is done, self-monitoring remains a powerful, if under used, tool for understanding and changing behavior patterns. Self-monitoring helps you determine the times of day that are most problematic (usually later in the day, after 6:00 p.m.), whether overeating at meals rather than snacking is an issue, to what degree becoming overly hungry is a factor in overeating, where eating takes place (cues), who may be involved (stress factors, which are also cues), and what thoughts and feelings (internal or private events that may influence behavior) play a role in inappropriate eating.

Changing Cues

Some people don't think they need to self-monitor because they already know what triggers their eating. They are aware that they skip breakfast and, perhaps, lunch and then overeat at dinner because they are so hungry. By that time, hunger is a powerful cue to eat and hard to deny. Or they may know that emotional eating is their problem or, alternatively, that mindless snacking is the real issue. They may recognize that just the sight or smell of food can trigger the urge to eat—for example, seeing food in a movie or in an ad, walking by the window of a bakery, or smelling meat grilling at a fast-food restaurant. Perhaps they know that having food readily available and in view is a cue to munch without much thought.

Other cues can trigger eating. Not thinking—that is, not staying conscious of behavior—can also lead to inappropriate eating. Eating without thinking and in the absence of hunger is mindless eating. Mindless snacking that starts in late afternoon and extends into the evening is common. Using food to alleviate sadness, boredom, anxiety, loneliness, and other emotions is a big contributor to emotional overeating. Even fun social occasions are common times for overeating or making poor food choices. For some women, the time just before their menstrual period is a time fraught with bad eating choices—eating may be a way to deal with the anxiety, touchiness, and hypersensitivity that can accompany monthly hormonal changes. Likewise, transition times—the time when you finish one task and before you start another—can serve as a cue to eat.

Cues are numerous but there are many ways to address their presence in your life. Most importantly, you need to consistently refer to your values and guiding principles regarding health and well-being. If you are not clear on your values, you need to reexamine what gives your life meaning and purpose. With your values in mind, you need to decide for yourself that "This is what I eat and what I do with regard to exercise and physical activity." Shifting your view of yourself to a new definition in relation to food and exercise will help you act in accordance with a higher level of value focused on making healthy choices.

Time of Day

Watch for a particular time of day that snacking or overeating starts. For many people, this is late in the afternoon or early in the evening. Take Vera. She finished work at 4:30 p.m. When she got home, she got something to eat, but her eating continued into the evening. Vera solved this problem by bringing an appropriate and satisfying snack to work and eating it in the afternoon before going home. Once she got home, she made sure to get busy with other tasks or she just relaxed with a book.

Another woman defeated inappropriate eating by talking back to the refrigerator. When she passed it, she would say, "You're not going to get me now." Her spouse thought this was funny at first, but eventually he recognized that she needed to make the refrigerator an "external threat." In due time, she managed this and other cues and succeeded in losing weight.

Evening snacking in front of the TV or the computer is a problem for many people. One solution, of course, is not to have snack foods available in the house. Another approach is to plan a snack for later in the evening. Make it something substantial and enjoyable, but still healthy. Decide that after finishing dinner, your next eating will be at the appointed snack time and stick to that schedule. Also tune into the function of this snacking. Is it to give your mouth and hands something to do? Or could you be using snacking at these times to stay awake? Eva, a college student, was able to pull all-nighters by snacking while studying.

Some people eat dinner late in the evening and find themselves overeating when they finally sit down to their meal. If your dinner is likely to be late, be sure to have a late afternoon snack to carry you through. Also, be careful about snacking in unhealthy ways before a late dinner. A couple of glasses of wine with cheese and crackers can add a lot of calories to your day.

Hunger and Fatigue

Being overly hungry is often a cue to overeat. To overcome such eating, be sure to eat three regular meals a day, including breakfast, lunch, and dinner, as well as planned snacks as needed. Don't let yourself become overly hungry. You probably will have to plan for food, especially if you work a stressful job that demands overtime. Some bariatric surgeons advise having only three meals a day with no snacking whatsoever. For some people, eating four, five, or more small meals a day works best. All experts agree that breakfast is an essential meal that should never be skipped.

Some people say, "I *can't* eat breakfast," meaning, "I don't have time to eat breakfast," or "I just can't face food in the morning." Such excuses only mean that you overate late last night, didn't get enough rest, or didn't plan ahead (or all three). For some people, knowing they overate the previous night, together with the attendant guilt, can reduce the desire for breakfast in the morning. Others may use the excuse, "Once I eat, I'm hungry all the time." If this is you, you need to learn to live with food, and that means breaking the fast of the night and feeding yourself regularly throughout the day with healthy food choices. Trying to stave off overeating by not eating is a strategy that inevitably leads to mindless eating or overeating later in the day. Eventually, hunger makes itself known and it will cause you to ingest excess calories.

Likewise, fatigue will make you vulnerable to overeating. Be sure to get enough rest at night—eight hours is usually recommended. Practice good sleep "hygiene": be sure your room is quiet and dark, don't eat or watch TV in bed, and have set regular times for going to sleep and rising. Don't do anything too stimulating before bed, such as vigorous exercise or watching a scary movie. Remember that alcohol disturbs sleep, so be careful about what you drink before bed. Alcohol might help you fall asleep, but it is likely to make it harder to get restful sleep. If you wake in the middle of the night, have a glass of water if you like, but go back to bed. Don't even *think* about eating in the middle of the night. (If you find yourself eating in the middle of the night and barely remembering it the next day, check with your doctor; you may have a sleep disorder or be having a reaction to medication.)

Location

Location can be a cue to snack inappropriately or eat mindlessly. Keeping food in your desk at work or in the car is ill advised unless it is part of a planned snack program. Planning about what you will eat and when and where you will eat can lead to success. Some people have access to a refrigerator at work and can keep planned snacks such as yogurt or cottage cheese handy. Items like apples and nuts packed in portioned bags don't need refrigeration. Candy and chips, however, are not part of a healthy planned snack program. At work, avoid the vending machines. At home, passing through the kitchen and snacking haphazardly as you go is mindless eating. Don't fool yourself: standing at the kitchen counter for a quick snack adds unwanted calories. Eat your planned snack sitting down at a place appropriate for eating, like the kitchen table.

Distractions

Don't leave food in sight; this means no cookies set out for the kids and no candy dishes for passers-by. Sit down while you eat and avoid multitasking, such as reading the paper or watching TV, while you eat. Eating without the TV on or without something to read at hand promotes mindfulness of eating and is a healthy habit to adopt. Take time to savor your food and eat without guilt. Eating in front of the TV may make you feel like you are not alone, but it robs you of the pure experience of enjoying your food. The distraction of the TV or reading while eating can lead to eating too fast and overeating—plus you miss the full enjoyment that food should bring. Don't eat food while you are surfing the internet or working on the computer; such snacking contributes to excess calories.

Social Influences

What if your spouse or a family member buys and leaves tempting food around the house? How do you avoid those cues? This presents a difficult problem, but one that has several solutions. First, request that food not be left out for you to see. Stay out of the kitchen if that is where food is on display. Distract yourself by getting involved in a project.

What if you are not the one who does the shopping or the cooking? You need to speak up and ask for what you want or need. Be respectful, of course; you want to maintain the goodwill of others. If all else fails, decide to eat smaller portions, and make the healthiest choices possible from what is available at the time. Let your values guide you.

Of course, sometimes drastic action is needed. Erin's mother, who was overweight, always had chips, dip, cookies, ice cream, and other tempting foods in the house. For two years, Erin refused to eat any of this or even the healthy foods her mother sometimes served. At age 19, she became anorexic; she was afraid to eat anything with fat in it. Eventually, the presence of all this tempting food broke her resolve and Erin started binge eating. Her solution was to move out of the house and do her own shopping. With time, she was able to overcome her disordered eating, shop for fresh and unprocessed foods, and live a healthy lifestyle by avoiding the undue influence of her family's food preferences.

Sometimes what you need most is for other members of your household to *not* comment on your weight-loss efforts. If others are sharing opinions that dishearten you, thank them for their concern and request that this topic not be brought up. Ask them not to make comments or allusions to your weight, your eating habits, or your weight-management efforts.

Some people's families or friends believe they have the right to question you about your eating and exercise, which can make you feel pressured and, perhaps, guilty. In that case, you will need to be more assertive with them. People commonly comment on weight loss they observe in others, and usually they mean it as a compliment. This can bring unwanted attention to you and may make you uncomfortable. You may feel that people shouldn't do this. Unfortunately, they do, so you need to be prepared with what you will say when it happens. Learn to be more assertive about your needs. (Assertiveness skills for weight management are addressed in chapter 13, "Managing Stress.")

Stress and Emotions

Managing stress and coping with emotions is covered more thoroughly in subsequent chapters. For now, be on the lookout for situations or feelings that trigger overeating. Binge eating is often triggered by unpleasant emotions such as sadness, anxiety, loneliness, and boredom. Eating is a way to avoid experiencing these feelings. You know you are a binge eater if you feel you lose control over food. (If this is your problem, be sure to read chapter 14, "Stopping the Binge-Eating Cycle.") When assessing your cues for eating, note how others may be causing you to engage in stress eating. Perhaps the stress of a boss who micromanages is driving you to the vending machine too often. Review the previous information given in this chapter as well as chapter 13, "Managing Stress" for more assistance.

Managing Cravings

A craving is an intense desire or longing for a particular substance. About 50 percent of obese binge eaters report having cravings for sweet and sugary foods. Both hunger and negative emotions can set off food cravings. Likewise, just imagining and thinking about something that would "taste good" can trigger a craving. When your desire overpowers your determination, you are in the grips of a food craving. The desire for sweet, rich foods results from the all-too-human drive for pleasure. A craving can be triggered (cued) by any manner of things: seeing an advertisement for desirable food, seeing food depicted in a delicious way, having an attractive leftover available (like surplus birthday cake), or just thinking about food. The more you dwell on the idea of eating a particular food, the more intense the craving becomes. The saved food seems to "call to you" from the kitchen or refrigerator. Tables 7.1 and 7.2 provide tips for coping with cravings and urges to eat.

Shopping for and Storing Food

You can manage your environment in other ways to reduce your vulnerability to existing cues around eating or acquiring problem food. When shopping, take a list and buy only items that are on the list. Don't go shopping when you are hungry or really tired. Plan to avoid the aisles that are problematic for you—like the ice cream or candy

Table 7.1 Tips for Coping with Cravings

1. **Catch a craving early.** Cravings need to be interrupted early on before they get out of control. As you start ruminating about eating something, turn your attention to something else. Think about a project you are working on or a recent vacation; don't let yourself focus more and more on eating. If you continue thinking about eating a particular food, your mouth will begin to water, and your attention will narrow until you lose control.

2. **Interrupt your taste buds.** Brush your teeth and gargle with strong mouthwash. It's difficult to feel like eating afterward. Or put a strong mint in your mouth—anything to spoil your taste buds. Alternatively, try dabbing some cologne or strong-smelling ointment under your nose. These are Band-Aids to stop a craving in its tracks. To avoid cravings altogether, you need to revise your self-definition. If you think of yourself as someone who lives by the words "I make healthy choices," you are less likely to experience or give in to cravings.

3. **Leave temptation behind.** Get out of the area of the temptation. Cross the street if you see a bakery looming in the distance. Stay away from the food table at a party. Hang out anywhere but in the kitchen.

4. **Substitute, substitute, substitute.** Drink water—lots of it. Take a walk. Take a shower. Get on the internet. Do whatever it takes to distract yourself from wanting something to eat. Avoid the refrigerator and the kitchen entirely.

5. **Manage your environment.** Put away leftovers, and don't keep tempting food in sight. If you don't buy it, you are less likely to eat it.

6. **Manage your self-talk.** Don't get persuaded by defeating self-talk; stay in touch with your goals and values.

7. **Indulge a craving with moderation.** If all else fails, let yourself eat in moderation. Watch your portions. If you indulge, do it with considered permission and without guilt.

8. **Remember that cravings pass.** Cravings peak and subside like waves in the ocean. Learn to "surf an urge"—that is, ride it out. It will pass. Tell yourself to wait ten minutes and then decide whether to eat. In the meantime, get busy doing something else. Tell yourself something like, "It won't kill me to wait. I can handle it."

9. **Avoid becoming overly hungry.** Don't skip meals. Eat at least three meals a day and planned snacks if necessary. Never go more than three to four hours without eating.

Table 7.2 The Five Ds for Coping with Cravings

1. **Delay** at least ten minutes before eating so that the impulse can pass.

2. **Distract** yourself in the meantime by getting involved in a project or doing something engrossing.

3. **Distance** yourself from the food or temptation; ruin it or put it in the trash if you really shouldn't eat it.

4. **Determine** how important it is for you to eat this food. Does it fit with your values? Are you making a conscious choice? (Remember: occasional treats are okay.)

5. **Decide** whether to go ahead and eat it, and if you do, choose a moderate amount to eat. Be mindful; enjoy it slowly and without guilt if you decide to eat it.

aisle. Ignore the candy displays at the checkout counter. If you don't have unhealthy food in the house, you are less likely to eat it. Yes, you could still go out and get it, and certainly some people do—even in the middle of the night—but if you "sanitize" your pantry and your refrigerator and discard problematic food, you reduce your vulnerability to eating it. And don't forget the freezer. You know in a pinch you might microwave frozen food or even resort to eating it frozen!

Remember to remove food stored in other places, like the family room or den. (Some people hide snacks in unlikely places, like the dirty laundry basket. One woman even hid her full-calorie Cokes in the toilet tank; it kept them cold as well as concealed from her family, who often criticized her food choices!) The idea of not having food in the house "just in case" frightens some people. Usually, these are the people who use food to deal with stress and emotional overwhelm. Or they grew up in a depriving environment. In either of these cases, consulting a therapist for help is a good idea. Others say, "I can't deprive others in my house just because I can't handle food." If this is the case for you, you can try repackaging food into portions. Put cookies in ziplock bags containing a few cookies (an appropriate child-sized portion) to hand out to the kids as needed. (Of course, this begs the question: Why not give them fruit instead of cookies? Why train them to eat foods made of white flour or sugar?) Put the kids' foods on a separate shelf or in a separate cabinet defined as "not mine," just as you would do if you were sharing living quarters with a roommate.

Mealtimes

Mealtimes are full of cues. There are things you can do to make some cues less bothersome, though. Serve food on smaller plates so it looks like you are getting more than you are. (Trick your eyes and your stomach!) Make eating meals an event rather than something you rush through or wish you could avoid. Set a nice table, put on some classical music, light candles. Invite friends to share a pleasant meal.

When sharing a meal with others, don't snack off their plates. Don't leave food out after a meal (especially desserts) for people to help themselves to more, because you may be the one taking extra. And beware the clean-up phase of meals. If possible, ask someone else to clear the table so you won't be tempted by scraps. Either throw away leftovers or save them in appropriate containers (not see-through) for another meal. Don't snack on scraps or leftovers because you don't want to waste food. Remember: *you can **waste** it, or you can **waist** it.* Be aware that your mind may obsess about tempting food you saved for later and may make you want to eat it sooner. If in doubt, trash it and take out the trash.

Review table 7.3, Winning Behavior-Management Strategies, to keep in mind the best way to manage cues in your environment.

Substituting Healthier Responses

Planning how to handle situations that can be troublesome is a good idea. Some common situations that require healthier responses include eating out in restaurants or at the homes of friends or family, entertaining guests, holidays, and vacations. Learning to slow down the pace at which you eat and redefining your relationship to food and eating are also essential for success.

Table 7.3 Winning Behavior-Management Strategies

❖ Always shop from a list.

❖ Don't shop when you are hungry or overly tired.

❖ "Sanitize" your pantry; remove tempting foods.

❖ Discard leftovers or store them in opaque containers.

❖ Put away reminders of food like the cookie jar or the partially full chip bag.

❖ Keep problem foods out of sight.

❖ Divide problem foods into portions before storing.

❖ Serve food on small plates so it looks like more.

❖ Choose and prepare healthy foods. Avoid frying—broil, bake, or poach instead.

❖ Slow down the pace of at which you eat.

❖ Let someone else clear the table and clean up.

❖ Dispose of problem foods.

❖ Brush your teeth before clearing the table.

Eating Out in Restaurants

Eating in restaurants or at the homes of friends or family can be a big challenge to weight management. Business meetings over lunch or dinner can sabotage one's best intentions, unless you have redefined how and what *you* eat. Plan ahead. Choose or, if you must, insist on a restaurant where you can order food that works for you, especially if you eat out frequently. Salads can be good choices, but be careful of the toppings like bacon bits and cheese and be sure to ask for the dressing on the side. Try dipping your fork in the dressing and then take a bite of salad, or only add a little dressing at a time to the salad. Order your meat or fish broiled, grilled, roasted, or baked plain without a high-calorie sauce or ask for the sauce on the side. Avoid breaded or fried foods, which are loaded with fat and calories. Consider choosing more meatless meals. Ask the waitperson not to bring bread.

Check the menu for the "heart healthy" items but don't rely solely on the restaurant's recommendations. Use good judgment as well;

cottage cheese and a meat patty are not necessarily a good "diet" choice. If you don't know what's in a dish, ask. Consider ordering an appetizer or two instead of a full entrée. Plan to take a portion of an entrée home or ask your dining partner to share an entrée with you. Before you begin eating, separate the entrée into two portions on your plate. If you get the take-home container right away, you can put the half to take home in it before you even begin. Limit alcohol, which adds calories but no nutrition to your meal. Remember that alcohol reduces your resolve. Avoid or minimize your visits to fast-food restaurants.

Eating at Friends' or Relatives' Homes

When you will be a guest in someone's home, you can call ahead and let the host or hostess know any special needs you have, including a preference for sauces on the side. Don't be afraid to say you are try-ing to cut back on calories and would prefer smaller portions. Make it known what you prefer not to eat. Offer to bring an appetizer and make sure it is one you feel comfortable eating. Forget the chips and dip; try a fresh fruit plate or vegetable crudités. Plan ahead and have a snack before you go out, especially if you think dinner might run late. Also decide ahead of time to manage your portions and forgo the butter or oil if bread is served. If you plan on drinking at all, have mineral water or just plain water initially and save your glass of wine for dinner. Skip the hard liquor—and the attendant calories—entirely. Alcohol undermines inhibitions and makes it easier to give in to the temptation to overdo.

Entertaining Guests

Entertaining at home tends to be easier because you are in charge of what is served. Don't think you have to serve high-calorie food to guests. They are typically delighted just to enjoy your company. Salads or light soups are generally appreciated for a first course or light supper, and it is okay to omit bread. Choose a lean protein or fish as your entrée. Keep portions appropriate. Fresh fruit is often a welcome dessert. The key to successful entertaining is in the details: nice presentation, pretty table, flowers or an attractive centerpiece for the table—whatever shows your creativity. Don't be afraid to try out new recipes, even those lower in calories. The internet is a good source for recipes.

Eating During the Holidays

Trying to lose weight during the holidays may be expecting too much (although some people manage it). Not gaining weight during the holidays may be a more achievable goal. To prepare for the holidays, think about what makes the season special for you. Your list might include the smell of a fresh pine tree or your family's traditional fruitcake. Maybe making cookies with the kids is your special thing. If there are foods that really represent a specific holiday for you, plan to have them in moderation. Go ahead with the turkey and dressing, but exercise portion control.

Holidays are often a time when some people feel sad, blue, or depressed. Perhaps there are missing loved ones, and those losses are accentuated during holidays. In addition, during the winter holidays, days are short and nights are long. Some people are vulnerable to a type of depression related to a reduced amount of sunlight called seasonal affective disorder or SAD. Holidays are also a time when expectations run high, with many people envisioning what the holidays "should" be based on their family traditions. If these expectations are not fulfilled, they may experience feelings of disappointment and depression. Knowing this about yourself beforehand can help you plan how to make this holiday season memorable or rewarding. Having a positive attitude is important. In addition, be sure to keep up your exercise, which will help you ward off feelings of depression.

Eating While on Vacation or When Traveling

Continuing to lose weight while on a vacation is a reasonable goal, especially if you plan to leave your desk job behind and get plenty of exercise. Choose carefully where you will go and what you will do on vacation. Consider what food temptations you might face and how you will cope with them. You need not deprive yourself of special food treats that are part of the local color, just exercise good portion control and be aware of foods with lots of sugar, fat, or salt that are likely to make you want to eat more. Exercise forethought and you won't feel guilty.

These days, most hotels have fitness centers, so take your gym shoes and plan to include exercise in your day. Sightseeing often involves lots of walking, which is good. Continue your exercise even when visiting friends. Plan to go for walks. Taking a cruise can increase the risk of overeating unless you employ good choices and portion control. Just because food is unlimited in quantity and seems "free" (avoid the common excuse that "I paid for it, so I'm going to eat it") doesn't mean you should eat more. Even on a cruise, you can still get in lots of exercise by walking or working out in the gym.

When you are traveling on a tour vacation, you have less control over your schedule and, as a result, the times when you eat or what you eat. This can expose you to becoming overly hungry. Plan to take prepackaged snacks such as power bars or nuts that fit into your eating plan. Likewise, traveling on airplanes presents food and eating challenges. They may serve free salted nuts or pretzels, but you usually must supply other food by either purchasing it from the airline or bringing prepurchased food on board. The airline food is prepackaged and often includes chips or cookies that might not fit your new eating pattern. A better idea might be to purchase a sandwich or salad to take on board with you.

Driving long distances by car presents other challenges. If possible, identify ahead of time the restaurants you could stop at for food. Take along food in a small cooler—healthy snacks such as fresh fruit or a picnic lunch—to enjoy at a pleasant rest stop. When you do make rest stops, go for a ten-minute walk, if possible. Stretching your legs will help refresh you and help you enjoy the ride more.

Eat Slowly

Eating slowly—not gulping food—helps your brain catch up with what is going into your stomach. Putting your fork down between bites is one way to do this. Another is to take sips of water between bites. (Bariatric patients are advised not to drink anything during eating to avoid prematurely emptying their smaller stomach pouch.) Take smaller bites. Chew food thoroughly. Pause during the meal. Practice mindfulness: notice whether the food is satisfying as you eat or whether you are getting full. Stop when your stomach is partly full or when the food no longer tastes really great. Resign from the "clean plate" club.

Redefining How You Eat

Developing a set of internal, guiding principles that redefine how you eat on a day-to-day basis is a good tool for long-term weight management. Consider putting foods you eat into these categories:

1. Foods I *usually choose* to eat

2. Foods I *sometimes choose* to eat

3. Foods I *rarely choose* to eat

4. Foods I *choose to treat with care* because they have been dangerous in the past and can cause me to binge or eat too much (for example, bread, cereal, chips, ice cream, peanut butter, trail mix, candy, and so on)

The key here is the word *choose*. What you eat must be a choice, not a "have-to," for you to succeed in keeping a healthy weight and a healthy lifestyle. What you choose is personal and should be guided by your values and your experience. Choices should not be guided by your momentary preferences. That doesn't mean you never have ice cream, or prime rib, or one of those molten chocolate desserts. It does mean that you put these in categories 2 or 3.

You want to develop *your own menu of choices of healthy foods and your way of eating* that is different from the way you choose foods now. Avoid a diet mentality; don't restrict any foods unless you know they might set off a binge. The new way of eating that you need to define for yourself is one in which you are mindful of healthy choices, you are guided by your values, and you are committed to choosing food with its legitimate purposes in mind—to sustain life and provide pleasure—not for escaping life's tribulations. Your new way of eating is guided by the overarching principle of living a healthy lifestyle.

Here's some helpful advice: never make any foods forbidden because doing so makes those foods even more tempting. People with an eating disorder are likely to pronounce certain foods off limits—especially foods containing fat. While no foods should be absolutely forbidden, for overeaters or binge eaters there are often one or two foods that are "dangerous." For instance, some people say they cannot have peanut butter in the house because they will end up eating an entire the jar in one sitting. If you have a danger food, you may have to put in category 4, the "foods I choose to treat with care" category. Such foods must be chosen with caution.

Using Rewards to Change Behavior

No doubt you've heard the story of someone buying a dress in a smaller size as an incentive to lose weight, only to give the dress away some time later, never having been able to fit into it. This was putting the cart before the horse. A reward must come *immediately after* the behavior is performed or the goal is reached, not before. (And as for the new dress being a cue, it is more likely that it will be a cue to feel guilty for not losing weight—and you may end up eating to forget about the guilt you feel.) There are several ways rewards can be used to change behavior, however. Providing incentives is one.

Consider two friends who got into a contest with each other to see who could lose the most weight. Each wagered some money, winner take all. The idea was that winning money would be an incentive to achieve weight loss and the possibility of losing money would be painful enough to stimulate good behavior. This is the carrot-and-stick approach to weight loss. Probably one of these gamblers did lose more weight than the other and collected the bounty. (Or neither of them lost much weight and they called off the bet.) But for the one who lost the money, in all likelihood, neither the potential prize nor the threatened punishment worked. The one who lost the bet just went back to eating as usual. And the winner? Did they keep it off or regain it in due time?

Punishment

Incentives for "good" behavior can work, but punishment for "bad" behavior does not work very well. No doubt the loser of the bet just mentioned shrugged it off and got another piece of cake. In the past, some misguided groups that formed to lose weight have punished members using public humiliation for not adhering to a diet. That didn't prove to be successful; those who were humiliated just quit the group. Well-meaning spouses or family members may try looking disapprovingly or making critical remarks about what they see as bad eating behavior to try to change another's behavior, only to have the dieter get so upset that they eat to spite the critics. Some overeaters even punish themselves with self-criticism to make themselves ashamed enough to change. That doesn't work either.

Punishment involves suffering, pain, loss, or an unwanted event or circumstance that usually results in the "wrongdoer" feeling they do not measure up, they are "less than," or they are unworthy. Punishment is not an effective tool for changing human behavior. Positive reinforcement or reward is more effective in incentivizing change. Reward that influences behavior best includes getting something desirable (like a fun sticker, a desired compliment, or perhaps money) or it involves the removal or avoidance of something undesirable (like hunger or painful feelings).

Making Choices

One way to encourage good self-behavior is to give yourself a choice between two options. The first choice would be to do something healthy in exchange for a reward you want with the reward occurring soon after the desired behavior. The second choice is to make a less-than-healthy choice and lose the reward. This is known as the *Premack Principle*. It involves the voluntary use of a highly desirable and frequently occurring event (such as watching a favorite TV show each night or reading a book in bed before going to sleep) and making its occurrence contingent on the performance of a desired behavior change. For example, you might make a bargain with yourself either to avoid second helpings at dinner and then watch your favorite TV show afterward, or to eat with abandon and forgo your favorite TV show. Giving yourself a choice between consequences can be powerful. Notice that the consequences must follow very soon after the behavior. Another part of making this work is to give yourself a mental pat on the back for succeeding with the desirable behavior. Not only do you get to watch your favorite program, but you also take pride in your accomplishment and feel good.

Shaping Behavior

Rewarding behavior that approximates "good" behavior helps shape a positive behavior pattern in yourself and others. Don't wait for the "big" win for the reward; instead reward small approximations of the goal. For example, Emma, the woman mentioned in the introduction to this chapter, wanted to reach a goal of walking for sixty minutes five days each week. Instead of waiting until she reached the final goal to reward herself, she set up smaller, easily reachable goals, and rewarded herself for accomplishing them. Her smaller initial goal was to walk twenty minutes a day, three days a week. When she accomplished this, she allowed herself a small reward. When she was able to achieve her smaller goal adequately and regularly, she set a new goal of walking 30 minutes three days a week, again followed by a reward. Then thirty minutes four days a week and so on until she reached her final goal. She rewarded herself for each of the smaller subgoals as she attained them. (She used the calendar-and-stickers method of self-reward, which is discussed on the next page.) Rewarding approximations to the desired behavior pattern is called *shaping*. (By the way, you can use positive thoughts and compliments as rewards too. Learn more about this in chapter 11, "Managing Thinking and Self-Talk," and chapter 12, "Challenging Your 'Inner Voices'.")

Using Self-Reward

Almost anything that is valued can be used as a reward. There are several ways to use self-reward to reinforce a new behavior habit or pattern. Remember, though, you are the one who sets the rules, and only you can enforce them. If you are going to reward yourself for good behavior, what you use as a reinforcer must have three characteristics:

1. You must perceive it as *valuable*, either symbolically (like a fun sticker) or in reality (for example, if it is money, it is enough money to really mean something to you).

2. The reward must be *presented as soon as possible*, if not immediately after the healthy behavior occurs. Planning a vacation as a reward is too far in the future. Instead, putting a small amount of money in a fund toward a vacation each time a desirable behavior occurs can be an effective reward.

3. The reward must be *contingent* upon your behavior occurring. You should receive the reward if and only if the healthy behavior occurs. If your spouse agrees to do the dishes if you avoid snacking before dinner, and he or she does them anyway even though you snacked, the reward (your partner doing the dishes) occurs without the behavior occurring; the reward is not contingent on your behavior. If you put money in the piggy bank for vacation even if you didn't make the healthy choice, this isn't a contingent reward.

Using rewards, such as money or putting stickers on a calendar, is intended to be a way of creating interest in and motivating behavior change in the short run. What will make the behavior take root is when you experience feelings of competence and effectiveness in taking charge of your health and your lifestyle. When your behavior is in line with your values, it is less of a struggle to maintain change.

Calendar-and-Stickers Method of Self-Reward

Remember how pleased you were to get a star or other sticker on something you produced—artwork, an essay, or a report—when you were in grade school? Well, stickers are still a great method to symbolically reward behavior, even for adults. Although you may initially be put off by the idea of giving yourself a sticker each time you engage in a desired behavior, it can be fun and motivating. To use the calendar-and-stickers method, you need a month-at-a-glance calendar, preferably a large wall calendar. Another option is to find a book-style month-at-a-glance calendar that is about 5 x 7 inches or, if necessary, use a week-at-a-glance calendar. Then you can use actual metallic stars or some other kind of small sticker (e.g., hearts, red-lip kisses, happy-face decals) to reward yourself for performing a desired behavior each day. Decide what each individual sticker will represent on your calendar. Each sticker would represent something related to the behavior you want to change. Maybe the heart sticker indicates thirty minutes of walking a day, or perhaps a star sticker represents a day you ate three regular meals. Whatever behavior the sticker signifies, apply it to the calendar for the day the behavior occurs. Post the wall calendar in a prominent place (e.g., on the refrigerator door, or somewhere in the kitchen or bathroom where you will see it) or carry the book calendar in your purse or briefcase and display it prominently when you get home. Not only will the stickers signal daily successes, the absence of stickers as days go by should motivate you to get back on track if you have strayed. (Stickers are a form of self-monitoring as well as a symbolic reward.) Each

Figure 7.2 **Calendar-and-Stickers Method**

July						
Sunday	Monday	Tuesday	Wednesday	Thursday	Friday	Saturday
	1 😃	2 😃	3	4	5 😃 ⭐	6 😃
7 😃	8	9 😃 ⭐	10 ⭐	11 😃 ⭐	12 ⭐	13
14 ⭐	15	16 ⭐	17 ⭐	18 😃	19 ⭐	20
21	22	23 ⭐	24 😃	25 ⭐	26 ⭐	27 😃
28	29	30 😃	31 ⭐			

😃 = Eating breakfast   ⭐ = Thirty-minute walk

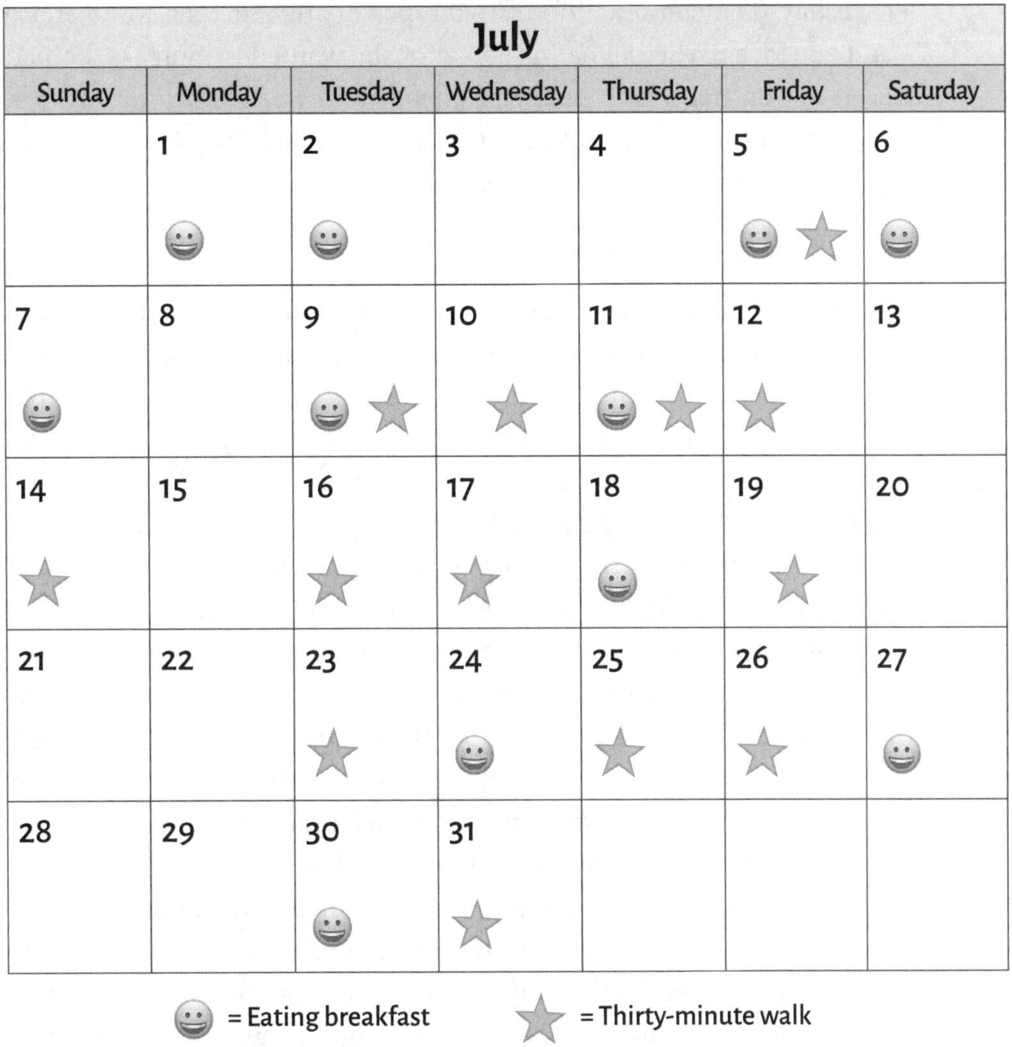

month (or each week) you get to turn over a "new leaf" and start with a clean slate. See the calendar in figure 7.2 using this method.

Emma used the calendar-and-stickers method to motivate and reward her behavior. She bought smiley-face stickers to reward herself for each day she she ate breakfast. She also bought some little stars that signified a thirty--minute walk along a beach boardwalk near her home. She also bought some little stars that signified eating breakfast each day. The combination of two types of stickers, one for exercise and one for a particular eating behavior she wanted to increase, helped keep her on track with behavior change and was rewarding and fun for her at the same time. It can be fun to use different stickers—like red lips, American flags, or anything that works for you.

Money as a Self-Reward

Money can be used as a way to reward yourself, but the difficulty is that the money you want to reward yourself with is yours already, so you need to use special rules to make it work. Take the example of Theo who wanted to reward himself with money for each day he did not binge and then use the money to go to the theater in a few weeks. You already know that a reward must follow promptly after the desired behavior, so having to wait to go to the theater several weekends from now wasn't a very powerful reward, especially when he was faced with a bag of chips and dip he could easily overeat now. So, here's what he did. He created two envelopes: one was to hold his reward money to go to the theater; the other was addressed to a person or organization he did not especially want to support or give money to. His bargain was that for each day or time the healthy behavior occurred, he put a predetermined amount of money in the theater envelope. On those times when he binged, the predetermined amount of money instead went in a stamped and addressed envelope for a disliked organization. Of course, it was the *idea* of supporting a cause he disliked that led him to do the right thing in the first place.

Now maybe you would say having to send money to a disliked organization is punishing. Actually, it does not meet the criteria of causing pain, suffering, and loss of self-esteem unless you berate yourself for "failing." (There's a hint here: what you say to yourself—your self-talk—can be punishing or reinforcing. More about this in chapter 11, "Managing Thinking and Self-Talk.") Is giving money away unpleasant? Yes. That's the idea. But it isn't catastrophic to your sense of self. Note that it doesn't work to give the "failure" money to someone you like. In that case, you can't "lose" the money to someone you like because you could rationalize that it is okay to give money to a good person or cause. Of course, the alternative is not to use money as a means of reward. Instead of losing money to a disliked organization, you could write a short note praising them. Or you could use the calendar-and-stickers method just discussed. Using a symbolic reward like stickers may be more motivating and less anxiety-producing than losing money.

Tracking Progress

Another part of behavior management involves tracking progress. The calendar-and-stickers method tracks progress in behavior change by showing both one's accomplishments and where you are falling behind in your goals. In addition to tracking weight loss, it's important to track progress toward goals.

Tracking Weight Loss

One frequently asked question is "How often should I weigh myself?" People want to know whether they should be keeping track of progress by weighing themselves regularly. Some research suggests that weekly weighing can be helpful. Other research advocates daily weighing. Daily weighing is probably not helpful for those who get upset by numbers because fluctuations in daily weight can be misleading and demotivating. Likewise, being weighed at a doctor's office and finding a discrepancy between the doctor's scale and your scale can be disheartening. (In that case, it is best to rely on the trend you see in your weight loss on your own scale and not the numbers on the doctor's scale.) There is no hard and fast answer to the question of how often to weigh. You should decide what works best for you.

Tracking changes in hip and waist measurements using a flexible tape is also an option. Some internet fitness programs allow you to input and track your measurements as a way of judging progress.

Tracking progress with exercise, perhaps using something like a Fitbit or your iPhone, can also be very motivating, and chapter 10,

"Exercise and a Healthy Lifestyle," goes into this in more detail. For example, you might use a fitness tracker to assess your progress, or even use the calendar-and-stickers method to show your exercise.

Some people assess their progress by the fit of their clothes. Noticing changes in the fit of your clothing can be a helpful indicator of progress, though it is not as readily apparent as tracking weight shown on a scale.

Other people prefer to focus on behavior change to assess progress. This is probably a good strategy for many people. Using the calendar-and-stickers method is a good way to track behavior change, as is self-monitoring—keeping a record of your behavior.

Tracking Goals

To determine if you are making progress with weight loss or behavior change, it is necessary to know what your goal or aim is. That is, what are you trying to achieve? (Remember: a goal is something that can be obtained, whereas a value is a direction in which you are heading.) What is your goal directed toward? For the purposes of weight and behavior change, a goal is a concrete, identifiable end point that can be measured or quantified. Thus, it could be the goal of adopting healthier eating by, for example, not using salt at the table, or exercising five times a week for thirty minutes each session. It is better to define goals in terms of behavior to change—what you will do or not do—and not in terms of pounds to lose. (You have control over behavior, but discernable weight loss is subject to many other factors.) However, some people need the reinforcement of seeing progress on the scale.

Short-term goals are usually those set up to reach larger end goals. *Shaping* means creating successive approximations of a behavior to achieve a final goal. Exercising three times a week for thirty minutes may be a short-term goal that is followed by additional goals that finally bring you to your long-term goal, which may be to participate in regular sixty-minute exercise sessions five times a week. Focusing on short-term achievable goals is more motivating than becoming too concerned about long-term goals that may feel too hard to achieve. The idea here is gradual change.

Avoiding Behavior Fatigue

If you have ever been on a diet before, even one with moderate success, you know that you can reach a time when it just seems too difficult to keep on trying. This phenomenon is known as *behavior fatigue.* The importance of your goal to lose more weight fades in the face of competing needs and progress that may seem too slow. Boredom can set in. Interest and excitement wane. The "high" that might have been present at the beginning of the endeavor evaporates in light of the vigilance and self-conscious monitoring of behavior needed for ultimate success with a diet. This is another reason why diets don't work in the long run.

People are motivated toward taking action to achieve a goal because they want to feel effective, competent, and self-determining. The problem is that people are also prone to disinterest and stagnation. You may remember a time at school or work when you just couldn't bring yourself to finish a project. It was as if you had an internal brain lock-up. The task just seemed too difficult or too boring, and you couldn't seem to keep your attention on it. No doubt you experienced anxiety about your behavior and lack of incentive. You may even have called yourself lazy. You had succumbed to behavior fatigue.

Motivation is vulnerable to the encroachment of common and socially sanctioned environmental forces. Remember the time you were "watching your weight" and you went to a party that had tempting food, so you went off your diet? Or perhaps you once got caught up in the latest dietary craze that everyone was talking about and even lost some weight. Then, after a while, interest in the craze faded, usually because people stopped doing it and regained weight, so you dropped it too. If something like this has happened to you, you know what behavior fatigue is.

Diets are inherently boring and difficult. People need and look for stimulation, and dieting does not provide that. Sooner or later, behavior fatigue is likely to set in for almost everyone who just goes on a diet. That's why success depends on more than just cutting calories; it is predicated on assessing your values and changing your attitude, your self-concept, and your lifestyle. The attitude you need is one of seeing small changes as successes—that is, you choose to see small changes as rewarding and take credit for the success. On a diet, perceived small "failures" can lead to ultimate failure. If you expect to lose 2 pounds a week and "only" lose a half pound, you are likely to be disappointed and feel less competent, and enough of such experiences will erode motivation. On the other hand, if you see behavior change as a gradual and *permanent* shift toward a new lifestyle, you are more likely to feel effective and successful. For example, getting yourself to the gym twice a week on a regular basis when you have never regularly been involved in exercise before should feel like progress and success. The alternative and destructive attitude is feeling that you *have* to go to the gym and that you don't want to go. This produces resistance, annoyance, alienation, and, eventually, stopping. How you think about what you do is key. Remember, just because you have the thought that you don't want to go, doesn't mean you have to act on that thought. If you remember that exercise is just something you do, it is part of who you are, then you can ignore the momentary resistance.

To avoid behavior fatigue, you need to keep up your interest and your excitement for what you are doing by dedicating yourself to your goals and revising your self-concept. Defining yourself, for example, as "someone who exercises regularly" or "someone who eats healthy foods" is a different way of thinking about yourself and one that reinforces feelings of self-determination. You get to decide "what I eat" and "what I do" instead of following a diet. Choosing to adopt a lifestyle characterized by regular exercise and eating a variety of healthy foods in moderation provides feelings of competence and leads to persistence and success.

New Ways to Think About Food and Eating Behavior

The phrases *mindful eating* and *normal eating* often seem to be used interchangeably on the internet and by people who have adopted this concept. Mindful eating is the process of paying conscious attention to your eating experience, without judgment. While mindful eating is compatible with intuitive eating, also called *conscious eating* in some circles, intuitive eating is a broader philosophy that includes physical activity for the sake of feeling good, using nutrition information without judgment, and respecting your body regardless of how you feel about its shape. In short, intuitive eating is a form of attunement of mind, body, and food.

Mindful Eating

Do you sometimes eat when you are not hungry? Do you let yourself taste your food or often just mindlessly chomp away? Do you find yourself putting food in your mouth without thinking about it? If you are like most people, you are usually multitasking while eating—watching TV, reading, or working on a computer. Do you pay attention to your body's signals to stop eating, or do you ignore your body's feedback because you want to eat more or because your plate isn't empty yet? Do you eat to avoid feelings like sadness, boredom, or anxiety? Or do you eat more and more to keep feeling good for a while longer? When you are eating, are you scolding yourself or thinking you shouldn't be eating? Mindless eating involves not paying attention to eating, to the circumstances of eating, and to the body's signals of hunger or satiety. Mindless eating inevitably leads to overeating.

A concept first introduced in 1990 by Jon Kabat-Zinn, *mindful eating* is about being conscious of why and how you are eating. If you are eating mindfully, you are aware and attentive to all dimensions of eating, including mindfulness of the mind, body, thoughts, and feelings. Mindfulness is the moment-by-moment awareness—really paying attention—of all aspects of eating. There are four foundations of eating mindfully:

❖ **Mindfulness of the *process*.** Pay attention to what you are doing. Observe the taste, texture, and smell of food. Are you staying in touch with each bite? Can you feel yourself chewing? Swallowing? Wanting more?

❖ **Mindfulness of the *body*.** Listen to your body. Pay attention to hunger pains, a rumbling stomach, your energy level, and any muscle tremor. You may need to learn (or relearn) your feelings of hunger and satisfaction. You may be confusing appetite—meaning here a psychological desire for satisfaction without hunger being present—with actual hunger—a feeling of discomfort or weakness coupled with a strong desire to eat. Notice when your body signals satisfaction—a positive response to food accompanied by feelings of well-being.

❖ **Mindfulness of *feelings*.** Notice your feelings as you seek food, find it, and eat it. What are the emotions that are triggering the desire to eat? Are you upset and eating seems like a way to feel better? Or are you trying to prolong feeling good by eating more? Get in touch with the emotions that might be driving your need or desire for food.

❖ **Mindfulness of *thoughts*.** Listen to your thoughts. Observe whether you have "should" or "should not" thoughts, critical thoughts, food rules, "good" or "bad" judgments about food. Are you using excuses or rationalizations that allow you to eat something less healthy? Or are you blank—not thinking at all about eating or food? Are you on automatic?

Although the practice of mindfulness is centuries old, mindful eating is a relatively new concept on the weight and health management scene. It has the potential to transform your relationship with food and eating. Here are some suggestions for eating mindfully:

❖ Learn to make choices about beginning or ending a meal based on awareness of hunger and satiety cues. When are you ready to eat? When have you had enough?

❖ Value quality over quantity of what you're eating. Choose healthy food and avoid "junk" food. Use portion control.

❖ Appreciate the sensual, as well as the nourishing, capacity of food. Learn to enjoy food without guilt. Feel the deep gratitude that may come from appreciating and experiencing food. Become aware of the interconnectivity of earth, living beings, and cultural practices and the impact of food choices on those systems.

Mindful eating helps focus your attention and awareness on the present moment, which in turn helps you disengage from unhealthy habits and behaviors.

"Normal" Eating

Some people think "normal" eating means not having to think about food choices. In fact, people with "normal" eating patterns do make choices, they just don't obsess about them. They have internalized "the way I eat" or the food choices they typically make, and they monitor their behavior, but "lightly." Their relationship with food isn't automatic but it is easy because it is in alignment with their values and who they believe themselves to be. This is the secret of changing behavior: know your values and live by them, the rest will follow.

8

Healthy Eating Patterns

Tina, age 35, and weighing in at 190 pounds, decided it was time to get serious about changing her lifestyle. She wanted to lose 20 pounds, and she tried any new diet that came out. Tina just wasn't able to stick to any of them. Tina went to the internet and found the Dietary Guidelines for Americans *site, which said that gradual change—not dieting—was the solution to getting healthier. The healthy eating patterns provided on the site were not intended for weight loss, but Tina decided that being healthy was more important than dieting to lose weight. She adopted the healthy US-style eating pattern and discovered that healthy eating did indeed help her lose some weight.*

The Dietary Guidelines for Americans (DGA) are published every five years by the US Departments of Agriculture (USDA) and Health and Human Services. They are designed to help all individuals ages 2 years and older consume a healthy diet that meets nutrient needs. The focus of the *2015–2020 Dietary Guidelines* is on disease prevention and health promotion, and not specifically on losing weight, but it is a helpful guide for those wanting to manage their weight as well as improve their health.

Previous editions of the *Dietary Guidelines* focused mainly on individual components of the diet, such as specific food groups and nutrients. While food groups and nutrients are important, a growing body of scientific literature has examined the relationship between overall eating patterns, health, and risk of chronic disease. This literature was sufficiently well established to support recommendations on three healthy eating patterns. As a result, eating patterns are the main focus of the recommendations in the most recent *Dietary Guidelines*.

What Is a Healthy Eating Pattern?

An *eating pattern* represents the totality of all foods and beverages consumed. A *healthy eating pattern* includes grains, at least half of which are whole grains; fat-free or low-fat dairy, including milk, yogurt, cheese, and/or fortified soy beverages; and a variety of protein foods, including seafood, lean meats and poultry, eggs, legumes (beans and peas), and nuts, seeds, and soy products. It also includes a variety of vegetables, fruits, and oils. A healthy eating pattern limits saturated fats, trans fats, sodium, and added sugars. Additional recommendations for a healthy eating pattern include consuming less than 10 percent of calories per day in added sugar, less than 10 percent of calories per day in saturated fats, and less than 2,300 milligrams (mg) per day in sodium. If alcohol is consumed, it should be limited to one drink per day for women and two drinks per day for men.

Components of Healthy Eating Patterns

Healthy eating patterns support a healthy body weight and can help prevent and reduce the risk of chronic disease. Individuals should aim to meet their nutrient needs through healthy eating patterns that include nutrient-dense foods. There is more than one way to achieve a healthy eating pattern. The healthy US-style eating pattern is what most people consume. Other patterns include a healthy

Mediterranean eating pattern and a healthy Vegetarian eating pattern. Information on all three are included in this book.

General *Dietary Guidelines* for all Eating Patterns

❖ Follow a healthy eating pattern by *gradually* making permanent changes.

❖ Aim to consume mostly nutrient-dense foods.

❖ Note that some recommendations in the tables that follow are in terms of daily needs; others are in form of weekly needs.

❖ Tailor an eating pattern to your own needs and personal preferences.

❖ A helpful resource for understanding healthy eating patterns and tailoring them to your needs is MyPlate.gov. You can input your age, height, and weight to get more information on healthy eating patterns.

Shifts Needed to Be Healthy

Three-quarters of the US population consume diets that are low in vegetables, fruits, whole grains, dairy, seafood, and healthy oils, and high in refined grains, added sugars, saturated fats, sodium, and, for some groups, high in meats, poultry, and eggs. Young children and older Americans generally are closer to the recommendations than are adolescents and young adults.

> ### *Nutrient Density*
> Nutrient density identifies the amount of beneficial nutrients in a food product in proportion to, for example, energy content, weight, or amount of detrimental nutrients. Terms such as *nutrient rich* and *micronutrient dense* refer to similar properties. Candy, pastries, chips, bacon, and sugar-sweetened beverages are less nutrient dense. These foods contain added sugar, solid fats, and refined starch, and provide few essential nutrients. Aim to minimize nonnutrient-dense foods.

More than half the population is meeting or exceeding total grain and total protein foods recommendations. Most Americans exceed the recommendations for added sugars, saturated fats, and sodium. Eating patterns of many are too high in calories, as evidenced by the high proportion of the society who are overweight or obese.

The Healthy US-Style Eating Pattern

The healthy US-style eating pattern is one of three USDA food patterns (Mediterranean and Vegetarian patterns are included in this book as well) and is based on the types and proportions of foods Americans typically consume, but in nutrient-dense forms and appropriate amounts. Calorie needs vary based on age, sex, height, weight, and level of physical activity.

Table 8.1 shows the recommended amounts from each food group at twelve calorie levels to achieve a healthy US-style eating pattern. *Note that some quantities are for daily consumption while others are for weekly consumption.* As would be expected, most foods in their nutrient-dense forms do contain some sodium and saturated fatty acids. In a few cases, such as whole-wheat bread, the most appropriate representative in current federal databases contains a small amount of added sugars.

Calories and Weight Loss

Medical studies have proven that if a person reduces their calorie intake by 500 to 1,000 calories per day, they are likely to lose 1 to 2 pounds of weight per week. For most women, this comes down to an intake of 1,200 to 1,500 calories per day, and for men, 1,500 to 1,800 calories per day to promote weight loss at a healthy pace. Sedentary persons probably need to reduce their calorie intake by more, and active persons by less. Older persons generally have lower caloric needs and need to reduce caloric intake further to lose weight.

Energy needs decrease as we age. Between the ages of 46 and 65, moderately active men need an average of 2,400 calories per day to

Table 8.1
Healthy US-Style Eating Pattern:
Recommended Amounts of Food from Each Food Group at Twelve Calorie Levels

Calorie Level of Pattern[a]	1,000	1,200	1,400	1,600	1,800	2,000	2,200	2,400	2,600	2,800	3,000	3,200
Food Group[b]	Daily Amount[c] of food from each group (vegetable and protein foods subgroup amounts are per week)											
Vegetables	1 c-eq	1½ c-eq	1½ c-eq	2 c-eq	2½ c-eq	2½ c-eq	3 c-eq	3 c-eq	3½ c-eq	3½ c-eq	4 c-eq	4 c-eq
Dark-green vegetables (c-eq/week)	1/2	1	1	1½	1½	1½	2	2	2½	2½	2½	2½
Red and orange vegetables (c-eq/week)	2½	3	3	4	5½	5½	6	6	7	7	7½	7½
Legumes (beans and peas) (c-eq/week)	1/2	1/2	1/2	1	1½	1½	2	2	2½	2½	3	3
Starchy vegetables (c-eq/week)	2	3½	3½	4	5	5	6	6	7	7	8	8
Other vegetables (c-eq/week)	1½	2½	2½	3½	4	4	5	5	5½	5½	7	7

continues ▶

Table notes appear on page 142–144.

Table 8.1
Healthy US-Style Eating Pattern:
Recommended Amounts of Food from Each Food Group at Twelve Calorie Levels (*continued*)

Calorie Level of Pattern[a]	1,000	1,200	1,400	1,600	1,800	2,000	2,200	2,400	2,600	2,800	3,000	3,200
Food Group[b]	Daily Amount[c] of food from each group (vegetable and protein foods subgroup amounts are per week)											
Fruits	1 c-eq	1 c-eq	1½ c-eq	1½ c-eq	1½ c-eq	2 c-eq	2 c-eq	2 c-eq	2 c-eq	2½ c-eq	2½ c-eq	2½ c-eq
Grains	3 oz-eq	4 oz-eq	5 oz-eq	5 oz-eq	6 oz-eq	6 oz-eq	7 oz-eq	8 oz-eq	9 oz-eq	10 oz-eq	10 oz-eq	10 oz-eq
Whole grains[d] (oz-eq/day)	1½	2	2½	3	3	3	3½	4	4½	5	5	5
Refined grains (oz-eq/day)	1½	2	2½	2	3	3	3½	4	4½	5	5	5
Dairy	2 c-eq	2½ c-eq	2½ c-eq	3 c-eq	3 c-eq	3 c-eq	3 c-eq	3 c-eq	3 c-eq	3 c-eq	3 c-eq	3 c-eq
Protein Foods	2 oz-eq	3 oz-eq	4 oz-eq	5 oz-eq	5 oz-eq	5½ oz-eq	6 oz-eq	6½ oz-eq	6½ oz-eq	7 oz-eq	7 oz-eq	7 oz-eq
Seafood (oz-eq/week)	3	4	6	8	8	8	9	10	10	10	10	10
Meats, poultry, eggs (oz-eq/week)	10	14	19	23	23	26	28	31	31	33	33	33
Nuts, seeds, soy products (oz-eq/week)	2	2	3	4	4	5	5	5	5	6	6	6

Table 8.1
Healthy US-Style Eating Pattern:
Recommended Amounts of Food from Each Food Group at Twelve Calorie Levels (*continued*)

Calorie Level of Pattern[a]	1,000	1,200	1,400	1,600	1,800	2,000	2,200	2,400	2,600	2,800	3,000	3,200
Food Group[b]	Daily Amount[c] of food from each group (vegetable and protein foods subgroup amounts are per week)											
Oils	15 g	17 g	17 g	22 g	24 g	27 g	29 g	31 g	34 g	36 g	44 g	51 g
Limit on Calories for Other												
Uses, calories (% of calories)[e,f]	150 (15%)	100 (8%)	110 (8%)	130 (8%)	170 (9%)	270 (14%)	280 (13%)	350 (15%)	380 (15%)	400 (14%)	470 (16%)	610 (19%)

Notes to Table 8.1

[a]Food intake patterns at 1,000, 1,200, and 1,400 calories are designed to meet the nutritional needs of 2- to 8-year-old children. Patterns from 1,600 to 3,200 calories are designed to meet the nutritional needs of children 9 years and older and adults. If a child 4 to 8 years of age needs more calories and, therefore, is following a pattern at 1,600 calories or more, their recommended amount from the dairy group should be 2 ½ cups per day. Children 9 years and older and adults should not use the 1,000-, 1,200-, or 1,400-calorie patterns.

[b]Foods in each group and subgroup are:

- ❖ **Vegetables**
  - ◆ Dark-green vegetables: All fresh, frozen, and canned dark-green leafy vegetables and broccoli, cooked or raw: for example, broccoli; spinach; romaine; kale; collard, turnip, and mustard greens.
  - ◆ Red and orange vegetables: All fresh, frozen, and canned red and orange vegetables or juice, cooked or raw: for example, tomatoes, tomato juice, red peppers, carrots, sweet potatoes, winter squash, and pumpkin.
  - ◆ Legumes (beans and peas): All cooked from dry or canned beans and peas: for example, kidney beans, white beans, black beans, lentils, chickpeas, pinto beans, split peas, and edamame (green soybeans). Does not include green beans or green peas.
  - ◆ Starchy vegetables: All fresh, frozen, and canned starchy vegetables: for example, white potatoes, corn, green peas, green lima beans, plantains, and cassava.
  - ◆ Other vegetables: All other fresh, frozen, and canned vegetables, cooked or raw: for example, iceberg lettuce, green beans, onions, cucumbers, cabbage, celery, zucchini, mushrooms, and green peppers.

❖ **Fruits**

- ◆ All fresh, frozen, canned, and dried fruits and fruit juices: for example, oranges and orange juice, apples and apple juice, bananas, grapes, melons, berries, and raisins.

❖ **Grains**

- ◆ Whole grains: All whole-grain products and whole grains used as ingredients: for example, whole-wheat bread, whole-grain cereals and crackers, oatmeal, quinoa, popcorn, and brown rice.

- ◆ Refined grains: All refined-grain products and refined grains used as ingredients: for example, white breads, refined grain cereals and crackers, pasta, and white rice. Refined grain choices should be enriched.

❖ **Dairy**

- ◆ All milk, including lactose-free and lactose-reduced products and fortified soy beverages (soymilk), yogurt, frozen yogurt, dairy desserts, and cheeses. Most choices should be fat-free or low-fat. Cream, sour cream, and cream cheese are not included due to their low calcium content.

❖ **Protein Foods**

- ◆ All seafood, meats, poultry, eggs, soy products, nuts, and seeds. Meats and poultry should be lean or low-fat and nuts should be unsalted. Legumes (beans and peas) can be considered part of this group as well as the vegetable group, but should be counted in one group only.

cFood group amounts shown in cup-(c) or ounce-equivalents (oz-eq). Oils are shown in grams (g). Quantity equivalents for each food group are:

- ❖ Vegetables and fruits, 1 cup-equivalent is: 1 cup raw or cooked vegetable or fruit, 1 cup vegetable or fruit juice, 2 cups leafy salad greens, 1/2 cup dried fruit or vegetable.

- ❖ Grains, 1 ounce-equivalent is: 1/2 cup cooked rice, pasta, or cereal; 1 ounce dry pasta or rice; 1 medium (1 ounce) slice bread; 1 ounce of ready-to-eat cereal (about 1 cup of flaked cereal).

- ❖ Dairy, 1 cup-equivalent is: 1 cup milk, yogurt, or fortified soymilk; 1½ ounces natural cheese such as cheddar cheese or 2 ounces of processed cheese.

- ❖ Protein Foods, 1 ounce-equivalent is: 1 ounce lean meat, poultry, or seafood; 1 egg; 1/4 cup cooked beans or tofu; 1 tbsp peanut butter; 1/2 ounce nuts or seeds.

[d]Amounts of whole grains in the patterns for children are less than the minimum of 3 oz-eq in all patterns recommended for adults.

[e]All foods are assumed to be in nutrient-dense forms, lean or low-fat, and prepared without added fats, sugars, refined starches, or salt. If all food choices to meet food group recommendations are in nutrient-dense forms, a small number of calories remain within the overall calorie limit of the pattern (i.e., limit on calories for other uses). The number of these calories depends on the overall calorie limit in the pattern and the amounts of food from each food group required to meet nutritional goals. Nutritional goals are higher for the 1,200- to 1,600-calorie patterns than for the 1,000-calorie pattern, so the limit on calories for other uses is lower in the 1,200- to 1,600-calorie patterns. Calories up to the specified limit can be used for added sugars, added refined starches, solid fats, alcohol, or to eat more than the recommended amount of food in a food group. The overall eating pattern also should not exceed the limits of less than 10 percent of calories from added sugars and less than 10 percent of calories from saturated fats. At most calorie levels, amounts that can be accommodated are less than these limits. For adults of legal drinking age who choose to drink alcohol, a limit of up to one drink per day for women and up to two drinks per day for men within limits on calories for other uses applies.

[f]Values are rounded.

Source: *2015–2020 Dietary Guidelines*

maintain weight. To maintain their weight, men over 60 should eat as follows:

1. Sedentary lifestyle (little to no movement a day): 2,000 calories

2. Moderately active: 2,200 to 2,400 calories

3. Very active: 2,400 to 2,800 calories

On the other hand, for older women to *maintain* their weight they need:

1. Sedentary lifestyle (little to no movement a day): 1,600 calories

2. Moderately active: 1,800 calories

3. Very active: 2,000 to 2,200 calories

To ascertain how many calories you must cut back and how much you need to increase activity to lose weight, Google "how many calories per day does a woman need.

Healthy Mediterranean-Style Eating Pattern

There's no single Mediterranean-style eating pattern—many countries bordering on the Mediterranean Sea have similar cuisines. But in general, a Mediterranean style of eating would involve eating lots of fruits and vegetables, beans and nuts, hearty grains, fish, olive oil, and small amounts of meat and dairy, and red wine in moderation. You can have yogurt, cheese, poultry, and eggs in small amounts. You should eat fish and seafood at least twice a week. The emphasis is on fresh foods—no packaged foods or meals. You'll use herbs and spices for flavoring, rather than salt. The Mediterranean eating style doesn't qualify as a low-fat diet, but it is low in saturated fat.

Years of research has shown that the Mediterranean eating pattern is one of the healthiest around. For weight loss, try this way of eating for six months (or forever), but be careful with portion control and get regular daily exercise. Even if you don't follow this pattern faithfully, simply eating more of the foods on the plan, dining more leisurely (slowing down your eating), watching portion control, and being active can provide important health benefits.

The healthy Mediterranean-style eating pattern is associated with health benefits, especially lower saturated fat, a lower glycemic index, and it reduces the formation of inflammation markers. For weight management, eat smaller portions and engage in adequate physical activity. Be aware that soaking bread in olive oil adds calories.

In the Mediterranean-style eating plan, the majority of the fat content is from olive oil, which may help improve longevity.

Tips for Adopting a Mediterranean-Style Eating Pattern

1. Plan in lots of fruits and vegetables.
2. Select whole-grain foods more often.
3. Substitute plant protein for animal protein.
4. Eat fish or seafood at least twice each week.
5. Include calcium-rich foods, such as yogurt and cheese, in your daily eating pattern. (Note: cream cheese, sour cream, and butter are fat and not a good dairy source of calcium.)
6. Use olive oil for cooking and extra virgin olive oil for salad dressings. (Note: olive oil provides vitamin E.)
7. Limit consumption of sweets and foods containing solid fats—consume no more than twice a week.
8. Avoid processed foods; use fresh as much as possible.
9. Drink water or tea instead of sweet drinks like sodas and carbonated beverages that contain extra sugar.
10. Observe recommended limits for alcohol consumption.

Check table 8.2 for recommended amounts of food from each food group at twelve calorie levels for a healthy Mediterranean-style eating pattern. *Note that some quantities are for daily consumption while others are for weekly consumption.* Using this table, you can pick a particular calorie level you want to follow to lose weight.

Table 8.2

Healthy Mediterranean Style Eating Pattern:
Recommended Amounts of Food from Each Food Group at Twelve Calorie Levels

Calorie Level of Pattern[a]	**1,000**	**1,200**	**1,400**	**1,600**	**1,800**	**2,000**	**2,200**	**2,400**	**2,600**	**2,800**	**3,000**	**3,200**
Food Group[b]	**Daily Amount**[c] of food from each group **(vegetable and protein foods subgroup amounts are per week)**											
Vegetables	**1 c-eq**	**1½ c-eq**	**1½ c-eq**	**2 c-eq**	**2½ c-eq**	**2½ c-eq**	**3 c-eq**	**3 c-eq**	**3½ c-eq**	**3½ c-eq**	**4 c-eq**	**4 c-eq**
Dark-green vegetables (c-eq/week)	1/2	1	1	1½	1½	1½	2	2	2½	2½	2½	2½
Red and orange vegetables (c-eq/week)	2½	3	3	4	5½	5½	6	6	7	7	7½	7½
Legumes (beans and peas) (c-eq/week)	1/2	1/2	1/2	1	1½	1½	2	2	2½	2½	3	3
Starchy vegetables (c-eq/week)	2	3½	3½	4	5	5	6	6	7	7	8	8
Other vegetables (c-eq/week)	1½	2½	2½	3½	4	4	5	5	5½	5½	7	7
Fruits	**1 c-eq**	**1 c-eq**	**1½ c-eq**	**2 c-eq**	**2 c-eq**	**2½ c-eq**	**2½ c-eq**	**2½ c-eq**	**2½ c-eq**	**3 c-eq**	**3 c-eq**	**3 c-eq**

Table notes appear on page 149.

continues ▼

Table 8.2

Healthy Mediterranean Style Eating Pattern: Recommended Amounts of Food from Each Food Group at Twelve Calorie Levels (*continued*)

Grains	3 oz-eq	4 oz-eq	5 oz-eq	5 oz-eq	6 oz-eq	6 oz-eq	7 oz-eq	8 oz-eq	9 oz-eq	10 oz-eq	10 oz-eq	10 oz-eq
Whole grains[d] (oz-eq/day)	1½	2	2½	3	3	3	3½	4	4½	5	5	5
Refined grains (oz-eq/day)	1½	2	2½	2	3	3	3½	4	4½	5	5	5
Dairy[e]	2 c-eq	2½ c-eq	2½ c-eq	2 c-eq	2 c-eq	2 c-eq	2 c-eq	2½ c-eq	2½ c-eq	2½ c-eq	2½ c-eq	2½ c-eq
Protein Foods	2 oz-eq	3 oz-eq	4 oz-eq	5½ oz-eq	6 oz-eq	6½ oz-eq	7 oz-eq	7½ oz-eq	7½ oz-eq	8 oz-eq	8 oz-eq	8 oz-eq
Seafood (oz-eq/week)[f]	3	4	6	11	15	15	16	16	17	17	17	17
Meats, poultry, eggs (oz-eq/week)	10	14	19	23	23	26	28	31	31	33	33	33
Nuts, seeds, soy products (oz-eq/week)	2	2	3	4	4	5	5	5	5	6	6	6
Oils	15 g	17 g	17 g	22 g	24 g	27 g	29 g	31 g	34 g	36 g	44 g	51 g
Limit on Calories for												
Other Uses, calories (% of Calories)	150 (15%)	100 (8%)	110 (8%)	140 (9%)	160 (9%)	260 (13%)	270 (12%)	300 (13%)	330 (13%)	350 (13%)	430 (14%)	570 (18%)

Notes to Table 8.2

a,b,c,dSee Table 8.1 Healthy US-Style Eating Pattern: Recommended Amounts of Food from Each Food Group at Twelve Calorie Levels, notes a through d on pages 140–141.

eAmounts of dairy recommended for children and adolescents are as follows, regardless of the calorie level of the pattern: For 2-year-olds, 2 cup-eq per day; for 3- to 8-year-olds, 2½ cup-eq per day; for 9- to 18-year-olds, 3 cup-eq per day.

fThe US Food and Drug Administration (FDA) and the US Environmental Protection Agency (EPA) provide joint guidance regarding seafood consumption for women who are pregnant or breastfeeding and young children. For more information, see the FDA or EPA websites https://www.fda.gov/food/consumers/advice-about-eating-fish; https://www.epa.gov/choose-fish-and-shellfish-wisely.

Source: *2015–2020 Dietary Guidelines*

Healthy Vegetarian-Style Eating Pattern

Compared to the healthy US-style eating pattern, the healthy Vegetarian-style eating pattern includes more legumes (beans and peas), soy products, nuts and seeds, and whole grains. It contains no meat, poultry, or seafood, but otherwise is similar to the healthy US-style eating pattern in amounts of other food groups. It is somewhat higher in calcium and dietary fiber and lower in vitamin D.

Considerations When Adopting a Vegetarian-Style of Eating

When deciding to become a vegetarian, keep in mind that the more restrictive your diet is, the more challenging it can be to get all the nutrients you need. A vegan diet, for example, eliminates natural food sources of vitamin B-12 and some good sources of calcium and vitamin D, which occur in dairy products.

Eggs and dairy products are good sources of protein, which help maintain healthy skin, bones, muscles, and organs. Plant sources

Types of Vegetarian-Style Eating Patterns

Lacto-vegetarian: Excludes meat, fish, poultry and eggs, as well as foods that contain these products. Dairy products, such as milk, cheese, yogurt, and butter, are included.

Ovo-vegetarian: Excludes meat, poultry, seafood, and dairy products, but allows eggs.

Lacto-ovo-vegetarian: Excludes meat, fish, and poultry, but allows dairy products and eggs.

Pescatarian: Excludes meat and poultry, dairy, and eggs, but allows fish.

Vegan: Excludes meat, poultry, fish, eggs, and dairy products, and foods that contain these products.

of protein include soy products, legumes, lentils, nuts, seeds, and whole grains.

Omega-3 fatty acids are important for heart health. Eating patterns that do not include fish and eggs are generally low in omega-3 fatty acids. However, canola oil, soy oil, walnuts, ground flaxseed, and soybeans are good sources of essential fatty acids. It may also be good to consider fortified products or supplements or both for these.

Iron is a crucial component of red blood cells. Dried beans and peas, lentils, enriched cereals, whole-grain products, dark leafy green vegetables, and dried fruit are good sources of iron. Because iron isn't as easily absorbed from plant sources, the recommended intake of iron for vegetarians is almost double that recommended for nonvegetarians.

Like iron, zinc is not as easily absorbed from plant sources as it is from animal sources. Zinc is an essential component of many enzymes and plays a role in cell division and the formation of proteins. Cheese is a good source for zinc, if you eat dairy products. Also include whole grains, soy products, legumes, nuts, and wheat germ.

Iodine is an important component in thyroid hormones, which help regulate metabolism, growth, and the function of key organs. Vegans may not get enough iodine and may be at risk of deficiency and possibly even goiter. Adding just a quarter teaspoon of iodized salt a day can provide a sufficient amount of iodine.

Check table 8.3 for recommended amounts of food from each food group at twelve calorie levels for a healthy Vegetarian-style eating pattern. *Note that some quantities are for daily consumption while others are for weekly consumption.* A vegetarian style of eating is not itself a weight-loss approach unless it contains primarily vegetables, such as the lacto-vegetarian option.

Table 8.3

Healthy Vegetarian-Style Eating Pattern:
Recommended Amounts of Food from Each Food Group at Twelve Calorie Levels

Calorie Level of Pattern[a]	1,000	1,200	1,400	1,600	1,800	2,000	2,200	2,400	2,600	2,800	3,000	3,200
Food Group[b]	Daily Amount[c] of food from each group (vegetable and protein foods subgroup amounts are per week)											
Vegetables	1 c-eq	1½ c-eq	1½ c-eq	2 c-eq	2½ c-eq	2½ c-eq	3 c-eq	3 c-eq	3½ c-eq	3½ c-eq	4 c-eq	4 c-eq
Dark-green vegetables (c-eq/week)	½	1	1	1½	1½	1½	2	2	2½	2½	2½	2½
Red and orange vegetables (c-eq/week)	2½	3	3	4	5½	5½	6	6	7	7	7½	7½
Legumes (beans and peas) (c-eq/week)[d]	½	½	½	1	1½	1½	2	2	2½	2½	3	3
Starchy vegetables (c-eq/week)	2	3½	3½	4	5	5	6	6	7	7	8	8
Other vegetables (c-eq/week)	1½	2½	2½	3½	4	4	5	5	5½	5½	7	7
Fruits	1 c-eq	1 c-eq	1½ c-eq	1½ c-eq	2½ c-eq	2 c-eq	2 c-eq	2 c-eq	2½ c-eq	2½ c-eq	2½ c-eq	2½ c-eq

Table notes appear on page 154.

Table 8.3

Healthy Vegetarian-Style Eating Pattern: Recommended Amounts of Food from Each Food Group at Twelve Calorie Levels (continued)

Grains	3 oz-eq	4 oz-eq	5 oz-eq	5½ oz-eq	6½ oz-eq	6½ oz-eq	7½ oz-eq	8½ oz-eq	9½ oz-eq	10½ oz-eq	10½ oz-eq	10½ oz-eq
Whole grains[e] (oz-eq/day)	1½	2	2½	3	3½	3½	4	4½	5	5½	5½	5½
Refined grains (oz-eq/day)	1½	2	2½	2½	3	3	3½	4	4½	5	5	5
Dairy	2 c-eq	2.5 c-eq	2.5 c-eq	3 c-eq	3 c-eq	3 c-eq	3 c-eq	3 c-eq	3 c-eq	3 c-eq	3 c-eq	3 c-eq
Protein Foods	1 oz-eq	1½ oz-eq	2 oz-eq	2½ oz-eq	3 oz-eq	3½ oz-eq	3½ oz-eq	4 oz-eq	4½ oz-eq	5 oz-eq	5½ oz-eq	6 oz-eq
Eggs (oz-eq/week)	2	3	3	3	3	3	3	3	3	4	4	4
Legumes (beans and peas)[d] (oz-eq/week)	1	2	4	4	6	6	6	8	9	10	11	12
Soy products (oz-eq/week)	2	3	4	6	6	8	8	9	10	11	12	13
Nuts and seeds (oz-eq/week)	2	2	3	5	6	7	7	8	9	10	12	13
Oils	15 g	17 g	17 g	22 g	24 g	27 g	29 g	31 g	34 g	36 g	44 g	51 g
Limit on Calories for Other Uses, Calories (% of calories)[f,g]	190 (19%)	170 (14%)	190 (14%)	180 (11%)	190 (11%)	290 (15%)	330 (15%)	390 (16%)	390 (15%)	400 (14%)	440 (15%)	550 (17%)

Notes to Table 8.3

[a,b,c] See Table 8.1 Healthy US-Style Eating Pattern: Recommended Amounts of Food from Each Food Group at Twelve Calorie Levels, notes a through c on pages 142–144.

[d] About half of total legumes are shown as vegetables, in cup-eq, and half as protein foods, in oz-eq. Total legumes in the Patterns, in cup-eq, is the amount in the vegetable group plus the amount in protein foods group (in oz-eq) divided by 4:

Total Legumes (beans and peas) (c-eq/wk)	1	1	1½	2	3	3	3½	4	5	5	6	6

[e,f,g] See Table 8.1 Healthy US-Style Eating Pattern: Recommended Amounts of Food from Each Food Group at Twelve Calorie Levels, notes d through f on page 144.

Source: *2015–2020 Dietary Guidelines*

Nutrition and Weight Management

Abby was normal weight, married, with one child. Her mother and sister, however, were very thin and worried constantly about watching what they ate and getting a lot of exercise. Abby felt big next to them, and she was confused about what was right to eat. Her mother and sister told her that fat should be avoided and that carbohydrates were bad. Abby bought different books that gave advice on food and eating but they just caused more confusion. One book talked about how to choose foods to improve the immune system, and another about choosing high-density foods to lose weight. Some books gave specific advice on diets for athletes, while others focused on why diets don't work. Advice often differed depending on whether the author's focus was on losing weight or promoting a healthy lifestyle. Abby wasn't sure if she should try to lose weight to be more like her mother and sister, though she didn't want to obsess about food like they did.

Sometimes it can be a challenge to figure out the relationship between nutrition and weight management. You may recall there was a time when all carbohydrates were considered "bad." People were advised to avoid carbs and eat lots of protein to lose weight or avoid gaining weight. Then some carbohydrates, like vegetables and grains, were said to be "good" because they were reported to help lower cholesterol. (They do.) Eating a low-fat diet together with vegetables was also recommended.

Now the evaluation of carbohydrates and which diets are best for whom is giving way to new ideas. Healthy eating patterns take a more holistic approach to nutrition, but there are helpful ways to choose foods within patterns. Glycemic index and glycemic load are ways of assessing how carbohydrates affect blood sugar levels. This is important to diabetics, or prediabetics, or those becoming insulin insensitive, which includes many people who are obese and have metabolic syndrome. Then there is the fullness factor—a measure of which foods, including protein and fat foods as well as carbohydrates, produce higher satiety when eaten. Satiety refers to that pleasant feeling of fullness and the corresponding reduction of hunger you feel after you eat. This is important to know because we all want to minimize hunger, especially when cutting back calories.

Of course, the concept of applying nutrition knowledge to creating a weight-loss plan is not new. An old standard for making calorie counting easier is the food exchange system, which was originally developed to help people with diabetes manage their food intake but has since been adopted for more general weight-loss efforts. This is still a good option instead of calorie counting and is easy to learn. There will be more discussion about this later in this chapter.

Macronutrients

It is necessary to know a little bit about nutrition to make good choices and to understand weight management. In this chapter, we will cover some of the basics. Let's start with the macronutrients.

Food is divided into energy sources called macronutrients—carbohydrates, proteins, and fats. Carbohydrates contribute four calories per gram, as does protein, whereas fat provides nine calories per gram. All three of these energy sources are necessary ingredients in a healthy diet; the question is balance.

Carbohydrates

Your body relies on carbohydrates as an immediate and continuous energy supply. About 40 to 50 percent of your diet should come from carbohydrates and these should be mostly unrefined carbs (such as vegetables, fruits, whole grains, and legumes). Without adequate carbohydrates, the body must rely on less efficient sources of energy that involve converting fat and body tissue into energy. So unrefined carbs are generally a must in a healthy diet. However, nutritionists recommend keeping carbohydrates made up of simple sugars to a minimum (such as white bread, sugar, and pasta).

A popular myth is that it is necessary to avoid all carbs to lose weight. One woman went to a pizza parlor with her husband for dinner. They ordered a large pizza with cheese and pepperoni. She was trying to lose weight and had heard that cutting back on carbs was the way to do it. When they got the pizza, she picked off the cheese and pepperoni and ate that, but she didn't eat the crust. In a misguided effort to lose weight, she didn't want the carbs in the pizza crust. She didn't lose any weight, so she gave up trying.

Protein

Protein is needed to grow and repair your body's tissues. The recommended dietary allowance (RDA) for protein is a modest 0.8 grams of protein per kilogram of body weight. The RDA is the amount of a nutrient you need to meet your basic nutritional requirements, and the minimum amount you need to keep from getting sick. Although you only need about 45 to 60 grams of protein a day (the higher amount is for men), the average person eats about 70 to 100 grams of protein daily. Sources of protein include meat, fish, poultry, eggs, and dairy. Vegetables and legumes also provide some protein but are incomplete sources. For most people, only 10 to 15 percent of total daily caloric intake should come from protein.

If you want to lose weight, aim for a daily protein intake between 1.6 and 2.2 grams of protein per kilogram of body weight (.73 and 1 gram per pound). Athletes and heavy exercisers should consume 2.2 to 3.4 grams of protein per kilogram of body weight (1 to 1.5 grams per pound) if aiming for weight loss.

To determine your daily protein intake, multiply your weight in pounds by 0.36. For a 50-year-old woman who weighs 140 pounds and who is sedentary (doesn't exercise) that translates into 50 grams of protein a day. Older people need more protein. Aging bodies process protein less efficiently and need more of it to maintain muscle mass and strength, bone health, and other essential physiological functions. Even healthy seniors need more protein than when they were younger. (Bariatric surgery patients need more protein and certain diets recommend around 20 percent of daily intake.)

Fat

The role of fat in the diet is a little more complicated than the role of the other macronutrients. Saturated fats, the "unhealthy" fats, are found in animal products such as red meat and butter and contribute to heart disease. Monounsaturated fats and certain polyunsaturated fats, the "healthy" fats, come from vegetable sources such as olives, corn, soybeans, and peanuts and are good for your heart. A few vegetable fats, such as coconut oil and palm oil, are unhealthy and should be avoided. Trans fats are man-made by adding hydrogen to monounsaturated fats, turning them into more shelf-stable fats that help preserve food products but are unhealthy for your heart. Trans fats are so bad that some states, like California, have passed laws that restaurants must stop using them.

The right kind of dietary fat is needed by the body and the brain. In fact, the brain is the fattiest organ in the body, consisting of nearly

60 percent fat. Dietary fat helps transport certain necessary vitamins to the brain. Fat is very important for proper brain function, but it needs to be the right kind of fat. Omega-3 fatty acids are essential building blocks for the brain and are important for learning and memory.

Polyunsaturated fats vary in health benefit depending on the amount of certain omega fatty acids they contain. Omega-3 fatty acids, which are found in fatty, cold-water fish, such as salmon, tuna, sardines, herring, anchovies, mackerel, and lake trout, as well as from certain plant sources such as flax and walnuts, are promoted by some experts as being better than omega-6 fatty acids. Although both are good for you, omega-3s help lower cholesterol in the blood and, so, contribute to the reduction of heart disease. Some people take fish oil supplements to ensure they get enough omega fatty acids; eating real fish is generally a better alternative.

It's important to avoid the wrong kinds of fats in your diet too. The wrong fats can increase more than just your risk of coronary artery disease. A high intake of saturated or trans fats can double your risk of developing Alzheimer's (as compared to diets low in these fats). This is because harmful fats in food also increase blood cholesterol levels, which in turn cause inflammation of blood vessels around the brain. This inflammation impairs memory and can result in Alzheimer's disease.

Depending on who or what organization is making it, the recommendation for percentage of dietary fat can be between 10 percent of total calories (very low and hard to achieve) to 35 percent of total calories, the level recommended by the American Heart Association (AHA). The AHA advises limiting saturated fat to less than 10 percent of total calories, avoiding trans fats altogether, and getting most of your fat calories from monounsaturated and healthy polyunsaturated sources. It's recommended that you have at least two servings of fatty fish a week. It's also smart to toss a few cubes of tofu into veggie stir-fries and sprinkle some walnuts on your salad a few times a week because some of the nutrients in vegetables are more readily absorbed by the body if they are eaten with fat.

What About Proportions of Macronutrients?

Don't worry much about the proportions of carbohydrate, fat, and protein. Recent studies have found that when it comes to losing weight, results pretty much boil down to calories consumed. A two-year study by the Dietary Intervention Randomized Control Study (DIRECT) looked at success and adherence among 322 moderately obese subjects in one of three groups: a low-fat diet group, a Mediterranean diet (high monounsaturated fats) group, and a low-carbohydrates group. The researchers found that, overall, each group lost about the same amount of weight. That said, people tended to stick to the low-fat diets more readily than the low-carb diets. The study concluded that the amount of weight loss at the six-month point, not the type of diet, best predicted long-term success. In other words, early success is a good sign for being able to take it off and keep it off and is a better predictor of success than any one type of diet.

Australian researchers looked at a similar topic: whether macronutrient ratios of the diet played a role in weight maintenance after one year. For this study, people were divided into either a low-carb or a low-protein diet group. Both groups maintained an average weight loss of about 32 pounds with no significant difference between the two groups. Once again, the type of diet mattered less in terms of weight loss and maintenance success than the composition of the diet—in other words, it doesn't matter much where the calories come from when it comes to weight management; it matters how many calories are consumed.

In another trial of 811 overweight adults, people were assigned to one of four diets with varying percentages of total calories from fat, protein, and carbohydrates. Group and individual instructional sessions were offered. At six months, subjects assigned to each diet had lost an average of 13 pounds, but they all began to regain weight after twelve months. The researchers concluded that reduced-calorie diets all result in weight loss regardless of the macronutrient spread. The bottom line is that to lose weight and keep it off you must maintain a lower caloric intake for the duration. The choice of a diet, then, depends on your preferences and what you decide is healthier. Recent research studies, however, suggest that a low-carb diet—one that avoids pasta, bread, rice, and alcohol—maintained for six months or more is better for reducing cholesterol. But to maintain weight loss, it is necessary to make behavior changes permanent.

Food Addictions

In his book entitled *Breaking the Food Seduction*, Neal D. Barnard, MD, of the Physicians Committee for Responsible Medicine contends that certain foods—including chocolate, cheese, red meat, and practically any food that includes both sugar and fat—can become a *behavioral addiction*—that is, the behavior is repeated again and again because the rewarding aspects of the behavior are highly reinforcing. These foods cause the brain to release its own natural opioids and certain chemicals that stimulate the brain's pleasure center. Chocolate, for example, offers a range of compounds from mild cannabinoids (these are the main ingredient that causes people to get high from smoking marijuana) to amphetaminelike chemicals that provide yet another kind of high. Other foods are rewarding as well. Cheese is mostly fat, and the texture of fat pleases the mouth and brain. Many people snack on foods such as cheese and salty crackers (salt is another pleasuring substance for many palettes) after a stressful day. Doing this can be like a behavioral addiction.

And what about physical addiction? *Physical addiction* is predicated by an increased tolerance to a desirable substance, leading the person to need more and more over time to achieve the same reward, and they suffer withdrawal symptoms when they stop consuming it. Although research has found that excessive sugar does not cause the same physical addiction as drugs such as cocaine or heroin, sugary foods do activate the same pleasure centers of the brain as certain drugs. Indeed, Barnard's book points out that research suggests that sugar releases natural opiates and the neurotransmitter *dopamine* (neurotransmitters are chemicals in the brain that help transmit nerve signals) into the body and, thus, repeated forays into eating sugary foods do take on the appearance of an addiction

Some people really do seem to develop serious cravings for sweet foods, particularly if they eat them frequently. You may know people who call themselves "sugaraholics" or "chocoholics." You may be one yourself. These people feel they can't get through the day without a sugar fix or once they start eating sugar, they can't stop. They feel "addicted" to sugar and sometimes other comfort foods as well. Some women report experiencing sugar cravings in the ten or so days before their menstrual period.

Some research has also found that high and chronic intake of sugar results in resistance to *leptin*—the hormone that curbs appetite. Over time, a high intake of sugary foods blocks the leptin signal in the brain, so leptin can't extinguish hunger. To reinstate the function of leptin, high-sugar foods must be minimized or even avoided. In particular, sugary beverages such as Coca-Cola, Pepsi, and Dr. Pepper, as well as sugary foods from brands such as Cinnabon, Krispy Kreme, Dunkin' Donuts, Hostess, Sara Lee, and the like should be curtailed.

Sucrose—the sugar you find in the sugar bowl—is the man-made version of naturally occurring sugars, such as those found in fruit, but it is sweeter than naturally occurring sugars. As such, it is highly rewarding to the pleasure center of the brain and, when eaten frequently, can then cause the overeater to want more and more. It is as if the brain "learns" to crave sugar. Other names for sugar include high-fructose corn syrup, honey, maple syrup, natural brown sugar, molasses, maltose, turbinado sugar, evaporated cane juice, dark brown sugar, raw sugar, confectioner's sugar, crystallized fructose, dextrin, beet sugar, cane sugar, and corn syrup, to name a few. Sugary foods do not produce satiety—they produce yearning for more sugary foods. Eating high quantities of sugar or sugary foods causes a spike in blood sugar, followed by a sharp rise in insulin, and then a feeling of hunger again. On a scale of 0 to 5, in which the lower the number the less filling per calorie, sugar (or sucrose) ranks at

1.3—not filling at all. Nevertheless, sweet taste is compelling, and for some people, sugar binges can last for days.

There is no doubt that foods high in fat or sugar are very appealing to many people and can become a regular habit and a behavioral addiction. Fast foods are not only fast, they have lots of fat, and fat provides a pleasant texture in the mouth. Like sugar, fat-laden foods also make the brain release dopamine—the neurotransmitter that is associated with reward and craving. Even if not technically considered addictive, these foods are consumed more and more to provide quick meals and cheap satisfaction—and lots of calories. The best way to beat a behavioral addiction is to eat a good breakfast, one that contains protein, each day and to eat regularly throughout the day. If you must eat sugary foods, make them part of a regular meal.

Depression and Sugar Sensitivity

Sugar may present other problems besides addiction. Research suggests that depression seems to be related to sugar ingestion and sensitivity to sugar for *some* people. Although the exact relationship between fatigue, depression, and simple carbohydrates (sugary foods, as well as alcohol, white pasta, bread, and rice) is not entirely known, recent studies seems to suggest that eating a lot of these simple carbs can cause fatigue and that persistent fatigue may contribute to the development or maintenance of symptoms of depression.

Fatigue is a common complaint of those who are depressed. And some depressed people develop a preference for food that is high in both sugar and fat, such as ice cream, candy, cookies, pastries, and other simple carbohydrates such as sugary soft drinks or juice drinks. Others report feelings of fatigue and lack of vigor *following* consumption of foods high in simple sugar. Some people refer to this as a "sugar hangover." That is, like the binge eater, the sugar consumer feels mentally slowed and physically tired soon after eating a large amount of sweet foods. It often takes days to get over a sugar hangover, and only then, by returning to balanced eating.

According to Kathleen DesMaisons, PhD, a nutrition expert and author of *Potatoes Not Prozac*, many people, including those who are depressed, are "sugar sensitive." Sugar induces endorphin production and promotes the manufacture of *serotonin*—a neurotransmitter associated with feeling calm. Initially, the sugar makes the person feel better. But when the good feeling wears off—which can be fairly quickly—the aftereffect is to feel down and depressed, which usually leads to eating more sugar to feel better again.

If you think you are sugar sensitive, you should carefully read the information that follows regarding glycemic index and glycemic load. This nutritional tool could help you cope with an "addiction" to sugar or sensitivity to simple carbohydrates. If you don't think sugar is a problem for you, you may benefit more from the other nutritional tools discussed in this chapter.

Helpful Nutritional Tools

Having discussed the basics of nutrition and weight loss, it is now time to turn attention to some helpful nutritional tools. These include the glycemic index and glycemic load, the fullness factor, and the food exchange system. Each of these provides a different way of understanding and selecting foods so you can choose your individual guidelines for eating. Once you have decided that good health is an important value for you, you need to discover what works for your body and your preferences. These tools are intended to help you do that.

Glycemic Index

People who are diabetic or prediabetic (or who might have sensitivity to sugar) should consider learning to use the glycemic index (GI) and glycemic load (GL). The *glycemic index* is an established numerical way of measuring how much of an increase in circulating blood sugar any given carbohydrate triggers. The higher the number, the greater the blood sugar response (which is followed by a corresponding release of insulin). Low GI foods cause a small rise, while high GI foods trigger a more dramatic spike. A GI of 70 or more is high and is an indication that that carbohydrate causes a surge of sugar in the bloodstream. Some examples of high GI foods include white bread, potatoes, rice milk, rice crackers, and cornflakes. High GI foods should be avoided to prevent a sharp rise in blood sugar followed by increased hunger. A GI between 56 and 69 causes a "medium" rise in blood sugar, although these cutoff points are arbitrary. Carbohydrates with GIs of 55 or less are ranked as low because they cause a lower rise of blood sugar. Some examples of low GI foods include most fruits, legumes, barley, boiled carrots, milk, and yogurt. But GI alone is not enough to help you decide what to eat. You really need to know the glycemic load of foods as well.

Glycemic Load

The *glycemic load* (GL) of foods takes the glycemic index into account but gives a more complete picture than the glycemic index alone. A GI value tells you only how rapidly a particular type of carbohydrate turns into blood sugar, but it doesn't take into account the standard serving size. The GI needs to be translated into an ordinary serving size for you to know how big a rise in blood sugar an ordinary serving would cause. This is where glycemic load comes in. You need to know the GL to understand a serving of a food's effect on blood sugar. The carbohydrate in watermelon, for example, has a high glycemic index (GI = 72). But there isn't much of it in a single serving, so the glycemic load of watermelon is relatively low (GL = 8). In other words, the GL is about the quality of the carbohydrate *given a standard serving size.*

A GL of 20 or more is considered high, a GL of between 11 and 19 is medium, and a GL of 10 or less is low. Foods that have a low GL frequently have a low GI as well. Examples of low GL/low GI foods include peanuts, bean sprouts, and most fruits. Some foods with a high GL also have a high GI. For example, white rice has a GI of

64 (high) and a GL of 33 (also high). Another dish that is high in both is macaroni and cheese, which has a GI of 64 and a GL of 30. A baked potato has a GI of 85 and a GL of 28—all red flags for blood sugar surges. Foods with an intermediate or high GI range can have GL values that range from very low to very high. For example, white bread has a low GL of 10 (for one slice) but a high GI of 70 because this latter value is based on a larger quantity of bread than is usually eaten at one sitting. Likewise, one tablespoon of sugar or honey has an intermediate GI value of 68 (you would have to eat a whole lot of sugar to cause the surge in blood sugar—like you get in most sweets) but a low GL of 8 (this is what you would get in an occasional tea- spoon of sugar in your tea or coffee). Both watermelon and popcorn have high GIs of 72 but low GLs of 8 and 7, respectively.

The GIs and GLs for some common foods are listed in table 9.1, Glycemic Index and Glycemic Load for Common Foods. In the table, the calculation of GIs is based on the glucose index where glucose is set to equal 100. The glycemic load is determined by a formula that divides the glycemic index of each food item by 100, then multiplies this by its available carbohydrate content (i.e., carbohydrates minus fiber) in grams. The serving size column is in grams for calculat- ing the glycemic load. Most online sites providing this information include a column for intermediate GI and GL foods, but here, to sim- plify, we have provided columns only for low and high GI and GL foods.

A quick set of rules for managing blood sugar using GI and GL is provided below:

1. Include at least one food that has a low GI *and* a low GL (like fruit) at every meal. This will moderate the effects of consum- ing a high GI and a high GL food by diluting the rise in blood sugar.

2. Instead of white bread, substitute whole-grain or sourdough bread (research shows that the acid content of sourdough helps reduce blood sugar response).

Table 9.1 **Glycemic Index and Glycemic Load for Common Foods**

Food	GI	Serving Size	Net Carbs	GL
Peanuts	14	4 oz (113g)	15	2
Bean sprouts	25	1 cup (104g)	4	1
Grapefruit	25	1/2 large (166g)	11	3
Pizza	30	2 slices (260g)	42	13
Low-fat yogurt	33	1 cup (245g)	47	16
Apples	38	1 medium (138g)	16	6
Spaghetti	42	1 cup (140g)	38	16
Carrots	47	1 large (72g)	5	2
Oranges	48	1 medium (131g)	12	6
Bananas	52	1 large (136g)	27	14
Potato chips	54	4 oz (114g)	55	30
Snickers bar	55	1 bar (113g)	64	35
Brown rice	55	1 cup (195g)	42	23
Honey	55	1 tbsp (21g)	17	9
Oatmeal	58	1 cup (234g)	21	12
Ice cream	61	1 cup (72g)	16	10
Macaroni and cheese	64	1 serving (166g)	47	30
Raisins	64	1 small box (43g)	32	20
White rice	64	1 cup (186g)	52	33
Sugar (sucrose)	68	1 tbsp (12g)	12	8
White bread	70	1 slice (30g)	14	10
Watermelon	72	1 cup (154g)	11	8
Popcorn	72	2 cups (16g)	10	7
Baked potato	85	1 medium (173g)	33	28
Glucose	100	50g	50	50

The complete list of the glycemic index and glycemic load for more than 1,000 foods can be found in the article "International Tables of Glycemic Index and Glycemic Load Values: 2008," by Fiona S. Atkinson, Kaye Foster-Powell, and Jennie C. Brand-Miller in the December 2008 issue of *Diabetes Care* 31 (12): 2281–83.

Note: GL of 20 or higher produces a surge in blood sugar, while a GL of 10 or less is "low" and preferred. Note that white bread has a high GI but an acceptable GL, as does ice cream, but notice the serving sizes. More than a cup of ice cream (one scoop) is problematic.

3. Switch your morning cereal from corn flakes to an oat cereal or one that is less processed and is high in fiber as well as low in sugar.

4. Choose basmati rice, quinoa, or bulgur instead of white rice.

5. Cook your pasta al dente. Overcooking pasta raises the GI and GL by significantly breaking down more of the starch.

6. Include legumes in your diet: chickpeas, kidney beans, lentils, and dried beans.

7. Adding acid to your meal slows down blood sugar response. Have vinaigrette with your salad or yogurt on your cereal. Try lemon juice on vegetables.

8. Choose snacks low in both GI and GL such as fresh fruit, dried fruit mixed with nuts, low-fat milk, or yogurt.

9. Eat some lean protein at every meal.

10. Exercise portion control, especially with carbohydrate-rich foods. The glycemic load you consume is higher if you overeat foods high in both GI and GL.

GI and GL are most relevant to those at high risk for diabetes, which could include those who are seriously obese or have metabolic syndrome. Those who are struggling with sugar cravings might also benefit from paying attention to GI and GL. Despite the usefulness of the glycemic load and glycemic index scales for those who are diabetic or prediabetic, ultimately it is total calories that count for losing weight. Paying attention to GI and GL alone is not enough, though it could help with satiety and cravings. A multicenter study found that participants achieved and maintained comparable weight loss after one year, regardless of whether they were on a low-glycemic load diet or a high one as long as they adhered to a calorie-restricted diet. Understanding glycemic load can help you choose carbohydrates more wisely.

Fullness Factor

While the GI and GL are ways of assessing carbohydrates alone, the *fullness factor* (FF) can be used to evaluate all foods. NutritionData .com developed the FF index after studying the results of numerous satiety studies. Recall that *satiety* refers to the feeling of fullness you feel after you eat. Values for the FF range between 0 and 5, with the lower numbers indicating foods that are less filling per calorie consumed and the higher numbers pointing to foods that are more filling per calorie consumed.

The FF is calculated from the food's nutrient content using values from those nutrients that have been shown experimentally to have the greatest impact on satiety. Of course, there are lots of factors that influence a food's ability to satisfy the palette. A person's preferences for taste or texture are two such influences. Quantity consumed is another factor.

Foods that contain large amounts of fat, sugar, or starch have a low FF and are much easier to eat too much of, as any overeater can attest. Foods that contain large amounts of water, dietary fiber, or protein have the highest FF. These high FF choices, which include most vegetables, fruits, and lean meats, do a better job of satisfying hunger and are also known as *high-density* foods.

FF can also be calculated for liquids, including soups and drinks. These usually have an above average FF initially due to their high water content, and small quantities are satisfying in the short term. However, low viscosity fluids, such as juice or soft drinks, will empty from the stomach quickly and, if you don't consume much of them, can leave you hungry again in a relatively short time. Of course, drinking adequate fluids and water is important for hydration and good health, and drinking water throughout the day is recommended for helping you feel full. (Bariatric surgery patients are advised to avoid fluids when eating meals to avoid "washing through" the food eaten.) Choosing high FF foods is a good way to avoid hunger when reducing calories. Table 9.2, Fullness Factors for Common Foods,

Table 9.2 Fullness Factors for Common Foods

Food	FF
Bean sprouts	4.6
Watermelon	4.5
Grapefruit	4.0
Carrots	3.8
Oranges	3.5
Fish, broiled	3.4
Chicken breast, roasted	3.3
Apples	3.3
Sirloin steak, broiled	3.2
Oatmeal	3.0
Popcorn	2.9
Baked potato	2.5
Low-fat yogurt	2.5
Banana	2.5
Macaroni and cheese	2.5
Brown rice	2.3
Spaghetti	2.2
White rice	2.1
Pizza	2.1
Peanuts	2.0
Ice cream	1.8
White bread	1.8
Raisins	1.6
Snickers Bar	1.5
Honey	1.4
Sugar (sucrose)	1.3
Glucose	1.3
Potato chips	1.2
Butter	0.5

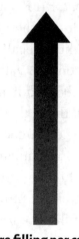

More filling per calorie

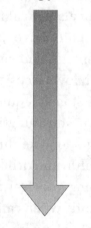

Less filling per calorie

Source: NutritionData.com.
Higher numbers indicate greater satiety.

lists the FF for some common foods. To learn more about FF, go to nutritiondata.self.com/topics/fullness-factor

Food Exchange Lists

Food exchange lists provide a way of grouping foods together to help people on special diets stay on track. Each group lists foods in a certain serving size. A person can exchange, trade, or substitute a food serving in one group for another food serving in the same group. A food exchange system is an easier way to calculate the caloric content of the foods you eat than keeping track with a calorie counting list, although some smartphone apps will do this for you. Initially, there were six exchange lists; now there are additional lists for categories such as alcohol and fast foods. You can find more information on all these lists by googling "food exchange lists" or checking out the American Dietetic Association's website.

Serving Sizes for Food Exchanges. For a given serving size, all choices on a particular list are approximately alike in terms of amount of carbohydrate, protein, fat, and calories per serving. Thus, one food choice on a list can be "exchanged" or traded for any other food on the same list. This approach was found to be helpful for weight control, and eventually was adopted by Weight Watchers early in the organization's history. It is the basis for methods such as counting points or other ways of choosing food that are still promoted by Weight Watchers, now called WW, and similar organizations. The basic food exchange system continues to be a good way to evaluate your food choices.

Review table 9.3, Food Exchange Lists, Calories per Serving, and Number of Servings. It shows six basic exchange lists (across the top), calories per serving, and serving sizes. The number of servings for various levels of caloric intake as well as for seniors is also provided.

Smart Nutrition Strategies

The nutritional tools discussed in this book can be helpful in making healthy food choices and developing personal guidelines for eating that are in alignment with your value of good health. The following

Table 9.3 Food Exchange Lists, Calories per Serving, and Number of Servings

Food Groups	Breads, Grains, and Other Starches	Vegetables	Fruits	Milk, Dairy	Meat, Meat Substitutes, and Other Proteins	Fats, Oils, Sweets, and Alcohol
Calories per serving	80 calories per serving	25 calories per serving	60 calories per serving	90 calories per serving for non-fat, 120 for low-fat, 150 for whole	35–55 calories per serving for lean, 75 for medium-fat, 100 for high-fat servings	45 calories per serving
What is a serving?	1 slice of bread; ½ cup of rice, cooked cereal or pasta; ¾ cup dry cereal; ½ English muffin	1 cup raw leafy vegetables, ½ cup other cooked or raw; ¾ cup vegetable juice; ½ cup potato, yam, peas, corn, or cooked beans	1 medium apple, orange, or ½ banana; ½ cup chopped, cooked or canned fruit; ¾ cup fruit juice	1 cup, milk ½ cup evaporated milk; ¾ plain non-fat yogurt	1 oz meat, fish, poultry, cheese; ½ cup dried beans; 1 egg; ¼ cup cottage cheese; ½ cup tofu	1 tsp oil, butter, margarine, peanut butter; 1 tbsp mayonnaise, regular salad dressing; ½ cup ice cream; 2 small cookies; 2 tbsp sour cream, half-and-half; 6 nuts; 1 slice bacon; 1 tsp sugar

Note: Women who are pregnant or breastfeeding, teenagers, and adults under 24 should have three servings of dairy a day.

Copyright © 2009 Joyce D. Nash.

Table 9.3 Food Exchange Lists, Calories per Serving, and Number of Servings (*continued*)

Food Groups	Breads, Grains, and Other Starches	Vegetables	Fruits	Milk, Dairy	Meat, Meat Substitutes, and Other Proteins	Fats, Oils, Sweets, and Alcohol
Total caloric intake of about 1,600	6 servings	3 servings	2 servings	2–3 servings	5 servings	Use sparingly
Total caloric intake for about 2,200	9 servings	4 servings	3 servings	2–3 servings	6 servings	Use sparingly
Total caloric intake for about 2,800	11 servings	5 servings	4 servings	2–3 servings	7 servings	Use sparingly
For seniors (70+)	6 servings	3 servings	2 servings	3 servings	2 servings	Use sparingly

Note: Women who are pregnant or breastfeeding, teenagers, and adults under 24 should have three servings of dairy a day.

Copyright © 2009 Joyce D. Nash.

173

smart nutrition strategies can also serve to guide weight-management behavior. Healthy snacking can help bridge the hunger gap between meals. Exercising portion control is crucial for weight management. Likewise, learning to read food labels and how to plan meals are important skills for controlling your weight and making good choices. Minimizing fast foods is the best bet for your health and weight. Finally, self-monitoring, as emphasized in previous chapters, is a proven powerful weight-loss strategy.

Snacking

Planned snacking between meals can help with weight management for many overweight and obese people (although most bariatric surgeons advise against it for their patients immediately post-surgery). Snacking can dampen rising hunger between meals and prevent overeating at meals. If you snack, stick to smart choices such as fresh fruit or raw vegetables; low-fat dairy products like cottage cheese, yogurt, or hardboiled eggs; snack-size low-fat popcorn; peanut butter (but not too much); and nuts and seeds in appropriate amounts. Always pack smart snacks for a road trip to avoid going too long without eating. Research has shown that people who eat a high-protein, moderate-calorie snack one hour before lunch automatically cut back their calories during subsequent meals on the same day. Remember the three-to-five rule: Be sure to eat between three and five hours after the last time you ate. Eating sooner is probably either stress-related eating or mindless eating, but also waiting too long to eat invites being overly hungry followed by eating too much.

Controlling Portions

Portion control is one of the keys to weight management. Keeping servings—portions—small is crucial. Many people overestimate the amount of food in a serving and, therefore, underestimate how many servings of foods they are consuming. It is important to have a mental image of serving sizes to succeed with portion control. One 3-ounce serving of meat or fish is about the size and thickness of the palm of your outstretched hand, an audiotape cassette, or a deck of cards. A single serving of hard cheese is the size of a pair of dice. A portion of pasta, rice, or mashed potatoes is about half the size of your fist. A portion of salad is the size of a baseball. A single portion of french fries, potato chips, nuts, or M&Ms is one small handful—filling up the center of a slightly cupped palm of the hand. Table 9.4, Typical Serving Sizes for Main Exchange Lists, lists some typical serving sizes and how they relate to the food exchange system.

Note that an ordinary portion may not be the same as a serving in a food exchange system. The definition of a single-serving size according to a food exchange list varies according to the food item. For example, the food exchange system refers to protein servings as single ounces, but most dietitians refer to a serving or portion of protein in terms of a 3-ounce serving. A 3-ounce portion size of protein is 3 exchanges. A 12-ounce steak, therefore, is four portions or 12 exchanges! Few people realize that a typical deli sandwich has 5 to 8 ounces of meat (5 to 8 exchanges) plus 2 servings of bread (2 exchanges) and 1 teaspoon of mayonnaise (1 exchange). This can easily add up to around 800 to 1,000 calories for a sandwich. A single baked potato can equal two to three vegetable servings or exchanges—plus a baked potato has a high GI and GL load and low satiety value!

Reading Food Labels

Food labels can help you make wise food choices. It is a good idea to learn how to read them. Most packaged foods in the grocery store list nutrition information on the package in an area called Nutrition Facts. The Nutrition Facts label lists the servings per container, the serving size, total calories (per serving), calories from total fat, fat broken down by saturated fat and sometimes trans fat, cholesterol, sodium, total carbohydrate including dietary fiber (sometimes soluble and insoluble fiber), total and added sugars, and protein. Next comes a list of vitamins and minerals as a percent of a reference diet (2,000 calories) followed by a list of ingredients. The list of ingredients shows the ingredients in descending order by weight, meaning

Table 9.4   Typical Serving Sizes for Main Exchange Lists

Exchange List	Contents	Calories per Exchange	Typical Serving Sizes
Starch	Cereals, grains, pasta, breads, crackers, snacks, starchy vegetables, and cooked dried beans,* peas,* and lentils*	80	▪ ½ cup cereal, grain, pasta, or starchy vegetable ▪ 1 ounce of a bread product, such as 1 slice of bread ▪ ¾ to 1 ounce of most snack foods (some snack foods may also have added fat)
Fruit	Fresh, frozen, canned, and dried fruits and fruit juices	60	▪ 1 small to medium fresh fruit ▪ ½ cup canned or fresh fruit ▪ ¼ cup dried fruit ▪ ¾ cup fruit juice
Milk	Milk and milk products, including skim (or very low-fat), 2%, and whole milk	90–150	▪ 1 cup skim, 2%, or whole milk, goat's milk, sweet acidophilus milk, or kefir ▪ ½ cup evaporated skim or whole milk ▪ ¾ cup plain nonfat or low-fat yogurt
Vegetable	Vegetables and vegetable juices	25	▪ ½ cup cooked vegetables or vegetable juice ▪ 1 cup leafy raw vegetables
Meat and Meat Substitutes	Red meat, poultry, fish, shellfish, game, cheese, processed meats, eggs, tofu, tempeh, soy milk, peanut butter, and dried beans,* peas,* and lentils*	35–100	▪ 1 ounce meat, fish, poultry, or cheese, ▪ ½ cup dried beans
Fat	Oil, butter, margarine, shortening, lard, cream, mayonnaise, salad dressing, nuts, seeds, nut butters, avocado, coconut, olives, and bacon	45	▪ 1 tsp regular margarine or vegetable oil ▪ 1 tbsp regular salad dressing

* Can be counted as either a Starch or a Meat Substitute.

that the first ingredient makes up the largest proportion of the food. Check the ingredient list to spot things you'd like to avoid, such as white flour, coconut or palm oil (both high in saturated fat), or hydrogenated oils (which are actually trans fats). Recall that high-fructose corn syrup is another name for sugar.

Note that if you eat more than the serving size listed on the Nutrition Facts label, (for example, 1 cup), you need to adjust the numbers from the Nutrition Facts section accordingly. For example, if you eat 2 cups and the serving size is 1 cup at 230 calories per cup, you are consuming 460 calories. Figure 9.1, How to Read a Nutrition Label, offers more suggestions.

How to Avoid Being Misled by Food Labels. A 2006 study published in the *American Journal of Preventive Medicine* found that only 32 percent of people studied could correctly calculate the amount of carbohydrates in a 20-ounce bottle of soda with multiple servings. Many were also confused by the nutrition label's complexity or they incorrectly interpreted information listed in the percent daily value column (the 2,000-calorie recommended daily allowance list). Not only is it hard to understand the nutrition information given, sometimes that information is misleading or just plain wrong.

The Center of Science in the Public Interest (CSPI), a nonprofit nutrition watchdog group, has thrown light on some of the misleading claims that manufacturers make to give their products a better image. One product, for example, claimed to be "whole grain" but only had 30 percent whole grain. The company was forced by the CSPI to change their labeling. In another case, Kraft, which claimed that such products as Crystal Light Immunity Berry Pomegranate help maintain a "healthy immune system," was challenged by the CSPI. Disease prevention claims on food labels require Food and Drug Administration approval before the product can hit the shelves, but manufacturers don't always comply. Some products have claimed to lead to weight loss, only to be withdrawn from shelves because the claim was found to be untrue.

Check the serving size. Is this the amount you normally eat? ————

How many fat calories come from saturated fat? ————

How many grams of dietary fiber are you getting? ————

Note the two levels of reference diets. ————

Check the ingredients list. ————

Nutrition Facts

Serving Size 1 cup (55g)
Servings Per Container about 9

Amount Per Serving	Cereal	with 1/2 cup Skim milk
Calories	190	230
Calories from Fat	10	10

	% Daily Value**	
Total Fat 1g*	2%	2%
Saturated Fat 0g	0%	0%
Cholesterol 0mg	0%	1%
Sodium 270mg	11%	14%
Potassium 220mg	6%	12%
Total Carbohydrate 44g	15%	17%
Dietary Fiber 4g	16%	16%
Sugars 20g		
Other Carbohydrate 20g		
Protein 4g		

	Cereal	Skim milk
Vitamin A	25%	30%
Vitamin C	0%	0%
Calcium	4%	20%
Iron	25%	25%
Vitamin D	10%	25%
Thiamin	25%	30%
Riboflavin	25%	35%
Niacin	25%	25%
Vitamin B6	25%	25%
Folic Acid	25%	25%
Phosphorus	10%	25%
Magnesium	10%	10%
Zinc	4%	8%
Copper	8%	8%

*Amount in Cereal. A serving of cereal plus skim milk provides 1.5g fat, less than 5mg cholesterol, 340mg sodium, 430mg potassium, 50g carbohydrate (26g sugars) and 8g protein.
**Percent Daily Values are based on a 2,000 calorie diet. Your daily values may be higher or lower depending on your calorie needs:

	Calories:	2,000	2,500
Total Fat	Less than	65g	80g
Sat Fat	Less than	20g	25g
Cholesterol	Less than	300mg	300mg
Sodium	Less than	2,400mg	2,400mg
Potassium		3,500mg	3,500mg
Total Carbohydrate		300g	375g
Dietary Fiber		25g	30g

INGREDIENTS: WHOLE WHEAT, RAISINS, SUGAR, HONEY, BROWN SUGAR, SYRUP, SALT, CORN SYRUP, TRISODIUM PHOSPHATE, VITAMIN...

Scan the calories and calories from fat. What proportion of total calories comes from fat calories?

Are the % Daily Values low for fat, saturated fat, cholesterol, and sodium?

Are the % Daily Values high for total carbohydrate, dietary fiber, vitamins, and minerals?

Note the qualifying footnotes.

Note additional information such as food exchanges.

Figure 9.1 How to Read a Nutrition Label

Still, labels can continue to mislead consumers about such things as fiber content or might be labeled "low fat" even if those are questionable claims. While fiber is known to be a heart-healthy nutrient that lowers cholesterol, a product may not necessarily provide those benefits if its fiber is derived from a source other than a whole grain, such as chicory root. Likewise, a low-fat food may sound healthy and even be a wise choice, but research shows that the average person concerned about his or her weight tends to consume up to 50 percent more calories when they eat foods labeled low-fat compared to eating the original full-fat version of the food. Many foods labeled "low fat" have only 30 percent fewer calories than the original.

A few rules can help you ferret out important information from a food label. First, check the list of ingredients. Pay close attention to the first three ingredients. If one of the first is sugar, honey, brown sugar, syrup, or high-fructose corn syrup (or any variation on that term), you are consuming mostly sugar. If it says hydrogenated anything, it contains trans fat and should be avoided. Keep an eye out for hard-to-pronounce ingredients, which tend to be chemicals for preserving shelf life. Look for healthy ingredients such as *whole-grain* wheat, oats, bran, or any other whole grain. Then check the serving size and calories per serving. Ask yourself this question and be honest with your answer: What is the amount I usually eat, and how does that compare to the serving size? Measure out a recommended serving to see what it looks like. Be sure to adjust the calories according to the number of servings you consume.

Check the sodium level of frozen entrees and canned foods and compare that with the recommended maximum of 2,300 mg per day. Such foods are often high in salt. Instead, buy the reduced sodium option. While purchasing a product that has reduced calories compared to the original might sound like a good idea, take a moment to think about what's been removed. For example, Welch's Light Grape Juice says "light" on the label, which translates to less sugar but more artificial sweeteners and 60 percent less juice. It would be better to buy the 100 percent grape juice and cut the portion size or add a little water. Another guideline used by some people is to buy foods with no more than three ingredients. If any of the ingredients are words you don't know or can't understand, put that food selection back on the shelf.

Check the total calories and the total fat. Fat should be no more than 30 percent of total calories in most instances. When you do the math, remember to keep the serving size in mind and how that compares to the amount you actually consume each time you eat this food. Examine the label in figure 9.1 to learn more about reading labels.

What Constitutes "Whole Grain"?

You may or may not be making the healthiest choice when choosing your bread. Most people know by now that whole grains are the best choice, but it is not always easy to tell which bread products include these healthy grains. If the first ingredient is "wheat," "enriched wheat," "enriched wheat bread," "unbleached wheat flour," or even "unbromated, unbleached wheat," the item is mostly refined white flour. To be a whole-grain product, the first ingredient listed must be a whole grain. Words to watch for include "whole" in front of wheat, rye, or oats. A whole grain must be listed as the first ingredient. The phrases "multi-grain" or "made with whole grain" on the label does not guarantee whole grain unless it is listed first in the ingredient list. Likewise, "high fiber" is not synonymous with whole grain. And you can't tell by color or texture. One good clue is to look for the "100% Whole Grain" stamp from the Whole Grains Council. Only products with at least 16 grams of whole grains per serving can display the "100% Whole Grain" stamp.

Meal Planning

Like smart snacking and good portion control, planning ahead for meals is another helpful strategy for managing weight. Many who struggle with weight issues don't plan ahead. They wait until they go to the grocery store after work to figure out what they feel like eating, often having skipped breakfast or lunch and feeling famished. Or they go to work without thinking ahead for lunch, only to be persuaded by colleagues to go to a restaurant where choices are problematic. Many people do not shop ahead for meals and, as a result, they eat what is handy regardless of its nutritional value, or they end up opting for fast food.

Meal planning can be as simple as making a note the day before of what type of food you will choose for each meal the next day. This is especially important for dinner. For many people, breakfast is simply cereal or something routine—that is, if they don't skip it altogether. Lunch can be more problematic: Will it be leftovers, or a sandwich, a salad, or what? And dinnertime is too often governed by expediency and hunger—what can I eat as soon as possible and what do I crave right this minute? This kind of approach to meals can result in poor choices.

One option is to use a week-at-a-glance type paper calendar and note the main dish for each day—for example, chicken on Monday, fish on Tuesday, a meatless entrée on Wednesday, and so forth. Whether you go low tech and simply write a note about the next day's meal each night before bed or go high tech and enlist your iPhone or a website, planning ahead is a proven key to successful weight management.

Limiting Fast Food

In a fast-paced society, fast foods and take-out are a convenience, but they are also unfortunately a source of high calories and bad fats. The healthiest choice, of course, is to avoid fast foods altogether. Fast foods have many nutritional shortcomings; still, they are part of the American scene. If you can avoid them, do so, or at least minimize your visits. If you must occasionally rely on fast foods, learn how to make healthier choices in these restaurants.

Some fast-food restaurants offer salads, which is a good choice provided you go easy on the dressing. Use half or less of the amount in the container provided. Avoid breaded choices in favor of grilled.

For example, get the grilled chicken sandwich, not the breaded and fried version. Choose a plain hamburger instead of a cheeseburger or a burger with all the fixings. Forget the fried mushrooms, onions, and bacon that can be added to hamburgers. Stick to lettuce and tomato on your burger. Try ordering the "junior" size instead of the larger size, if it's available. Avoid the french fries or, if you must, order the smallest size (or share a larger size) and don't add extra salt to them.

If ordering Mexican food, avoid the sour cream and guacamole; substitute salsa made from fresh tomatoes. Choose burritos, soft tacos, enchiladas, and tamales over cheese-stuffed chile rellenos and quesadillas, but be careful of added cheese or sour cream on any menu item. Cut your burrito in half and take the rest home for a later meal. Be careful with the tortilla chips too; they contain a lot of grease, and it is hard to control your portions when they are served in a constantly refilled community basket. (Put chips on a paper napkin for a few minutes and watch what happens to the napkin.)

When ordering pizza, order the thinnest crust available and top it with fresh vegetables. Skip the sausage, pepperoni, Canadian bacon, salami, and double cheese. At a salad bar, choose fresh vegetables and limit bacon bits and croutons, fried Chinese noodles, marinated vegetables, and cheeses. Order dressing on the side and try dipping your fork into it and spearing some salad, rather than pouring the dressing over the salad. Get the diet drink or simply choose plain water. If you don't like plain water, try carbonated water like Pellegrino. It gives the same "mouth feel" as carbonated, high-sugar drinks without the calories.

Self-Monitoring Caloric Intake

An important strategy for reducing calories is to keep track of them. This may not be a good idea for those who tend to become obsessed with such activities but, for most people, self-monitoring of caloric intake is a helpful strategy. Self-monitoring can keep you conscious of what and how much you are eating. There are many online programs, as well as smartphone apps, for tracking caloric intake, or you can do it the low-tech way by keeping a simple diary of what you eat and the calorie content.

The food exchange lists mentioned earlier in the chapter can be helpful when it comes to recording your calories. Instead of pouring over calorie lists of individual foods, you may prefer the simplicity of using the simple food categories and exchanges listed in table 9.3 on pages 172–173. In the food exchange system, for example, all fruits, depending on serving size, count for about 60 calories per serving. Likewise, all vegetables count for about 25 calories per serving. Starches, which include breads, cereals, and grains, and starchy vegetables such as corn, potatoes, dried beans, peas, and lentils, count about 80 calories per serving. Protein, which includes meat and meat substitutes, varies depending on fat content, for instance, 35 calories (very lean meat, such as skinless chicken breasts) per 1 ounce exchange to 100 calories per ounce for high-fat meat and meat substitutes (pork spareribs, cheese, hot dogs, and sausage). So, a 3-ounce serving of lean meat is a little more than 100 calories while the same size serving of high-fat meat is more like 300 calories per serving. Consult table 9.4, Typical Serving Sizes for Main Exchange Lists, on page 176 for more information on food exchange lists and serving size.

What Constitutes a Healthy Diet?

So, in the final analysis what constitutes a healthy diet? For weight loss, your diet should focus on protein and unsaturated fat and carbohydrates in the form of fruits, vegetables, and small amounts of whole grains. At least once or twice a week, choose a meatless main course. Keep saturated fat from red meats to a minimum. Don't overdo bread, pasta, and rice. If you do choose these foods, choose the whole-grain varieties and practice portion control. Minimize sugary foods and foods with added sugar (e.g., many salad dressings, marinades). Watch your sodium. Consume no more than

2,300 grams of sodium and preferably less. Read the labels on frozen, canned, and packaged foods to ascertain the sodium content, which is often high. Include beans and nuts in your diet. Eat more "real"— fresh and unprocessed—foods. Choose foods that are dense in water and fiber (e.g., apples). Be careful with liquids that contain lots of calories (e.g., sugary sodas, fruit drinks, smoothies). Remember: All foods in moderation. Occasional treats are okay.

10

Exercise and a Healthy Lifestyle

Jacob wanted to lose weight even though his wife, who was also overweight, was not concerned about her weight. Jacob worked out in the gym three days a week for an hour each time. He lifted weights and trained with machines. Jacob's workout routine was skewed toward building muscle mass and was light on aerobic exercise and stretching. His wife continued to buy tempting foods for herself and the kids, and Jacob struggled to stay in control of his eating. He started using a personal trainer who helped him adjust his exercise routine to achieve aerobic-endurance goals as well as strengthening goals and to get social support to motivate him to make healthy choices in the face of temptations at home.

Physical activity and exercise are nonnegotiable components of a healthy lifestyle and a successful weight-management plan. Physical activity is any body movement that works your muscles and requires that your body use more energy than it does at rest. Exercise is a subset of physical activity that is planned, structured, and repetitive for the purpose of conditioning any part of the body. An exercise program can include walking, jogging, running, swimming, bicycling, water aerobics, Pilates, working out in a gym or fitness center, doing floor exercises, following along with an exercise video, or working with a personal trainer or physical therapist. Exercise improves health, maintains fitness, and helps you recover from physical disabilities and such things as back pain. Activities of daily living are also a form of physical activity, including gardening, climbing stairs, cleaning, or parking farther away from, and walking to, your destination.

The quality and quantity of exercise you undertake is important for weight management as well as health. To achieve and maintain optimal health, a program of regular exercise most days of the week—six or seven—together with increased activities of daily living are the goals to strive for. Many obese people are sedentary or inconsistent exercisers, and they may or may not do much in the way of burning extra calories through activities of daily living. A beginning exercise plan for them may simply involve walking regularly for whatever time they can endure and gradually increasing the time and distance they walk as they become more fit. Later, they may set a goal to walk a set number of steps a day or plan to walk for a set time. For example, they may decide to walk for twenty minutes a day. After they achieve this, they could have a goal to walk for longer. Eventually, they may be able to take up hiking for both calorie burn and enjoyment. For adults in both the healthy weight range and those who are overweight, instituting a program of regular exercise that is of sufficient frequency, duration, and intensity (that is, raises heart rate) is essential for reducing health risks and managing weight. Optimal fitness is the goal for preventing premature loss of vital capacities.

A number of internet sites and smartphone apps are available to help a person get started with walking or exercising, and many of these allow the user to monitor food consumption, calories, weight, and exercise. There are also online programs and apps for those who already engage in exercise and want to challenge themselves more, perhaps by competing in fun-runs or marathons, or they may just want to share their fitness accomplishments with others.

Despite the well-established role of physical activity and exercise as a crucial component of a healthy lifestyle, many confirmed dieters go from diet to diet searching for the magic answer—the diet that will finally let them lose weight easily and keep it off without having to move much or do exercise. Of course, no such magic exists. Even if there were a diet that could make losing weight easy, the key to keeping weight off is to engage in regular physical activity and follow a healthy eating pattern that is low to moderate in calories and consists primarily of vegetables, fruit, and lean protein. Similarly, exercise alone, without reducing calories consumed, does not necessarily result in significant weight loss. An abundance of research has established that long-term success managing weight involves exercising regularly and eating moderately. Achieving optimal fitness should be a goal as part of your plan to live a healthy lifestyle.

Defining Fitness

Physical fitness is to the human body what fine-tuning is to an engine. It enables you to perform at your maximum potential. Fitness is a condition that helps you look, feel, and do your best. There are several definitions of *physical fitness.* One of them is the ability to perform daily tasks vigorously and alertly, with enough energy left over to enjoy leisure-time activities and meet emergency demands. It is the ability to endure, to bear up, to withstand stress, to carry on in circumstances where an unfit person could not continue; it is the basis for good health and well-being.

Another way of thinking about physical fitness is that it is the ability to function efficiently and effectively without injury, to enjoy leisure, to be healthy, to resist disease, and to cope with demanding situations.

Despite the evidence that physical fitness is essential for good health and that expending calories and maintaining muscle mass through exercise is essential for healthy weight management, millions of adults—and more and more children—are essentially sedentary. According to one survey of physical activity trends among residents of twenty-six states, roughly six in ten adults either were not active at all or were engaged in physical activity only on an irregular basis. Of the four in ten adults who did engage in regular physical activity, only one of those four got enough exercise to promote or maintain fitness.

People who want to lose weight but who exercise on an irregular basis not only don't lose weight, but they usually have a higher calorie intake than they realize. And often the calories they consume are about the same as, or more than, the calories they burn. Or they may engage in less exercise or the wrong kind of exercise than is necessary to lose weight. (For example, Pilates is good for strengthening the core and improving flexibility, but aerobic exercise is better for burning calories.)

Another potential problem for those who want to lose weight might be that they are not achieving sufficient intensity during their workouts to make a difference, or they simply aren't working out long enough or often enough. It takes months, if not years, of working out with sufficient intensity, duration, and frequency to obtain optimum fitness. Plus, exercise routines need to be changed regularly as muscles adapt. Paying a trainer to set up a single exercise routine is a waste of money; you need to have the trainer regularly change the routine. Muscles need new challenges to achieve fitness.

Working out with a qualified personal trainer can increase your likelihood of doing what it takes to achieve optimal fitness. Finding an internet program or a smartphone app that helps motivate you for greater fitness is also a good option.

Other than the elderly and infirm, those least likely to engage in exercise are the obese. One study found that of 1,172 American men and women, overweight females are most likely to find it hard to start or continue exercise. At the time of that study, two-thirds of subjects were not exercising regularly, and nearly one-quarter indicated they did not intend to start exercising in the next six months. Of those who tried to exercise, only 20 percent were able to maintain regular exercise for six months or longer.

Overcoming Barriers to Exercise

Clearly, many people encounter barriers to exercise, despite its well-known benefits. Barriers can include attitudes, schedules, fears, worries, and any number of "reasons." These must be overcome to achieve the goal of physical fitness. Starting and maintaining an exercise program can be a daunting task, especially if you embrace any of these, or other, perceived barriers. See table 10.1 for possible barriers you might experience. It is crucial to find ways to overcome barriers once you have identified them.

You may have to reevaluate your schedule to find time to exercise. Be aware that you may be giving yourself excuses for not

Table 10.1 Barriers to Exercise

❖ **Attitude:** "It's boring." "I just don't feel like it."

❖ **Excuses and rationalizations:** "I don't have anyone to exercise with." "I can't stick with it, so there's no point in trying." "Exercise makes me hungry." "Gyms are for young people."

❖ **Lack of time**: "Taking care of kids all day doesn't leave me with any time for myself."

❖ **Fatigue:** "I'm tired and want to relax after working all day."

❖ **Worry:** "Exercise just makes me hungrier."

❖ **Lack of success:** "I used to exercise, but it didn't seem to help."

❖ **Self-consciousness:** "I don't want others to see me looking like this."

❖ **Lack of knowledge:** "I don't know how to get started."

❖ **Age:** "I'm too old to start now."

❖ **Fear**: "What if I have a heart attack?"

❖ **Environmental barriers:** "Where I live, there's no room for me to exercise." "There are no fitness centers in my area." "It's not safe for me to walk in my neighborhood."

exercising that just aren't valid. One man who initially claimed he didn't have time to get out and walk admitted that he could spend less time with his ham radio activities in order to increase his physical activity.

Most people find that regular exercise is invigorating and gives them more energy for other things. Worries about suffering injury or a debilitating heart event as the result of exercise are usually not warranted, but it is a good idea to see your doctor first before undertaking vigorous exercise if you are concerned. Health problems arising from exercise are less likely if you do not do too much too soon. A common prescription for those who have had a heart attack is to get regular exercise to improve the strength of the heart as well as overall fitness.

Having the confidence that you can be more physically active and that doing so will help you achieve your health and weight management goals is important. With confidence, you are more likely to make every effort to overcome barriers to exercising. Part of this involves deciding that leading a healthy lifestyle, which includes regular exercise, is an important personal value for you. You must become committed to making regular exercise a part of your lifestyle. It must be "just what I do." When you make exercise a daily habit, you redefine your self-concept—how you think about yourself.

Undertaking exercise or intensifying your current exercise means starting from wherever you are now and setting small but challenging goals to get you where you want to be.

Addressing Reasons for Not Exercising

Lack of Time. Try scheduling exercise time in your daily calendar. Treat it as an important appointment that can't be missed. And remember, you can break up your exercise into ten-minute intervals over the course of the day and aim for the recommended number of minutes a week needed to lose weight. Get a friend to go for a walk with you. Get a smart watch such as the FitBit and make a game of getting more steps.

Fatigue. Lack of energy is often cited as a reason for skipping exercise, especially by women. Working full time outside the house and then coming home to tend to the family takes energy. Finding time for yourself can be hard. It can be tempting to simply sit down in front of the TV or read a book when you can steal precious minutes. Try delegating some of your household tasks to others in the family so you can make time for exercise. Try taking ten or fifteen minutes to clear your head by taking a short walk; you'll likely feel better and more energized afterward. The best way to incorporate exercise into your daily routine is to plan to do it in the morning—before your day starts. Make exercise a priority and let the family know you intend to make time for it.

Unfounded Worry. Some women worry that doing exercise will increase their appetite or add weight by building muscle mass. In fact, it is hard to build much muscle unless you work out hard and long and have the right hormones (i.e., testosterone). If you exercise regularly, you might improve your muscle mass, which is a good thing. It leads to a toned body with sleek muscles. Don't worry, though; it won't be so extreme that you'll be entering a body-building contest. Another good thing about increasing muscle mass is that you will increase your calorie burn. Men, who naturally have more muscle, burn more calories than women and, as a result, lose weight faster. Rather than increasing appetite, exercise usually decreases it. If you find that you feel like eating after exercise, plan to have a healthy snack afterwards.

Embarrassment. Some people worry they will look silly in exercise clothes, and so think they would be embarrassed to go walking in public or go to a gym. In fact, most people admire heavier people who are out walking or working out in a gym because they are showing dedication to better health. (One heavier woman wearing exercise clothes during her daily walk discovered that the drivers of passing cars often gave her a "thumbs up.") Of course, you could stay at home and use an exercise video, but it is hard to stay self-motivated to do this on a regular basis.

Lack of Knowledge. Brisk walking doesn't take any special knowledge, but you need a good pair of walking shoes. If you join a gym, they usually have people who will show you how to use the machines. It's worth investing in the services of a personal trainer to achieve fitness. A trainer can assess your capabilities and design workouts that are best for you. It is necessary to change up your exercise routine periodically, and a trainer can help you do that too. Another reason to keep working with a trainer is that they will make sure you are doing an exercise the right way—that is, using the right form so you get the most benefit from the exercise and do not injure yourself.

Age. Some older adults think they don't need much exercise or they're just too old to do it. Nearly a fifth of respondents who were over 40 years old responded to one survey saying they didn't think physical exercise provided health benefits. Many older adults, particularly women, did not grow up participating in or valuing exercise. When they do join an exercise program, they are more likely than younger women to drop out. Women often put the needs of the family before their own health needs, and this leads to not exercising or not even acknowledging the need for physical fitness.

Fear of Being Injured. Some people don't exercise because they have a "bad back" or another physical problem. They fear that exercise will make their problem worse. Naturally, beginning to exercise after having been sedentary for a long time is likely to bring some mild soreness. But with the right exercise—and with the help of a personal trainer—even a bad back can improve. Most injuries come from doing high-intensity exercise too soon for your fitness level or from doing it improperly. If you want to engage in a more vigorous program, get the help of a personal trainer. (For example, a man who was diagnosed with Parkinson's Disease was advised by his doctor to take up kick boxing. He needed the services of a personal trainer to do this correctly and safely.) For many older people, walking is a good exercise. In bad weather, you can walk in a covered mall. Another option is to join a water aerobics class.

Commitment to Exercise

Good intentions and an awareness of the benefits of exercise, though important, don't help much with getting you started or keeping you sticking to an exercise routine. More important is your commitment to being physically active and placing a high value on exercise. Confidence in persisting, even in the face of barriers like lack of time, fatigue, lack of knowledge, bad weather, or living in an unsafe neighborhood, will help you achieve the benefits of exercise.

Benefits of Exercise

Most people think that if they exercise, they must also cut back on calories and lose weight to get any health benefit from it. While exercising and cutting calories are certainly the best approach for losing weight, there are health benefits to exercising even if you don't lose much weight or aren't trying to. One study that illustrates this point included twenty-four middle-aged men who weren't in the habit of exercising. Eight were lean, eight obese, and eight had type 2 diabetes. For three months, they followed a fairly rigorous exercise program that consisted of an hour of aerobic exercise five times a week. The twist was that they were told to eat enough to compensate for the extra calories burned while exercising so that they would *not* lose weight. Two results stood out: in all three groups, the waist size of the men shrank by about an inch and the levels of *interleukin-6* (an inflammatory chemical produced by fat and certain other tissues) declined. The most important aspect of the study was the proof that exercise produced a measurable reduction in health risk despite the fact that the participants did not lose weight.

An important reason that being overweight is unhealthy is that fat tissues are metabolically active, producing hormones and chemicals that harm the cardiovascular system, the liver, and other systems. Getting and staying active with exercise helps cut down this risk. Of course, if you are overweight, exercise that brings about some weight loss is better than than doing nothing at all. Cutting calories and exercising more is necessary to lose weight, but even if you don't lose weight, staying fit and active promotes better health.

Not only does regular exercise offer improved health benefits and increased protection from heart failure as you age, but exercise can also boost your brain size and reduce the risk of developing dementia or less-serious memory loss. Research suggests that doing aerobic exercise—mostly brisk walking—three days a week for forty-five minutes a day increased the size of participants' brains. It makes sense that strength training would help too. Your best approach is to embark on an exercise program that involves aerobics, strength training, and stretching, leading to optimal fitness.

How Much Exercise Is Needed to Lose Weight?

A study conducted by the American College of Sports Medicine (ACSM) examined different recommendations for how much exercise is needed to lose weight. As a result of the research, the organization makes several recommendations. They advise that you should get between 150 and 250 minutes of moderate to vigorous exercise each week to lose weight. That's roughly 22 to 35 minutes of exercise per day to lose weight. But they also state that more is better. They found that more than 250 minutes per week of moderate to vigorous activity is associated with more substantial weight loss. That means an average of about 35 minutes per day.

When to See a Doctor Before Exercising

If you are over 35 years of age, especially if you have been sedentary and are obese, it is a good idea to check with your doctor before undertaking a relatively vigorous conditioning program. If you are 35 or younger, have not been completely sedentary for years, have no previous history of cardiovascular disease and no known disease risk factors for CD, and have had a medical evaluation within the past two years, you can probably begin an aerobic exercise program without special medical clearance. If you have any risk factors for cardiovascular disease—that is, if you smoke, are obese or sedentary, have high blood pressure or high cholesterol, or a family history of heart disease—a supervised exercise stress test may be appropriate before you undertake a vigorous exercise program. Table 10.2 on page 196 lists the factors that indicate a need for medical clearance prior to undertaking vigorous exercise.

Components of an Optimal Fitness Program

Optimal fitness means being the best that you can be physically given your age, gender, and body type. This should be the ultimate goal of your exercise program, although it will probably take time to reach optimal fitness. The components of optimal fitness include aerobic fitness (achieved with endurance training), strength training (by using muscles and resistance training—brisk walking, jogging or running, riding a bicycle, swimming), core strengthening (involving exercise for the midsection of the body and back), balance training (involving movement exercises aimed at improving stability), and stretching and joint flexibility. Two other important types of exercise that accelerate fat loss include interval training, which involves periods of high-intensity anaerobic exercise interspersed with rest, and circuit training, which is when you alternate between several exercises (usually five or ten) that target different muscle groups.

To achieve optimal fitness, you need to participate regularly in a variety of exercises that address all these components. Because exercise that develops one aspect of fitness generally contributes little to the other fitness components, different exercises should be chosen to meet individual needs and capacities. Table 10.3 on pages 197–198 provides you with guidelines for exercising by age and intensity.

Cardiovascular Fitness

Cardiovascular fitness is the cornerstone of good health. Aerobic or endurance exercises that promote cardiovascular fitness are a crucial part of a well-rounded exercise program. The term *cardiovascular fitness* refers to the heart's ability to pump oxygen-rich blood to the muscles. (The term *aerobic* means "in the presence of oxygen.") Any

Table 10.2
When to See a Doctor Before Undertaking Vigorous Exercise
Consult your doctor before beginning an exercise program if you:

- ❖ Are over 35 years of age.
- ❖ Have not had a medical checkup in more than two years.
- ❖ Smoke.
- ❖ Are more than 30 percent above recommended weight, a BMI over 30.
- ❖ Have any close male relatives (father, brother) who have had a heart attack or stroke before the age of 55 or any close female relatives (mother, sister) who have had a heart attack or stroke before the age of 65.
- ❖ Have heart trouble or a heart murmur or have had a heart attack yourself.
- ❖ Have irregular heartbeats or uneven heart action.
- ❖ Have uncontrolled high blood pressure or are on medication for hypertension.
- ❖ Have kidney disease.
- ❖ Have insulin-dependent diabetes.
- ❖ Have elevated cholesterol.
- ❖ Have bone, joint, muscle, or vein problems, such as arthritis, rheumatism, bad back, or bad leg veins.
- ❖ Have a resting heart rate (RHR) of more than 80 beats per minute.
- ❖ Easily become short of breath doing ordinary activities.
- ❖ Often feel faint or have dizzy spells.
- ❖ Often experience pain or pressure in the left shoulder or arm, mid-chest area, or left side of your neck during or right after exercise.
- ❖ Have any doubts about your health status.

activity that employs the large muscles of the body (especially the leg muscles) for a relatively continuous time or is rhythmic in nature and is done with sufficient intensity to elevate the heart rate and promote the body's ability to utilize oxygen efficiently is classified as aerobic or endurance exercise. Oxygen is your main energy source during aerobic workouts. Examples include brisk walking, running, swimming laps, bicycling, singles tennis, hiking, spinning, interval training, and circuit training.

Table 10.3 Physical Activity Guidelines for Americans

Children and adolescents should do 60 minutes (1 hour) or more of physical activity daily.

❖ Aerobic: Most of the 60 or more minutes a day should be either moderate-[a] or vigorous-intensity[b] aerobic physical activity, and should include vigorous-intensity physical activity at least three days a week.

❖ Muscle-strengthening:[c] As part of their 60 or more minutes of daily physical activity, children and adolescents should include muscle-strengthening physical activity on at least three days a week.

❖ Bone-strengthening:[d] As part of their 60 or more minutes of daily physical activity, children and adolescents should include bone-strengthening physical activity on at least three days a week.

Continues ▶

[a]Moderate-intensity physical activity: Aerobic activity that increases a person's heart rate and breathing to some extent. On a scale relative to a person's capacity, moderate-intensity activity is usually a 5 or 6 on a 0 to 10 scale. Brisk walking, dancing, swimming, or bicycling on a level terrain are examples.

[b]Vigorous-intensity physical activity: Aerobic activity that greatly increases a person's heart rate and breathing. On a scale relative to a person's capacity, vigorous-intensity activity is usually a 7 or 8 on a 0 to 10 scale. Jogging, singles tennis, swimming continuous laps, or bicycling uphill are examples.

[c]Muscle-strengthening activity: Physical activity, including exercise that increases skeletal muscle strength, power, endurance, and mass. It includes strength training, resistance training, and muscular strength and endurance exercises.

[d]Bone-strengthening activity: Physical activity that produces an impact or tension force on bones, which promotes bone growth and strength. Running, jumping rope, and lifting weights are examples.

Table 10.3 Physical Activity Guidelines for Americans (*continued*)

Children and adolescents should do 60 minutes (1 hour) or more of physical activity daily.

❖ It is important to encourage young people to participate in physical activities that are appropriate for their age, that are enjoyable, and that offer variety.

18 to 64 years: All adults should avoid inactivity. Some physical activity is better than none, and adults who participate in any amount of physical activity gain some health benefits.

❖ For substantial health benefits, adults should do at least 150 minutes (2 hours and 30 minutes) a week of moderate-intensity, or 75 minutes (1 hour and 15 minutes) a week of vigorous-intensity aerobic physical activity, or an equivalent combination of moderate- and vigorous-intensity aerobic activity. Aerobic activity should be performed in episodes of at least 10 minutes, and preferably, it should be spread throughout the week.

❖ For additional and more extensive health benefits, adults should increase their aerobic physical activity to 300 minutes (5 hours) a week of moderate-intensity, or 150 minutes a week of vigorous-intensity aerobic physical activity, or an equivalent combination of moderate- and vigorous-intensity activity. Additional health benefits are gained by engaging in physical activity beyond this amount.

❖ Adults should also include muscle-strengthening activities that involve all major muscle groups on two or more days a week.

65 years and older

❖ Older adults should follow the adult guidelines. When older adults cannot meet the adult guidelines, they should be as physically active as their abilities and conditions will allow.

❖ Older adults should do exercises that maintain or improve balance if they are at risk of falling.

❖ Older adults should determine their level of effort for physical activity relative to their level of fitness.

❖ Older adults with chronic conditions should understand whether and how their conditions affect their ability to do regular physical activity safely.

Source: Adapted from US Department of Health and Human Services. 2008 *Physical Activity Guidelines for Americans.* Washington, DC: US Department of Health and Human Services, 2008. Available at: https://health.gov/our-work/physical-activity.

Anaerobic Exercise

Anaerobic exercise involves quick bursts of energy performed at maximum effort for a short time. During anaerobic exercise, your body requires immediate energy, so it relies on stored energy sources, rather than oxygen, to fuel itself. This includes breaking down glucose. Examples of anaerobic exercise are heavy weightlifting, jumping, sprinting, kickboxing, or any exercise requiring high intensity and a high rate of work for a short period of time.

The term *anaerobic* means "without air" or "without oxygen," but it is still a component of cardiovascular and optimal fitness. It is good for building strength and muscle mass and benefits the heart and lungs. In the long run, increased muscle mass helps a person become leaner and manage weight, because muscle burns large amounts of calories. To achieve cardiovascular fitness, you need to start wherever you are on the fitness continuum and work toward optimal fitness. Your first goal should be aerobic exercise. Walking is a good activity to begin with and, later in this chapter, you will learn more about walking for exercise and good health. Walking is free and can be done whenever you can fit it in. If you have been sedentary, you should start at a comfortable level and gradually increase your walking until you can do more and more each day. If you've been exercising a long time or are trying to lose weight, add anaerobic workouts to your routine.

Muscle Strength and Endurance

Muscle strength is the ability to exert force. *Muscle endurance* is the ability to sustain an activity over a period of time. With adequate muscle strength and endurance, you can perform all activities, including those of daily living, with less stress and strain. Adequate muscle strength and endurance allow you to walk, stand, or sit without becoming overly fatigued or experiencing back pain. In the absence of this type of fitness, you tire easily, your efficiency suffers, and your productivity declines.

Muscle fitness and endurance is achieved through resistance, strength-building activities, and weight-bearing activities. These include lifting weights, which can involve using exercise resistance bands or tubes; working out with machines that isolate particular muscle groups; and doing a range of exercises, including floor exercises that use various body parts to provide the resistance. (Exercise resistance bands can be obtained from internet stores like Amazon as well as Target, and they are easy to take with you on vacations.) Floor exercises work various muscles or muscle groups; an example would be doing planks. The current trend in fitness is to use multiple groups of muscles at a time, rather than isolating a particular muscle group. Core fitness is the first order of business in strength and endurance training.

Core fitness is the basis for training all muscle groups. It focuses on developing strong abdominal, low back, pelvic, and hip muscles to encompass the whole "core" and these exercises should be done daily. Examples of core exercises include planks, reverse crunches, bridging (which involves lying on the floor, pushing the mid-body up from the floor using the feet and arms for support), and various other exercises focusing on the core muscles just mentioned. Learning to tighten the midsection of the body—known as "pulling the belly button to the spine"—is an important skill. Having a strong core reduces the likelihood of experiencing back pain.

Another advantage of striving for good, overall muscle strength is that, over time, it can build muscle mass. Men can do this more easily than women because they have more of the hormone testosterone. They also start off with more muscle mass than women. Muscles that are not exercised regularly *atrophy*—that is, unused muscles shrink in size over time—and thus the maxim "use it or lose it." (It's not true that muscle turns into fat, but it is true that muscles shrink and body fat is gained over time.) As men and women age, they tend to exercise less and be less active in general, and as a result muscle mass decreases, along with muscle strength and endurance. In addition, metabolism decreases along with muscle mass, leading to weight gain unless there is a corresponding decrease in caloric intake. The chronically sedentary person inevitably loses muscle mass without exercise and gains weight as their metabolism slows down, a natural process called *sarcopenia*.

To attain muscle strength and endurance in specific muscle groups, you need at least two or three sessions of resistance exercise per week to yield improvement. A range of exercises that work the muscle groups should be selected depending on your goal. Building strength requires gradually increasing resistance weight and stressing the muscles to fatigue. Endurance involves doing multiple repetitions at low weight. That is, high-resistance weight with few repetitions builds muscle, while low-resistance weight with high repetition encourages endurance.

The number of sets you do (a *set* being a specific number of repetitions, such as ten or twenty repetitions) depends on your goal. Start doing two to three sets of each exercise and gradually increase the number of sets or the number of repetitions per set. Proper form is key. Posture is important. You also need to move the resistance (for example, the dumbbells or resistance bands) in a slow, controlled manner and avoid going too fast or jerking the weights or bands. Maintain normal breathing; don't hold your breath. Exhale during exertion. Resistance training should be rhythmic, be performed at a moderate-to-slow pace, and should involve a full range of motion. Working with a personal trainer who is observing you and making corrections to your form as necessary ensures you will get the most out of your workout. Some gyms provide an initial workout and introduction to the weights and machines with a trainer at no additional cost. If you want to keep working with a trainer, there is a fee.

Weight training involving the large muscle groups should not be done on consecutive days. While it's a good idea to exercise often, it may not be beneficial to perform the same exercise on consecutive days. A day of rest between sessions involving large muscle groups allows the muscles to recuperate. Without recuperation time, the risk of injury increases. Some people do weight training five or six days a week, but they alternate muscle groups from day-to-day so that a specific muscle group is trained only two or three days a week. This is called a *split routine*. Those who want to do a full-body workout involving all the major muscle groups in one session should do this only two or three times a week on nonconsecutive days.

If you want help getting started with an exercise program focused on muscle strength and endurance, you don't necessarily have to hire a trainer. Check the internet for apps that act as your personal trainer. Some of these present more than two hundred exercises, all with clear photos, videos, and recorded instructions for how to do each exercise safely and correctly. You can browse by category or muscle group and follow a workout checklist with a suggested routine or create your own custom set of exercises. Most of these apps let you log and chart your progress in a journal with entry screens tailored for each exercise.

Types of Exercise

Different types of exercise provide different types of benefits. Joint flexibility focuses on movement to improve your range of motion during daily activities. Interval and circuit training are best for increasing calorie burn.

Joint Flexibility

Flexibility refers to how fully your joints or limbs are able to move. Being flexible allows for easier movement and reduced joint pain so it is easier to perform daily activities. Flexibility is a fitness goal overlooked by many people. Adequate flexibility helps you avoid muscle pulls and strains, while lack of flexibility usually contributes to sports injuries, lower back pain, and those annoying pains and injuries that often seem to occur out of nowhere when you reach for or pick up something. Any sudden stretching that forcibly extends a muscle beyond its limits can produce injury and pain. Regular stretching exercises, in addition to helping improve appearance by promoting good posture, protect against possible injury.

Static stretching, also known as *passive stretching*, is the most commonly recommended stretching exercise. It involves slowly stretching a muscle to the point of mild tension and then holding that position for a period of time—usually ten to thirty seconds or longer—until you feel the tension release or you no longer feel the tension at all. An example of static stretching would be to slowly and comfortably bend down to touch your toes (or as far as you can go) and hold the position for a few seconds. Don't bounce; that could cause injury. Static stretching has a low risk of injury, requires little time or assistance, and is quite effective.

Dynamic stretching, or *active stretching*, uses the momentum created by repetitive bouncing movements to stretch muscles and should be avoided by those who are not high-performance athletes since it can result in injury if not done properly. Also known as *ballistic stretching*, this method stretches muscles much farther and faster. For example, the ballistic method of touching your toes would be to bounce and jerk toward your feet. With this type of stretching, you do not hold a position. Repeat: unless you are a highly trained athlete, you should not use ballistic stretching.

Yoga and tai chi are two forms of exercise that involve gentle movement stretching. Check local listings on the internet for such classes. Another way to engage in these activities without having to join a class is to search the internet for "learning tai chi" or "learning yoga." YouTube has videos for beginning and more advanced classes in both. In addition, there are internet apps that demonstrate these movements.

Interval Training

In terms of losing weight, *interval training* produces more weight loss than steady, moderate-intensity aerobic exercise such as jogging or running and is a type of anaerobic exercise that should be part of any serious weight-loss effort. Interval training involves bursts of high-intensity exercise alternating with periods of rest or low-intensity activity—the "intervals" in interval training. The term refers to any cardiovascular exercise—such as spinning or using an elliptical machine—that can be done in brief, intense bouts (from 30 seconds to 2 minutes) at near-maximum exertion (measured by heart rate) interspersed with periods of lower-intensity activity. A bout of high-intensity exercise followed by a low-intensity exercise cycle is called a "set." Repeated sets done for about twenty minutes, three times a week, can produce significant fat loss. Part of the reason for this is that interval training drains the muscles of inbuilt energy sources and replenishment takes up to forty-eight hours to occur, resulting in prolonged fat burn, referred to as *afterburn*. Check the internet for information on interval training.

A popular type of exercise that lends itself well to interval training is spinning. Usually done in classes, spinning involves riding a stationary bike that allows for quick adjustments of tension. Spinning rates depend on heart rate (see the content later in this chapter about target heart rate) and is done in intervals. An instructor leads the class and sets the pace, but you can set the tension to your level of fitness.

Circuit Training

Circuit training is a combination of high-intensity aerobics and resistance training exercises designed for muscle building and heart–lung fitness. It also helps with fat burning. An exercise "circuit" is one completion of all prescribed exercises in the program, of which there can be five or more. When one circuit is complete, the exercises are repeated for another circuit. The duration of individual circuit-training stations can be between forty-five and sixty seconds and, in some cases, as long as two minutes, depending on the number of repetitions performed at each station. Higher repetitions put the exercise further toward the endurance end of the intensity continuum. Fewer repetitions and increased weight optimize muscle strength. Typically, circuit training boosts heart rate. Either a trainer or a smartphone app can assist you in composing your workout as well as timing your circuits. They tell you when to move on to the next exercise so you can focus on what you need to do.

Combining Exercises

To achieve optimal fitness, you will want to combine exercises focused on cardiovascular fitness exercises (aerobic and anaerobic), muscle strength and endurance exercise, and stretching exercise. Doing interval training or circuit training accelerates weight loss and fitness. It is helpful if you can combine exercises that are varied and that you enjoy. One woman who was committed to improving her fitness and losing weight did a spinning class on Tuesdays and a kickboxing class on Thursdays. On weekends she usually did a five-mile hike. Two of the other days she worked out with a trainer. That may seem like a lot of exercise if you are just starting out, but this routine is one that can lead to good physical fitness and weight loss.

Beginning Your Exercise Program

Having decided to undertake an exercise program that leads toward optimum fitness and health, you can now determine what you need to do to reach this goal. Warming up and cooling down are important parts of any exercise workout. This should be done each time you exercise. Learning to assess your target heart rate is another skill you need so you can know if you are exerting yourself enough while you exercise. You will learn how to assess your heart rate later in this chapter.

Warming Up

It is important to perform a proper warm-up before any type of physical activity. The purpose of a warm-up is to prevent injury by increasing the body's core and muscle temperature. Warm muscles increase the rate of energy production, which increases reflexes and lowers the time it takes to contract a muscle. A good warm-up should also increase range of motion and mentally prepare you for more exercise.

Types of Stretching

* *Static stretching* (also known as *passive stretching*) stays in one position and holds for ten to sixty seconds. An example of a static stretch is bending down at the waist to touch your toes (or as far as you can go) and holding it for ten to sixty seconds. Any stretch that holds a position for several seconds is a static stretch.
* *Dynamic stretching* (also known as *active stretching*) involves a stretch that keeps moving. It is not held in position. Dynamic stretches are active movements where joints and muscles go through a full range of motion. Examples include walking while raising the knee to the chest, straight-leg kicks, or heel-to-rear jogging.

Warm-ups should be specific to the type of exercise you are doing but should be a full body warm-up even if you only plan to work out a few muscle groups. For example, if you are planning to do a leg workout, you should do a warm-up with mostly lower body exercises, but also include a few upper body/full body exercises as well. If you plan to go for a run, start with a few minutes of jogging in place.

How to Warm-Up. A warm-up has certain key elements. (1) The general warm-up consists of five to ten minutes of light physical activity, which will allow the muscles to be stretched effectively afterward. An example would be walking at a moderate pace on the treadmill before stretching, which results in a light sweat. (2) After the general warm-up, gentle, static stretching should be done for all the major muscle groups for five to ten minutes. (3) After the general warm-up and static stretching, the body needs to be prepared for the demands of the specific sport or activity to be undertaken during the workout. This involves more vigorous exercise. Exercise at this time should reflect the movements and actions that will be required during the sport. For example, in anticipation of a bicycle race or a long bicycle ride, some short "joy riding" or light pedaling is a good idea. For a foot race, jogging for a short distance would be good preparation.

How to Cool Down. When you have finished your exercise, you need to cool down and stretch again. Cooling down is an essential part of your routine. *Cooling down* helps the heart rate and breathing return to normal and the muscles return to rest. The three elements of cooling down are gentle exercise (slowing down and gradually decreasing intensity), stretching, and refueling. If you have been jogging, you should drop back to a fast walk and then progressively slow down. If walking briskly is your chosen exercise, simply slow down gradually. Stretch the muscle groups you have been working. Finally, drink water and eat a small and healthy snack afterward.

Muscle fibers, tendons, and ligaments undergo a lot of strain during intense exercise. This produces *lactic acid*, a waste product that can cause muscle stiffness and soreness. A proper cool-down helps the body chemistry readjust and is vital for removing this lactic acid. Cooling down helps prevent Delayed-Onset Muscle Soreness (DOMS). DOMS is generally felt a day or two after a strenuous workout. Cooling down for about ten minutes can prevent, or reduce, the risk of it occurring.

Target Heart Rate Zone

Intensity of aerobic exercise can be measured by assessing target heart rate. The *target heart rate zone* is the percentage of maximum exercise heart rate (MEHR) at which you will benefit most from exercise. The American College of Sports Medicine provides guidelines that indicate the percent of MEHR that will allow you to reach your fitness goals. You should choose your limits based on your present level of fitness and your exercise goals.

Sedentary persons should strive to do exercise that reaches 50 percent of MEHR. Initially, the upper limit should be no more than 60 to 75 percent. These limits are also recommended for older or overweight people until their fitness level improves. Those who have been exercising and who have optimal fitness as a goal need to exercise at a level of intensity that produces a heart rate between 60 and 90 percent of maximum. However, benefits start to tail off with intensity greater than 85 percent. Unless you expect to compete in a sport that requires an exceedingly high level of fitness, you probably should not exceed 75 to 80 percent of maximum.

Calculating Your Target Heart Rate Zone. There are several ways to determine your target heart rate zone. One is to use the following equations, which allow you to calculate the lower and upper limits of your choice for your age:

Lower limit = (220 − your age) × 0.50 = beats per minute

Upper limit = (220 − your age) × 0.75 = beats per minute

Once you get these numbers, you can divide by six to get your beats for every ten second interval. Alternatively, look up your target heart rate limit in table 10.4. Or you can find a smartphone app that measures heart rate. If you have a fitness tracker such as a FitBit, you can use it to measure heart rate. Check the internet for other options.

Staying in the Zone. Before you begin your aerobic exercise or interval training, you should determine your target heart rate zone based on your age and the upper and lower limits you have chosen using the methods above. As a beginning exerciser, you need to take your pulse (figure 10.1) three or four times or more during an exercise session, or about every five to ten minutes, until you learn what your body feels like in the zone. Take it first after you have finished warming up. After your warm-up, when you are ready to begin your exercise session, your heart rate should be approaching the lower limit of your target heart rate zone, although it may not yet be in the zone.

Next, take your pulse about five minutes into the aerobic part of your exercise session. By then, you should be in your target heart rate zone. If you are below the lower limit, increase your level of effort (e.g., increase your speed or intensity). If you are above the upper limit, slow down or reduce the intensity so that your heart rate falls back into the zone. Continue to take your heart rate periodically

Table 10.4 Limits for Target Heart Rate Zone

Age	50%		60%		75%		85%		90%	
	Beats Min.	10-sec. Count	Beats/ Min.	Count 10-sec.	Beats/ Min.	10-sec. Count	Beats/ Min.	10-sec. Count	Beats/ Min.	10-sec. Count
20	100	17	120	20	150	25	170	28	180	30
25	98	16	117	20	146	24	166	28	176	29
30	95	16	114	19	143	24	162	27	171	29
35	93	15	111	19	139	23	157	26	167	28
40	90	15	108	18	135	23	153	26	162	27
45	88	15	105	18	131	22	149	25	158	26
50	85	14	102	17	128	21	145	24	153	26
55	83	14	99	17	124	21	140	23	149	25
60	80	13	96	16	120	20	136	23	144	24
65	78	13	93	16	116	19	132	22	140	23

1. Locate your carotid artery with the tips of your third and fourth fingers. (The carotid artery is in the front strip of muscle that runs vertically down your neck.) Press your fingers on one side only of the neck. Press lightly with your fingers until you feel the blood pulsing beneath your fingers.

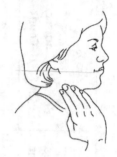

or

Find your radial artery by pressing your fingers on the inside of your wrist just below your wrist bone.

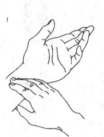

2. Using a watch with a sweep hand or with a digital readout of seconds, count the number of times your heart beats in ten seconds.

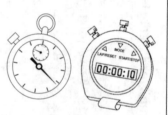

3. Multiply the number of beats you feel for ten seconds by six to get your heart rate (pulse) per minute. Compare this to your target heart rate zone. Adjust your exercise intensity up or down so you are in your target heart rate zone.

Figure 10.1 **How to Take Your Pulse**

throughout your exercise session and adjust your level of effort up or down so you stay in your target zone.

Check your heart rate again immediately after stopping the aerobic part of your exercise session. As you become more physically fit, your heart rate will become lower for the same amount and intensity of exercise. Eventually you will need to adjust the intensity of the exercise to get your heart rate back up in the zone. Finally, check your heart rate near the end of your cool-down phase (when you are walking slowly or exercising with less intensity). Over time, as you reach your goal of optimum fitness, your heart rate will return to your baseline—where you heart rate is usually—more quickly. (In fact, recovery heart rate is one measure of fitness.)

Perceived Exertion Method

Unfortunately, not everyone can use target heart rate zone to assess intensity. Some people have a naturally high or naturally low heart rate. Certain medications, such as those containing beta blockers (including some high blood pressure medications), can also increase or decrease heart rate. Pulse monitoring may not be appropriate for cardiac patients, diabetics, or pregnant women. Such people may need to use the perceived exertion method.

Perceived exertion is how you feel when your body is working. It is based on the physical sensations you experience during physical activity, including increased heart rate, increased respiration or breathing rate, increased sweating, flushing of the face, and muscle fatigue. Using perceived exertion to assess intensity of exercise involves paying attention to your physical sensations. Even though this is a subjective measure, research suggests that there is a high correlation between a person's perceived exertion rate and actual heart rate during activity. Check the internet for more information on the perceived exertion method.

Choosing Your Exercise Program

Now that you have learned about warming up before exercising and cooling down afterward, and you know how to use target heart rate or perceived exertion as methods to assess intensity of the exercise you are doing, it is time to decide on what exercise to begin with on your way to optimum fitness and weight management.

The easiest and most readily available exercise is walking. All you need is a good pair of walking shoes. Or you might decide to join a gym or work with a personal trainer. If you are seriously obese, you may need to start with less taxing exercise and use resistance bands for working out by using your arms only, or get your exercise in a pool. If you are sufficiently motivated, you might choose to exercise at home. Also, everyone can increase activities of daily living.

When to Exercise

If you are undertaking an exercise program for the first time, you probably have several questions: When is the best time to exercise? How much exercise do I need to do? How do I cope with challenging weather conditions?

There is no "best" time to exercise. Some people prefer to start off the day by exercising in the morning. Others claim that their body isn't ready to move until later in the day, while others like to go to the gym after work. The hour just before the evening meal is popular for other people. Some people even work out late at night at a twenty-four-hour fitness gym or facility. When you work out is up to you, although studies have shown that, from a motivational point of view, most people find it is easier to work out sooner rather than later in the day. Waiting to exercise later means that other demands can preempt exercise and move it off your calendar for that day. Making exercise an appointment on your calendar or setting off a certain hour for exercise makes it more likely to occur. Likewise, having an appointment with a personal trainer will motivate you to show up. Similarly, agreeing to meet a friend to walk or go to the pool will increase the likelihood that you keep the appointment.

It is generally advisable to wait an hour or so after eating a big meal before exercising, but having a light snack beforehand is a good idea. If you exercise in the morning, you should have something light to eat first, such as yogurt.

Be aware that doing stimulating exercise just before bedtime may make it harder to fall asleep. To decide the best time for you to exercise, consider the demands of your schedule and listen to your body.

How Much to Exercise

According to the National Heart, Lung, and Blood Institute, regular exercise is one of the best things you can do for your health. It has many benefits. It can improve your overall health and fitness and reduce your risk for many chronic diseases. To get the most benefit, here's how much physical activity you should get:

For adults: Get at least 150 minutes of moderate-intensity or 75 minutes of vigorous-intensity aerobic physical activity each week. Or you could do a combination of the two.

❖ Try to spread your physical activity out over several days of the week. That's better than trying to do it all in one or two days.

❖ Some days, you may not have long blocks of time to do physical activity. You can try splitting it up into segments of ten minutes or more.

❖ Aerobic activities include walking fast, jogging, swimming, and biking.

❖ Moderate intensity means that, while you are doing that activity, your breath is such that you can only say a sentence while doing the activity.

❖ Vigorous intensity means that, while you are doing that activity, you won't be able to say more than a few words without stopping for a breath.

Also, adults should do strengthening activities twice per week.

❖ Strengthening activities include lifting weights, working with exercise bands, and doing sit-ups and push-ups.

❖ Choose activities that work all the different parts of the body—your legs, hips, back, chest, stomach, shoulders, and arms. You should repeat exercises for each muscle group eight to twelve times per session.

For preschool-aged children (ages 3–5): Preschool children should be physically active throughout the day to help with their growth and development. They should get both structured and unstructured active play. Structured play has a goal and is directed by an adult. Examples include playing a sport or a game. Unstructured play is creative free play, such as playing on a playground.

For children and teens (ages 6–19): Get sixty minutes or more of physical activity every day. Most of it should be moderate-intensity aerobic activity.

- ❖ Activities should vary and be a good fit for the child's age and physical development.
- ❖ Moderate-intensity aerobic activities include walking, running, skipping, playing on the playground, playing basketball or soccer, and biking.

Also, children and teens (ages 6–19) should try to get each of these at least three days a week: vigorous-intensity aerobic activity, muscle-strengthening activity, and bone-strengthening activity.

- ❖ Vigorous-intensity aerobic activities include running, doing jumping jacks, and fast swimming.
- ❖ Muscle-strengthening activities include playing on playground equipment, playing tug-of-war, and doing push-ups and pull-ups.
- ❖ Bone-strengthening activities include hopping, skipping, doing jumping jacks, playing volleyball, and working with resistance bands.

For older adults, pregnant women, and people with chronic health problems: Older adults, pregnant women, and people who have special health needs should check with their healthcare provider on how much physical activity they should get and what types of activities they should do.

Exercise tips: People who are trying to lose weight may need to get more physical activity. They also need to adjust their diet, so they are burning more calories than they eat and drink.

FITT and the Overload Principle

The *overload principle* is based on the idea that when muscles are exercised at a level above that at which they normally operate, they adapt so that they function more efficiently. Overload can be accomplished in several ways: by increasing the *frequency* of your exercise (how often you exercise), by increasing the *intensity* of your exercise (how hard you exercise), or by increasing the *duration* of your exercise (how long you exercise). Frequency, intensity, and time spent depend on the *type* of exercise involved—whether it is cardiorespiratory or resistance exercise. This is referred to as the *FITT principle*.

Your individual FITT prescription depends on your goal. For example, if your goal is to run a 5K race, your FITT prescription must focus primarily on your aerobic capacity, which involves cardiorespiratory activity. If, on the other hand, you want to be a better golfer, you will adjust your FITT prescription for muscle strength and endurance exercises that attack those muscles you most need to play golf—resistance exercises that focus on the core, the back, and the arms. Snow skiing requires doing exercises that mainly focus on leg muscles. Of course, the core and other muscle groups should not be neglected.

Exercising in Every Type of Weather

Cold weather, precipitation, very hot and humid weather, and darkness can pose unique problems for exercising safely outdoors. Rather than giving up, you can take the following precautions to promote safe exercise under adverse conditions.

On cold days:

❖ Wear several layers of clothing rather than one heavy layer. The inner layer should be a material that wicks away moisture, such as polypropylene or wool. Do not wear cotton next to your skin because it loses its ability to insulate when it gets wet as you perspire. Some of these materials absorb body odors readily and should be washed frequently.

❖ Avoid using cotton socks for the same reason given above; choose wool socks or socks that help moisture evaporate.

❖ Use mittens, gloves, or socks to protect your hands.

❖ Wear a hat and scarf. Up to 40 percent of your body's heat is lost through your neck and head.

On rainy, icy, or snowy days:

❖ Be aware of reduced visibility for both yourself and drivers. Be careful around cars and traffic. Wear bright clothing or apply reflective tape to your workout clothes. Consider wearing ski glasses or goggles that enhance your ability to see contrasts, especially in snow.

❖ Be aware of reduced traction on sidewalks and roads. You could slip and fall, or a car may not be able to stop quickly.

❖ Consider investing in exercise clothing made of special material that repels water but allows moisture produced by the body to escape (see the *on cold days* list above for more information on wicking fabrics).

On hot, humid days:

❖ Exercise during the cooler hours of the day, such as early morning or early evening after the sun has gone down.

❖ Drink lots of cold water. Hydrate with water before you start to exercise. Avoid using electrolyte-replacement drinks (they slow down the absorption of fluids from the stomach) unless you drink lots of water too.

❖ Wear minimal light, loose-fitting clothing so sweat can evaporate easily.

❖ If you are exercising when the sun is out, wear sunblock and a hat to prevent overexposure to the sun.

❖ Avoid clothing that makes you sweat, such as sweatpants.

❖ Watch out for signs of heat stroke—dizziness, weakness, lightheadedness, or excessive fatigue.

At night or on dark days:

❖ Wear bright, reflective clothing, preferably with special reflective tape or markings.

❖ Carry a flashlight or wear a headlamp.

Coping with Discomfort

Some discomfort is natural when you first begin to exercise, but the maxim "no pain, no gain" is outdated. The overload principle of fitness states that a greater than normal stress or load on the body is required for training adaptation to take place. What this means is that to improve fitness, strength, and endurance, you need to increase the workload accordingly. This does not mean pushing muscles to the point of experiencing pain, however. Pain is the body's signal to stop, and it should always be heeded.

When you first start an exercise program, you may find that you are easily fatigued, and sometimes after the session you may feel muscle stiffness and soreness; adequate warm-up, cool-down, and stretching should reduce the risk and intensity of the discomfort. By starting exercise moderately and gradually increasing frequency, intensity, and duration, discomfort will be minimized, especially if you take time to stretch before and after your workout.

At the beginning of an exercise session, you may sometimes find your body is slow to get moving. You must push through that feeling: tell yourself how important it is to exercise and that it will be over before you realize it. Usually positive self-talk will help overcome inertia. Working out with a personal trainer (or a friend) can help you stay motivated. Realize that even highly trained athletes have days when their bodies don't want to cooperate. Your attitude is important at this point—you don't have to want to exercise or enjoy it, you just have to do it. Accepting a bit of discomfort and overcoming resistance are the dues you pay for better health.

Occasionally, you may experience a little pain during exercise. A cramp or "stitch" in your side while running or doing aerobic exercise just means you need to stop and stretch. To manage a stitch, simply slow down and focus on deep breathing and relaxing until it goes away. This is different than pain that comes from an injury. You need to learn the difference between tolerating the natural discomfort that can come from exercising and pain that warns you to stop all together.

Coping with Injury

Injury is a risk during exercise, but it need not signal the end of your exercise efforts. Injury usually occurs because of lack of flexibility, muscle imbalance, or simple overexertion. Flexibility injuries— muscle pulls, ankle sprains, Achilles tendinitis, and shin splints— account for 90 percent of exercise-related injuries. You can usually prevent such injuries by warming up properly. Injury, in general, can be prevented by taking care to work opposing muscle groups, varying your exercise routine, and not attempting too much too soon.

If you do experience an injury, apply the *RICE principle*—rest, ice, compression, and elevation. Immediately apply ice to the injured area, avoiding direct contact of ice to skin by using a towel or other material as a barrier. Cold causes damaged blood vessels to constrict, which limits swelling. Continue to apply ice for twenty-minute periods, followed by twenty-minute rest periods without ice. Do this a minimum of three to four times a day for two or three days after

Table 10.5 Warning Signs to Stop Exercising

❖ Pain in the chest, shoulders, arms, or abdomen

❖ Irregular heartbeat

❖ Sudden, very fast heart rate

❖ Shortness of breath when you aren't exercising very hard

❖ Unexplained dizziness

❖ Fainting

❖ Nausea

❖ Leg cramps

❖ Lack of coordination, confusion, or visual disturbances

❖ Pale, blue, or clammy complexion

sustaining the injury. Take it easy for a while and rest while your injury is healing. See table 10.5 for warning signs to stop exercising.

Walking for Health and Weight Loss

A great way to begin an exercise regime is to walk. Walking can be fun as well as health enhancing. Although walking is not an exercise that necessarily elevates the heart rate, it still provides many benefits, including calorie burn. Because hiking takes place on trails and involves walking up and down hills and on uneven ground, it can burn quite a few calories (more so than a neighborhood walk or using a treadmill), especially if your hike lasts several hours.

Starting from Zero

Some obese people have trouble walking at all. If that is your case, start by walking a block, or as far as you can. Keep this up and gradually increase the number of blocks you can walk. Try several short walking sessions of ten minutes each (or whatever you can do) if you have been sedentary and walking is difficult. You may have to do this for several weeks until you build up your stamina. (It's possible that you'll have to cut back on calories to lose some weight before you can walk very far.)

As your ability to walk increases, start walking around the neighborhood or on a high school track. Work on extending your time until you can walk at least twenty minutes at a time three days a week on a regular basis. Then begin to add days and extend your time so you are exercising thirty to sixty minutes a day most days of the week. As you become better conditioned, your goal is to complete sixty minutes of walking most days of the week.

If you have access to a treadmill or stationary bike, you might want to start with ten to twenty minutes of walking or pedaling at a comfortable pace. Learn to use your target heart rate or the perceived exertion method as discussed earlier in this chapter to assess the intensity of your exercise. On the treadmill, you can vary the intensity by varying the angle of the machine and increasing the speed. The more intense your pace and the longer you walk, the more calories you will burn. Consider progressing from walking or using the treadmill to hiking, which is more vigorous. As you improve your walking, you will be able to engage in a regular exercise program at a gym or at home.

Runners and walkers can easily measure pace and distance using the app iTreadmill, which uses a motion detector on an iPhone or iPod. The device also turns into a pedometer that counts the number of steps you take. "Start," "stop," and "pause" buttons trigger iTreadmill to start measuring your run or walk, tracking your pace, distance, or steps. You can even enter your weight to have it estimate the number of calories you've burned. Before starting, tap the "cal" button on the top right to calibrate your stride. Then set your pace using the dial at the top right. When you turn on the pacer, the app makes a ticking rhythmic sound to keep pace with your footfalls.

Another approach to exercise for people who find walking too difficult is to join a water aerobics class. The water supports you, while an instructor provides the class with exercise instructions. Buoyant "dumbbells" and plastic tubes are often used for different exercises.

Walking as an Exercise

Walking is a popular and easy way to become physically active, and pedometers or step counters like the FitBit are useful ways to track progress. Popular advice, such as walking 10,000 steps a day, is one way people may choose to meet the physical activity guidelines given in the *2015–2020 Dietary Guidelines*. It's helpful to use a pedometer to help meet the key guidelines by setting a time goal (minutes of walking a day) and then calculating how many steps are needed each day to reach that goal. Or, check the internet for apps that help with walking measurements, including the Health app for the iPhone or Google Fit for Android devices.

Moderate- or vigorous-intensity physical activity, such as brisk walking, counts toward meeting the key guidelines. You need to plan episodes of walking if you want to use step goals to progress toward meeting key physical fitness guidelines. Time spent walking is more important than trying to achieve 10,000 steps a day (although this would be a good long-term goal). As a basis for setting step goals, it is preferable to know how many steps you take per minute of a brisk walk. A person with a lower fitness level, who takes fewer steps per minute than a fit adult, will need fewer steps to achieve the same time of walking. One way to set a step goal is:

1. To determine your usual daily steps, use a pedometer or fitness tracker to count the number of steps taken on several ordinary days with no episodes of walking for exercise. Suppose the average is about 5,000 steps a day. (Most of those steps are light-intensity activity.)

2. With the pedometer or fitness tracker, you should measure the number of steps taken during a ten-minute walk. Suppose this is 1,000 steps. For a goal of twenty minutes of walking, the goal would total 2,000 steps (1,000 times 2).

3. To calculate a daily step goal, add the usual daily steps (5,000) to the steps required for a twenty-minute walk (2,000) to get the goal of total steps per day (5,000 + 2,000 = 7,000).

Then, each week, you should gradually increase the goal of the number of total steps a day until the next higher goal is reached. Rate of progression should be individualized to your walking. Some people who start out at 5,000 steps a day can add 500 steps per day each week. Others who are less fit and are starting out at a lower number of steps should add a smaller number of steps each week until they reach their long-term goal.

Keeping Track of Your Progress

You can make a fun and rewarding game out of tracking your progress as you increase your daily mileage or number of steps. Let's use the example of a pedometer (you can buy an inexpensive one at a sporting goods store or, if you prefer, invest a small fee for a smartphone app, or use a Fitbit as discussed earlier). Set the pedometer for your stride. Be sure the pedometer stride is set correctly and that it is measuring distances accurately by wearing it for a set measured distance. Then simply wear it daily and record your progress. Always wear the pedometer correctly; usually they are designed to be worn on your hip over the side seam. (It is a good idea to pin it to your clothes to prevent losing it.)

After your pedometer has been adjusted for your stride and you are sure it is measuring reasonably accurately, determine your *baseline*—that is, the distance (miles or steps) you normally walk in a day. The best way to do this is to wear the pedometer over the course of a week or over several *representative* days (days in which you do not walk much more or less than normal.) Each day during the baseline period, wear your pedometer and record the distance displayed at the end of the day. Using graph paper such as that shown in the sample graph in table 10.6a (or use the blank graph provided in table 10.6b), determine how much each block or square represents. For example, if your pedometer or Fitbit measures number of steps, you might decide that each square represents some number of steps. If your pedometer measures mileage, you might set each block to a quarter mile or if digital, .2 miles (as shown on the sample graph).

Divide the graph into seven-day blocks to represent each week. Note that on the graph shown, quarter miles walked is on the left-hand scale and on the right-hand scale digital miles are shown. Then total up your miles or steps for each week (all seven days). You can even take an average of those seven days by dividing the total by seven at the end of the week. Your goal is to increase either your total miles per day, per week, or your average mileage or steps over the course of time.

Each week, set a goal for the following week that is a little above your average, or total miles or steps, for the current week. Strive to increase your walking each week. Be reasonable in setting your goals. Don't overestimate how much you can increase your walking in one week. Remember, the idea is to increase your walking gradually at a pace that will allow you to sustain progress.

Selecting a Gym or Health Club

Fitness facilities vary considerably in the equipment they have available, the programs and services they offer, the atmosphere and experiences they provide, and cost for use or membership. Some facilities are minimalists, providing nothing more than the basics, while others are more "high-end" establishments that cater to a clientele that can afford to pay for amenities such as childcare or a juice bar. Increasingly, workplaces are providing workout facilities for employees.

Some facilities define themselves as "serious" gyms and cater primarily to bodybuilders, while others are intended to provide social interaction as well as workout opportunities. Other facilities with gyms, such as YMCAs, are family oriented. Still others provide access only with a personal trainer to guide you. Some gyms have a pool or sauna, while others offer on-site massage or nutrition counseling. Fees are typically commensurate with the extent of offerings.

In choosing a gym or fitness facility, consider your needs and preferences. Consider the ease or difficulty in commuting to the facility from your home or workplace. Having to travel more than

Table 10.6a Sample Graph for Tracking Walking Mileage

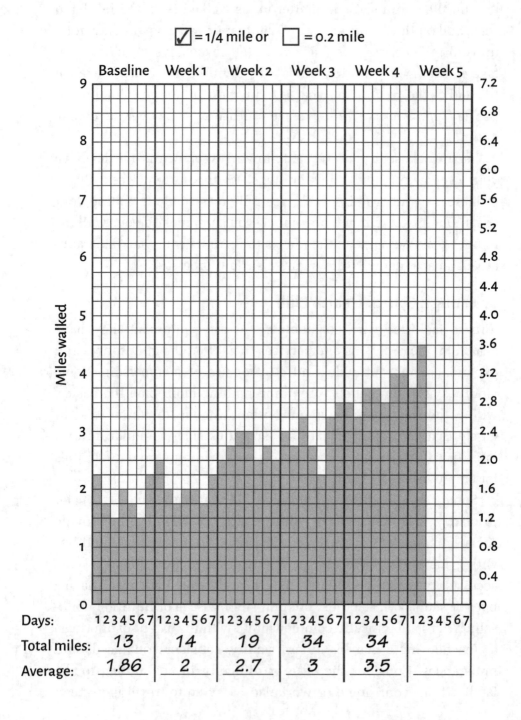

☑ = 1/4 mile or ☐ = 0.2 mile

Miles walked

	Baseline	Week 1	Week 2	Week 3	Week 4	Week 5
Days:	1234567	1234567	1234567	1234567	1234567	1234567
Total miles:	13	14	19	34	34	
Average:	1.86	2	2.7	3	3.5	

Table 10.6b Graph for Tracking Walking Mileage

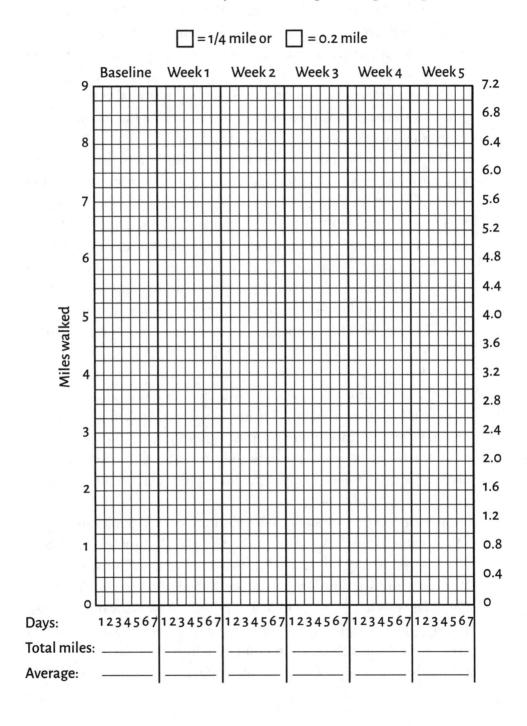

☐ = 1/4 mile or   ☐ = 0.2 mile

twenty minutes is likely to decrease your motivation to go to the facility. To decide on a gym, locate the fitness facilities nearest to you and arrange for a tour of each—preferably a tour that includes a trial workout or gives you a free pass for a later trial workout. Ask about hours, hours of most use, refund policy, vacation closings, and fees, and whether the gym employs certified personal trainers. Also ask about classes and programs available for beginners, or special programs such as spinning classes or kickboxing.

Notice the type of equipment and its condition. Is there a variety of equipment as well as duplicates of popular equipment such as treadmills and StairMasters? Are there time limits on the machines? How many "Out of Order" signs do you see? Do seats and padding of machines have tears or worn places? Is the free weights area littered or tidy, cramped or roomy? Check out the floor space. Avoid gyms where machines are jammed together taking up most of the floor space, leaving little room for floor exercises. Do you notice any personnel whose job it is to keep the place clean? Does the pool water seem clear and appropriately maintained? Is the club well lit and is the temperature set at a comfortable level for exercise? Are the locker rooms clean and spacious? Are there telltale signs of overuse or poor maintenance, such as burned out lights, broken lockers, torn or soiled carpets, dirty floors, or peeling paint?

Ask patrons or members how they feel about the facilities and about their experience using different aspects of the club. See table 10.7 for suggested questions to ask them.

Be sure to notice the image the club projects. What kinds of people use the facility? All sizes and ages? Mostly buff athletes? Singles who seem more interested in one another than in working out? Women who wear makeup, jewelry, and the latest workout fashions? Consider whether you would feel comfortable working out in a particular gym. Remember that fitness training is not just about building muscle; the focus needs to be on functionality as well as preservation, or building of, lean body mass, and, when appropriate, corrective

Table 10.7 Questions to Ask Current Members About a Facility

❖ Are the showers temperature controlled, or does the water temperature fluctuate when others are taking a shower or flushing the toilet?

❖ Do members think there are enough lockers and other personal amenities like towels?

❖ Is working with the trainers a positive experience?

❖ Is it easy to get an appointment with a trainer?

❖ When is the club most crowded?

❖ What is the longest wait to use a piece of equipment?

❖ Are other patrons friendly?

❖ Is there adequate parking, especially at peak hours?

❖ Is the club's vacation schedule convenient? Is it open when you want to work out?

❖ Is there a policy for excused absences?

❖ What is the membership cancellation policy?

exercise. Ask yourself, is this gym a place where you could accomplish your personal goals?

When you settle on a gym or club, read the contract carefully, if one is required. You should have the right to cancel membership within a few days of first signing. Find out what your rights are for terminating membership if you move or are permanently disabled. What is the refund policy? Can you extend your contract to make up time if you become sick and cannot work out for an extended period? Make inquiries about the financial health of the club and avoid facilities that may be experiencing economic difficulties, especially if there is an upfront membership fee. Remember that fees may not be refunded if the club or gym ceases operations.

Working with a Personal Trainer

Personal fitness trainers work one-on-one with clients, usually by appointment. Clients may exercise at the trainer's studio, or they may work out with the trainer in a gym or health club. Some trainers will come to your home and bring their own equipment, usually handheld free weights.

Some trainers offer nutrition analysis in addition to exercise training. Care should be taken to make sure a trainer who offers such advice and services is qualified to do so—that is, they have had education toward an advanced nutrition certification other than just having read a nutrition book. Some trainers, or others who call themselves nutritionists, attempt to implement nutrition advice given in books written by other unqualified "experts." Others may have simply taken a single course that offers a "certificate" for completion and, subsequently, call themselves nutritionists. In fact, the term *nutritionist* is unregulated and does not imply any special qualifications; anyone can use this label. But you should ask what sort of training and education any person who claims to be a nutritionist has—they should have a degree in a food science field. A sure tip-off to a bogus expert is if they attempt to sell you vitamins or supplements as part of your "nutrition" program.

A good trainer will do an assessment of your flexibility and your current fitness level before you start a program of exercise. The assessment should cover your flexibility, cardiovascular fitness, gait, strength, and your ability to push and pull. Protocols for flexibility assessment are readily available, but the trainer needs to be trained and supervised in the use of these protocols. Similarly, some trainers do body-composition assessments using a tape measure or skin calipers. This requires adequate training to avoid errors that could contribute to serious mismeasurement. A few trainers claim to do body work involving massage or muscle and bone manipulation. Do not hesitate to ask any trainers you are considering where they received training for this and whether they are certified to do such assessments.

Trainer Certification

A variety of organizations provide certification for trainers. These include the American College of Sports Medicine (ACSM), the

National Strength and Conditioning Association (NSCA), and the Aerobics and Fitness Association of America (AFAA), among others. A trainer should have at least a bachelor of science degree in exercise and sport science or kinesiology. Another important level of experience would be work in a rehabilitation facility or as an assistant to a physical therapist. Beware of those who are doing personal training as an avocation (a hobby), in addition to another job, or whose only qualifications are that they now play, or did play, various sports. Not all health and fitness clubs require certification or prior relevant experience. Once you obtain names and contact information, take time to interview and assess each person before making your selection.

Choosing a Personal Trainer

Ask a prospective personal trainer questions about motivation, education and training, certification, and fees. This will help you get to know the person better and help you decide whether you want to work with them. Table 10.8 provides questions you might ask.

Warning Signs When Selecting or Working with a Trainer

Heed the warning signs that indicate trainers who may not be a good choice for you. If the trainer promotes or sells supplements, protein drinks, or nutritional products as part of their fitness recommendations, understand that they may have an agenda that could conflict with your needs. Beware of a trainer who wants to sell you multiple advance sessions that are nonrefundable. Don't work with a trainer who is, or has been, a professional or semiprofessional athlete unless they have other credentials as well. Just because a person once played sports in high school or college is not enough to qualify them to be a personal trainer. Avoid clubs that don't require certification for their trainers. Most especially, don't work with a trainer who seems distracted while working with you or fails to explain the reason for doing particular exercises. Trainers should be able to describe which muscle groups are involved in an exercise and why you are doing that exercise. Personality is important too; you will be

Table 10.8 **Questions to Ask a Potential Trainer**

❖ Why are you a personal trainer? Is this your profession or is it a second job or a hobby?

❖ What is your education on health and fitness assessment and instruction? Have you worked in a rehabilitation facility or as an assistant to a physical therapist?

❖ By what organization and at what level are you certified to be a personal trainer?

❖ Does the gym or health club you work in require certification for trainers? What kind?

❖ How many years of experience as a personal trainer do you have?

❖ Are you trained in CPR and first aid?

❖ What are your fees?

❖ How long is each session?

❖ How many sessions must I commit to initially?

❖ What is your cancellation and refund policy? What commitment am I expected to make?

working closely with this person. Make sure you get along with your trainer and feel safe and comfortable asking questions. See table 10.9 for qualities to look for in a personal trainer.

At-Home Exercise

Some people do not frequent a gym for exercise, or they combine working out at a gym with exercise at home. More and more people are choosing to invest in home fitness equipment and turning one room of the house into their workout room. Some people have a personal trainer come to their home. (Others just put on their walking or running shoes and head out the door for their workouts.) A wide variety of home equipment options are available in the marketplace ranging from inexpensive (and often useless) gadgets to expensive multipurpose, multistation machines. Whatever machine you choose, it must provide resistance to be useful. For example, riding

Table 10.9 Qualities to Look For in a Personal Trainer

Look for a personal trainer who exhibits certain behaviors. The trainer should:

- ❖ Spend time at the introductory session getting to know you and your exercise goals.
- ❖ Do an assessment of your current flexibility and fitness status.
- ❖ Demonstrate a sincere interest in you.
- ❖ Be able to design a program to achieve the goals you specify while considering your physical abilities and personal preferences.
- ❖ Introduce you to the gym and locker room and make sure you feel comfortable and relaxed and help you to feel a sense of belonging.
- ❖ Ask for an emergency contact for you.
- ❖ Ask you to provide information on your medical history and possibly provide you with a health-risk appraisal.
- ❖ Be enthusiastic and personable.
- ❖ Support your training efforts with positive feedback while still correcting your form.
- ❖ Counsel you on proper exercise apparel (shoes and clothing) as necessary from a functional (not fashionable) standpoint.
- ❖ Talk to you in terms you can understand.
- ❖ Suggest exercises to do at home in between training sessions.

a stationary type bicycle without resistance provides no fitness benefits. Before buying, consider whether you will really use it.

Home equipment can provide fitness benefits, but these benefits may depend on how easy it is to use the equipment and how familiar you are with the movements required. One study found that, compared to other options, the best choice for burning calories and improving cardiovascular fitness was a treadmill. The other good options in this study included a stationary bicycle, a stair climber, a rowing machine, and a stationary bicycle with push-and-pull levers for one's arms. Least effective in producing fitness benefits is, ironically, the conventional stationary bicycle with the push-and-pull levers included in the study. This is not because these machines are ineffective, but because users liked using them the least.

Walking and running on a treadmill were movement patterns people in the study were already familiar with, whereas rowing equipment required a level of skill not everyone possessed. Even so, more and more people today are using rowing machines because these machines allow for both cardiovascular exercise and muscle strength and endurance development without the impact of a tread-mill.

The reason why treadmills were "better" for some people in this study is that people tend to exercise more vigorously and stick with the exercise longer when they are more familiar with the movement required. Intensity and duration were therefore maximized on the treadmill and users found it more enjoyable than the other options. Treadmills for the home are available in fold-up versions so they don't take up much room.

In choosing home fitness equipment, consider your current level of fitness, your likes and dislikes, your skill level, the space available for such equipment, your budget, and, of course, your motivation to work out on your own. To ease the strain on your wallet, check internet sites such as eBay and Craigslist for used equipment, or shop at a store that specializes in used equipment. Or you can buy exercise resistance bands, which are inexpensive, usually under twenty dollars (available through Amazon and Target). You can also easily pack resistance bands in a suitcase for workouts on the road. Less expensive options like these are useful for those assessing their motivation for working out at home, and for people who don't want to invest in expensive equipment or have limited space.

Some people enjoy doing various workouts in the privacy of their home with the aid of videotapes, DVDs, or streaming content. These sources provide convenient options when the weather is inclement, or you just want a change of pace. Fitness programs can also be viewed through the "on demand" feature of some cable television providers or you can record television fitness shows to play and work out to at a convenient time. The internet and smartphones can also provide programs and apps for exercise and workout routines, many of which are free. When using streaming or video workout content, it's important to take care that you participate at your own fitness level and within your limitations.

Increasing Activities of Daily Living

Whether you exercise outdoors, at a gym, with a trainer, or at home, you can achieve additional calorie expenditure by focusing on burning calories through activities of daily living. These include routine physical activities such as gardening or cleaning the house. Even once you have begun to do regular exercise, increasing activities of daily living will help you burn additional calories. Table 10.10 on the next page lists suggestions for increasing your daily activity outside your regular exercise regime.

Table 10.10 Suggestions for Increasing Activities of Daily Living

- ❖ Take the stairs instead of an elevator or escalator.
- ❖ Walk instead of driving short distances.
- ❖ Park farther away and walk to your destination.
- ❖ Get off public transportation a stop or two early and walk.
- ❖ Ride your bicycle instead of taking the car.
- ❖ Take a walk at lunchtime or on your coffee break.
- ❖ Deliver items yourself rather than sending someone else.
- ❖ Stand and talk on the phone or pace the floor if you have a handheld phone.
- ❖ Pedal a stationary bicycle while watching television.
- ❖ During television commercials, get up and walk around or march in place.
- ❖ Replace cocktail hour with exercise.
- ❖ Get things yourself instead of sending your children.
- ❖ Clean the house more often.
- ❖ Sweep the sidewalk in front of your house—and even in front of your neighbor's house.
- ❖ Rake the leaves, trim the hedges, and do the gardening yourself.
- ❖ Wash the car by hand instead of taking it to the car wash.
- ❖ Mow the grass with a push lawn mower or a power mower you don't ride.
- ❖ Play golf without a golf cart or caddy.
- ❖ When on vacation, take walking tours.
- ❖ At the sports stadium, climb the stairs and walk during intermissions.
- ❖ Go dancing more often.
- ❖ Put a pair of walking shoes in the trunk of your car and look for opportunities to walk.

11

Managing Thinking and Self-Talk

Emily asserted that she "should" be able to manage her weight. After all, she was effective in her job and ran a tight ship at home. "I know what to do. I just don't do it." Instead Emily kept finding excuses: "I'll start on Monday." "I'll have just one." "It's been a stressful day and I deserve a treat." When tempting food was present, she just couldn't say no. Emily was a perfectionist, and when she failed to live up to her own expectations, she saw herself as a failure. It took a while for Emily to recognize that her thinking and self-talk were undermining her weight-management efforts. She realized she had to stop believing her hindering self-talk and stop allowing herself to make unhealthy choices. She needed to take stock of her values and commit herself to leading a healthy lifestyle. Emily changed her thinking and that helped her let go of some of her "fat talk" and she started reaching out to others with positive messages that increasingly helped her be more positive about herself and her efforts to make her life more satisfying.

The act of thinking is something you probably don't give much thought. Yet *thinking* (also called *cognition*) plays a big role in feelings, behavior, and weight management. How you think—what you say to yourself and how you process the information your senses gather—helps you understand the world around you and informs how you act. Cognition consists of representing and transforming information from your senses into knowledge. This can be done by sensing something directly through the five senses, or indirectly by reasoning. Thinking includes the mental process of knowing and aspects of knowing, such as awareness, perception, reasoning, and judgment.

What you say silently to yourself is one type of thinking called *self-talk*. Self-talk is thinking that involves words, sentences, and phrases. You may not be aware that you talk to yourself, but everyone does. Self-talk is that little voice in your head that is chattering most of the time. It is the little voice that just said, "What little voice?"

To succeed in adopting a healthy lifestyle and managing weight, you need to identify and challenge "fat talk." Caitlin Boyle's book entitled *Operation Beautiful* proposes a unique way to build and maintain a positive attitude. The stated mission of the editor and her website and blog of the same name is to shift negative self-talk, or what she calls "fat talk," to more positive thinking by taking certain actions. The idea behind Operation Beautiful is simple: post anonymous positive notes in public places like a public restroom or an elevator for women and young girls to find. The process of creating the uplifting messages helps you and whoever reads the note you post to become aware of how certain thoughts can produce positive feelings and to inspire others to participate in this positive movement. To spread the word, participants are asked to include the website URL (http://www.operationbeautiful.com) in the messages they post. Think how good most people feel coming across a message such as "Smile and someone might smile back." Check out Boyle's book or her website to find daily positive messages and blog with others about life-affirming accomplishments.

Self-Talk

Self-talk can involve mulling over something in your mind—talking silently to yourself to decide what you think about something. For example: "Let's see, the steak is probably pretty high in calories. Maybe the fish would be a better choice." Usually, self-talk is internal and silent, but sometimes you may talk to yourself out loud: "Where are those keys?" When you have a conversation with yourself, you use self-talk. Sometimes your internal conversation can be an argument—as if one part of your mind is trying to persuade another part of your mind to accept an alternative action or idea. For example:

> YOU: "I shouldn't eat that."
>
> INNER VOICE: "Why not? I've been really good in watching what I eat."
>
> YOU: "But if I give in now, I'll hate myself."
>
> INNER VOICE: "Maybe I can have just one."

This is an example of "fat talk." The parts of you that carry on the argument are sometimes called subpersonalities or *voices*. Chapter 12, "Challenging Your 'Inner Voices,'" is devoted to identifying these voices and understanding how they can affect behavior.

At times, you may have an imagined dialogue with another person; perhaps you mentally review a previous, real interaction, or you imagine an encounter you are anticipating. Can you recall a time when you had an argument or sharp words with someone and later kept reviewing it in your mind? You were using self-talk to ruminate about what happened. Another example of using self-talk can occur when you think about what you want to say to another person, and you rehearse it first in your mind.

Often self-talk is internal stream-of-consciousness thinking—the continuous, disconnected flow of thoughts through your mind: "Nice car, wish I had one of those." "I feel fat today." "I wonder if he'll call tonight." "Maybe I should get to the gym." "How long do I have to wait for this light to turn green?" These are examples of mind chatter. Random thoughts seem to come automatically, as if from nowhere. Another example of thinking—one that can get stuck in your mind—is when you hear a jingle or a word, and it keeps running in your head like a track of a CD that keeps repeating. Sometimes unwanted thoughts come unbidden into your head.

Feelings—that is, emotions—are another function of the mind— the amygdala section of the brain, to be specific—and these can be influenced by, or contribute to, self-talk. *Feelings* are products of the mind and are another way of "knowing." They should be thought of as nonverbal signals telling the rational mind to bring its attention to something and decide what to do. Feelings can trigger self-talk, and self-talk can influence feelings.

What Influences Self-Talk?

Self-talk is influenced by several components: information that comes to your *awareness* and that you *focus on*; your *experiences* in life and how you *understand*, or interpret, them; your underlying *beliefs*; and the way in which you *process information*. Although much information comes to your senses, your brain's processing allows only a portion of it to come into your awareness. Once you are aware of something, you may or may not direct your thinking to focus on it. When you focus on something, you use your beliefs and perhaps emotions to try to make sense out of the experience at hand. As a result of how you process the information, you behave in a certain way. And all the while, you are probably talking silently to yourself.

For example, imagine that you go to a party where there is a table heaped with food. Soon after you arrive, you notice the food table. When you approach the table, your mind scans the choices available and focuses in on the desserts. Perhaps you become so focused on them that you don't even pay attention to the other options, even though at some level you "know" they are there. The appearance of the desserts causes you to anticipate the sweet taste. You imagine how good a particular one would taste. Past experience with sweets and an attractive presentation direct your thinking to what you want to eat. At this point, you may abandon conscious thinking altogether and indulge your taste for sweets.

Take another example: Suppose your friend tells you about a new diet that is working for her. You may get excited and think it might work for you too. You might ask for more details and perhaps buy the new diet book she recommends or search the internet for more information. If you try the new diet and you don't lose weight, you could decide nothing you do is going to help you lose weight. Instead of deciding the diet was poorly conceived or that you started the diet without really being ready, you blame yourself. This conclusion could give rise to self-talk such as "I can't do it," and reinforce an already existing thought that losing weight is too hard. Failing sets up the expectation of failure in future efforts to manage your weight, which is reinforced by negative self-talk.

Becoming Aware of Your Self-Talk

It may not be immediately obvious to you that you engage in self-talk until you reflect on or listen in to your thinking. The best way to do this is by keeping a journal and writing down your thoughts. In that way, you can become aware not only that you are talking to yourself, but also what it is you are saying. Keeping a record of your thoughts, together with the situations in which they occur and the emotions that accompany them, is called *self-monitoring*. (You learned about this in chapter 7, "Changing Behavior," where monitoring of cues and reinforcers was discussed.) By writing down your self-talk, you will probably discover that certain themes reoccur. For example, you may find that you criticize yourself harshly or that you have a lot of worry thoughts. Other themes may involve how you think things "should" be or that it's not fair that you struggle with your weight while others seem to be naturally thin.

Sometimes these themes fall into the category of *cognitive distortions*, which are ways of thinking that distort understanding in such a way that you end up feeling bad and perhaps choose behaviors that are not healthy. These interpretation errors may contribute to painful emotions that could impair your emotional well-being. We discuss these sorts of interpretations in more detail later in this chapter. First, let's rethink thinking.

A New Way of Thinking About Thinking

The new way of thinking that ultimately influences behavior is known by the acronym ACT. The letters stand for Accept, Choose, and Take Action:

❖ **A**ccept your reactions to events (thoughts and feelings), while staying mindful (aware) of your here-and-now experience with openness, interest, and receptivity (that is, without judgment).

❖ **C**hoose a valued direction for your life and goals that support your values.

❖ **T**ake committed action in accordance with your values and goals.

ACT is a practical approach to life. The idea is to live life in the present, more focused on important values, and less focused on painful thoughts, feelings, and experiences. ACT is not about stopping pain or fighting emotions—it's about embracing all that life presents. It offers a way out of suffering by encouraging you to choose to live a life based on what matters most to you. Through the processes of acceptance, mindfulness, and values, ACT helps people cope with obstacles in life and experience greater satisfaction. For example, a person diagnosed with multiple sclerosis might want to give up on living. But if he accepts what is—his chronic disease—and chooses to make the best of it, he will focus on making the most of his life. Consider the meaning of each letter.

Accept. The "A" in ACT refers to the idea that we get hooked into the *content* of our thoughts and feelings (that is, our reactions to events—both external and private) and we need to learn to accept those thoughts and feelings rather than react to them. We become *fused* or joined with the content of our thoughts. For example, although thinking "What she said hurt my feelings" may be accurate, you don't have to hold onto the hurt. You can accept that you feel hurt in the moment and then let it pass. We often believe thoughts and feelings represent the "literal truth" that must be acted upon, or are rules that must be obeyed, or are important events that require our full attention, or threatening events that must be gotten rid of. In the example just given, the remark is an event, but you don't have to fuse with it. The ability to *defuse* is the remedy. *Defusing* means to "make less potent" or "make less harmful." Defusing involves being able to step back and observe our thoughts and feelings without being caught up in them. When we can defuse, we can recognize that thoughts and feelings are transient—that is, they come and go. Thoughts are an ever-changing stream of words, sounds, and images. (So, feeling bad because of someone's hurtful remarks will pass if you don't obsess over them and just let them pass without buying into them as a "truth.") As we defuse and distance from our thoughts, they have much less impact and influence. So, in the example just given here, you might say to yourself, "Okay. She said something I don't like. That makes me feel bad, but that's just her opinion. I'm not going to let her get me down." Notice that you are feeling hurt and just let the feeling pass without acting on it.

Take another example: after looking in a mirror, you might think to yourself, "I'm fat." This is a painful thought. As a result, you feel bad. Soon afterward you may get something to eat to feel better. That is, you do something to avoid or escape feeling bad. This is called *experiential avoidance*—trying to escape bad feelings. It may be true that you need to lose weight to be healthier or because you want to feel better about yourself, but when you come face-to-face with your dissatisfaction about your weight, it feels bad. Instead of trying to escape the bad feeling, it is better to accept that you just had a thought about being fat (notice the thought) and this led to painful feelings (your reaction to the thought). Now you need to carry on with life. This would be a good time to redirect your focus on doing something pleasant—like reading a book or going for a walk.

Instead of getting fused with the content of thoughts and feelings that are painful and trying to avoid the experience of pain and upset, it is better to "just notice" the thought or feeling in a mindful way. You need to defuse from the unpleasant thought and see it for what it is—a painful thought, and that's all. If, for example, you are feeling anxiety, just acknowledge that that is what you are feeling at the moment and don't fight it. Remember, the feeling of anxiety will pass given a little time.

Mindfulness is the practice of living in the present moment and experiencing thoughts and feelings, rather than getting lost in them, overwhelmed by them, or trying to control them. Just because you have a painful thought doesn't mean you need to act on it or blot it out. *Acceptance* means observing thoughts and feelings and allowing them to come and go without struggle and without fusing with them.

Let's return to the example of the thought "I'm fat." You may realize you have this thought often, and it hurts. It does hurt but trying to escape the pain of the thought (the hurt emotion) is not the solution. What you need right at this moment is to take care of yourself and not try to feel better by escaping the thought or feeling by eating. Tell yourself "At this moment, I need to go on with some activity. I need to . . . finish the laundry . . . make dinner . . . take a shower," and so forth. "And I need to make healthier choices with food and exercise. If I accept my situation as it is now, which is unsatisfactory to me, and focus on changing my lifestyle, my weight will eventually arrive at a healthier place." In other words, refocus your thinking on what you can do in the immediate future—your food choices or your physical activity.

Acceptance is analogous to the Serenity Prayer, which talks about accepting those things (thoughts or feelings) we cannot change (like a bad experience in the past or a painful current situation), and taking actions toward living a valued life (like making healthier choices or getting exercise). Remind yourself that changing behavior takes time. Acceptance does not mean accepting untenable situations—an abusive relationship, for example. It does not mean accepting obesity as inevitable. In ACT, acceptance relates to unpleasant private experiences—painful thoughts and feelings such as worries and anxiety (which may be prompted by current difficult situations). Acceptance is not about external situations or circumstances for which there is no immediate action available. For example, it is not about having trouble with a micromanager boss; it is about realizing you have *upsetting thoughts and feelings* about having trouble with a micromanager boss. Accept that you are annoyed with the boss and focus on what you need to do at the moment.

Choose. The "C" in ACT refers to making a commitment to higher values and choosing goals that serve those values. Values give meaning to life. As mentioned in an earlier chapter, a *value* is a belief or philosophy that is personally meaningful to you. Though most people don't think a lot about what their values are, every person has a core set of personal values that guide his or her behavior. Values are the overarching principles that give direction to your behavior, and should not be confused with goals, which are things that can be obtained. The person with multiple sclerosis mentioned earlier realized that what he most valued was his relationships with his family.

Take Action. Finally, the "T" in ACT means taking action in accordance with your values and goals. It means doing what matters, even if it is difficult or uncomfortable. To do this, you need to discover what is important to your true self. Consider that you already have many values, some of which are more conscious than others. Perhaps you value dressing nicely to present a professional appearance or for your own satisfaction. You may value your general health, and therefore you do things like brushing and flossing your teeth regularly and visiting the doctor as needed. You may not have given as much attention to having a healthy lifestyle. When you decide what truly matters to you, you'll focus on what you want your life to stand for and what you want out of life. Then you will more easily act in ways that move you forward in life, even if that means bringing cravings and urges to eat along for the ride. Of course, people can differ on exactly what they believe constitutes a healthy lifestyle. You might consider referring to the definition of *optimal fitness* offered in chapter 10, "Exercise and a Healthy Lifestyle," as one possible description of a healthy lifestyle, adding to it the idea of making healthy food choices. The person with multiple sclerosis discussed earlier made it a point to tell family members how much he appreciated them.

The Observing Self

Another important concept in ACT is that of the observing self. There are two parts to the mind: the *thinking self*—the part that is responsible for all your thoughts, self-talk, beliefs, memories, judgments, fantasies, and so on, and the *observing self*—the part of your mind that is able to be aware of what you are thinking, feeling, or doing at any moment without getting caught up in the content. Without your observing self, you couldn't develop mindfulness skills. And the more you practice being mindful, the more you'll become aware of this part of your mind and be able to access it when you need it. The observing self is neutral and doesn't judge; it merely notices.

Let's go back to the thought "I'm fat." The observing self notices that this thought occurred just after you looked in the mirror, and the observing self notices you have mixed feelings of frustration and sadness—that is, you feel bad. The observing self just notices; it doesn't try to make the thought or feelings go away. It is your thinking and experiencing self that wants the feelings to go away. Adopting the perspective of the observing self is a good idea. When you can stay in that neutral place and are mindful—open to whatever is happening in the present moment—you are less likely to get caught up in

> **Mindfulness**
> *Mindfulness* is a mental state achieved by focusing on the present moment, while calmly acknowledging and accepting your feelings, thoughts, and bodily sensations without judgment.

painful emotional turmoil. It is a good idea, then, to be an observer of your own thoughts and feelings, not to escape them, but to accept them and ride them out. So, for the person who thinks, "I'm fat," their observing self notices the thought and accepts that it is painful. Then, if they use the ACT approach, they remember they are trying hard to make healthy choices and resolve to go for a twenty-minute walk later today.

Common Cognitive Distortions

We tend to believe that our thinking is always correct—that is, that it doesn't mislead us in most cases (except when we get the wrong information). In fact, the mind can be a trickster. We can't always trust what we think. In *obsessive-compulsive disorder*, or OCD, for instance, the mind tricks the person with the disorder into believing certain repetitive and intrusive thoughts, and the person acts on them as if they were objective truths. The mind tricks the person with OCD into feeling fearful.

Likewise, the mind can develop bad habits—ways of interpreting or understanding the information from your senses that are misleading. For example, one woman believed other people were critical of her. She expected to be criticized and, as a result, she often felt bad, even when no one meant to hurt her.

The mind also erroneously attributes causes to things that occur close together in time. So, for example, if you got sick after going to a restaurant, you are likely to think it was something you ate. (That may or may not be true.) We tend to think that when one event occurs close to another event, one caused the other. The mind can make mistakes, so it is a good idea to step back and notice your thoughts with a bit of skepticism.

Researchers and clinicians have explored how the interpretive errors we call *cognitive distortions* affect weight management and living a healthy lifestyle. People are generally not aware of making these errors; cognitive distortions are unconscious, bad habits that most people would reject if they were conscious of them. When you make these errors, you are processing the evidence from your senses in a distorted or biased way. As a result, you come to conclusions that make it harder to act in your own best interest or to feel okay about yourself. Learning to recognize these errors in thinking can help you avoid them.

Dr. David Burns identified common cognitive distortions in his book *The Feeling Good Handbook*. Some cognitive distortions include all-or-nothing thinking, catastrophizing, overgeneralization, jumping to conclusions, mind reading, fortune-telling, filtering and disqualifying the positive, emotional reasoning, "should" thinking, taking things personally, and labeling. These are described in table 11.1, and the material that follows goes into more detail about each type of cognitive distortion.

All-or-Nothing Thinking

All-or-nothing thinking is polarized thinking—seeing things in stark contrasts like good or bad, black or white, right or wrong, perfection or failure. There is little to no room for grays or a middle ground. Examples of all-or-nothing thinking would include: "I ate something 'bad.' The whole day is ruined so I may as well keep eating." To avoid making the error of all-or-nothing thinking, you need to recognize this error and challenge it with a more helpful thought. This is a good time to use the ACT method: "Okay, I wish I hadn't eaten that. Now I need to refocus and make the best of the rest of the day."

Catastrophizing

Catastrophizing involves thinking that if a future, negative outcome does occur, it will be terrible and awful, overwhelming, unmanageable, or intolerable. It involves both overestimating the threat and underestimating your ability to cope. Catastrophizing is your mind's way of trying to control the future. To avoid catastrophizing, practice staying in the moment—focus on whatever is at hand now.

Table 11.1 **Overview of Cognitive Distortions**

❖ **All-or-nothing thinking** involves seeing things in only two completely opposing categories: black and white, right or wrong, perfection or failure. An example of such dichotomous thinking might be, "If I have just one cookie, it is terrible and awful, and I am a failure." Or, "If I make one unhealthy choice, then I have blown it and I can't change."

❖ **Catastrophizing** involves focusing on potential problems in the future. Worry thoughts that assume the worst will happen and usually start with the words, "What if": "What if I gain all the weight back and then some?" "What if I can't do it?"

❖ **Overgeneralization** involves using a single piece of evidence from an isolated experience or a series of negative events as proof that a never-ending pattern of defeat exists. For example, "She criticizes my work so she must hate me."

❖ **Jumping to conclusions** involves making an interpretation based on minimal facts or misinterpretation of the evidence. One woman decided that she could not make behavior changes because she had too much to do during a day.

❖ **Mind reading** involves thinking you know what someone else is thinking without checking with the person. "I know my husband is bothered by my weight even though he doesn't say anything."

❖ **Fortune-telling** involves anticipating that things will turn out badly and feeling convinced that a prediction is an already-established fact. "I know I won't enjoy the party."

❖ **Filtering** involves picking out a single detail and dwelling on to the exclusion of all else such that your vision of reality is distorted. "I'm upset that I only lost a pound this week. Obviously, I'm not succeeding."

❖ **Disqualifying the positive** involves rejecting positive experiences by insisting they don't count for some reason outside your control. "It was just luck that I lost two pounds this week. I really didn't do anything to deserve it."

❖ **Emotional reasoning** involves judging yourself or your circumstances based on your emotions. For example, one woman used emotional reasoning to conclude that she was worthless, and that way of thinking led her to an eating binge.

continues ▶

Table 11.1 Overview of Cognitive Distortions (*continued*)

❖ **"Should" and "shouldn't" thinking** involves relying on your own (perhaps) irrational internal rules about how things "should" be to pass judgment; not being willing to accept a situation as it is. "I shouldn't have to set limits on my eating. Other people don't." Sometimes people use "should" thinking as a whip to motivate themselves with guilt. "I should be able to resist sweets." When the judgment is directed at others, "should" thinking often results in frustration or anger and resentment. "You should listen to me." "You should not feel that way."

❖ **Taking things personally** involves blaming yourself or someone else for a situation that, in reality, involved many factors and was out of your control. "They are whispering. They must be talking about me because I'm so overweight."

❖ **Labeling** involves describing a person or situation in a narrow, derogatory, or negative way. Labeling is simplistic and judgmental and prevents further analysis. It is dismissive and suggests that little can be done or nothing more needs to be understood. "She's an idiot." "He's a workaholic." "That driver is a jerk."

Overestimating the Threat. When you catastrophize, you tend to *overestimate the threat* or the negative consequences of events that haven't even happened yet. Often catastrophic thoughts can be identified by the stem question: "What if . . . ?" "What if I gain weight?" "What if I can't stop thinking about the ice cream in the freezer?" "What if I can't resist?" "What if I make a mistake?" "What if they think I'm stupid?" Often the threat is imaginary or minimal at most, but it feels real and huge. Sometimes the threat is actual and serious. Usually, it is something beyond your immediate control. If you can't do anything about it now, there is no point in worrying. If there is something you can do immediately to influence the situation, then take action. For example, instead of worrying about losing weight, pay attention to making healthy choices and getting regular exercise. Your weight is the long-term result of immediate choices, so focus on what you can do now. (*Hint*: If you can't take action right away, put it on a to-do list and let the list do the worrying.)

Underestimating Coping Ability. Another part of catastrophizing is the tendency to *underestimate your ability to cope*. In this case, you worry that you won't be able to handle a future problem or cope with the expected consequences of an anticipated threat. The overestimation of threat coupled with an underestimation of your ability to cope usually results in emotional overload and an attempt to retreat from the problem—often by eating to avoid thinking about it or to squelch feelings of anxiety or other emotions that the threat causes. Examples of this thinking include: "If I don't lose weight this time . . . then I couldn't stand what people would think," or ". . . then I'd be too ashamed to even try again," or ". . . that would mean I really can't ever control my eating." The problem is that the worry thought you are trying to forget keeps coming back again and again. So, the best thing to do is just let the thought be there, acknowledge it and the unpleasant emotions that accompany it, and focus instead on the here and now and whatever you need to do at this moment, like making the bed or taking the dog for a walk. Don't try to make the thought go away; accept it for what it is—just a worry thought—and recognize you don't need to do anything but let it be.

The more you deem a threat to be catastrophic, the less likely you are to feel you can cope. In most cases, you are more capable than you give yourself credit for. In fact, people almost always do cope. In the worst situations—tsunamis, hurricanes, bankruptcy, deaths in the family, divorces—people find a way to cope and survive. You might think you should think ahead, "If such-and-such happens, how will I cope?" Too often you think about what you would need to do, trying on different potential solutions over and over again. Don't do this. You are trying to control the future and your anxiety with misdirected planning. Such thinking leads nowhere except to more anxiety. Instead, acknowledge to yourself that whatever the imagined catastrophe, you will handle it at the time. In the meantime, figure out what you need to do at this moment to live your life.

Overgeneralization

When someone *overgeneralizes*, they decide after a single event or series of events that what has happened will be a never-ending pattern. The use of the words *always* and *never* in your thoughts or speech are clues that you are overgeneralizing. Because you have not succeeded in losing weight in the past, if you overgeneralize, you might decide you can never control your weight. To avoid making this interpretive error, check all the possibilities before making an informed decision. Separate facts from feelings. Try to be even-handed in evaluating the facts and take into consideration evidence for and against the conclusion you came to: perhaps you haven't lost weight in the past because you kept trying fad diets that didn't work, so you resumed bad eating habits. Before you decide it is impossible for you to maintain regular exercise because one time you joined a gym and only went once, consider that there are other ways you might successfully make exercise a regular part of your lifestyle.

Jumping to Conclusions

When you *jump to a conclusion*, you decide what something means by relying only on an intuition or a suspicion with no concrete evidence to support your conclusion. Or you believe unreliable sources. You may make unwarranted connections between ideas or events that are unrelated or are related in a much different way than you assume. Take the following examples: "My trainer didn't comment on my weight loss, so he doesn't really care." "It must be true. I read it on the internet." Check out the facts and keep an open mind about the situation until you have more evidence to support a conclusion.

Mind Reading

Like jumping to conclusions, mind reading also involves making assumptions. In the case of mind reading, the assumptions are about another person's thoughts or feelings. *Mind reading* is assuming you know what is in someone else's mind without checking it out, and then acting as if what you think is true and proven. For instance, if you're eating alone in a cafeteria, you may assume everyone thinks you are a loser and that you have no friends. Or, if you get to work a few minutes late, you may think everyone is thinking about your tardiness. If you engage in enough distorted mind reading, you will feel pretty miserable after a while.

To avoid mind reading, stop and check yourself when you believe you know what someone is thinking or what their behavior means. What is the evidence for your assumption? What have you done to check out your conclusions? For example, when your spouse doesn't say anything about your ordering dessert, don't assume they're thinking you should have skipped dessert. Ask them what they think. Do they, in fact, care about what you eat?

Fortune-Telling

Fortune-telling involves predicting the future, usually with little or no evidence to support the prediction. You engage in fortune-telling when you predict a negative outcome without realistically considering the actual odds of it happening. Deciding ahead of time that you won't enjoy a party virtually assures that you won't. It becomes a self-fulfilling prophecy. It is better to be open to possibilities and consider how your behavior influences your feelings about an outcome. Having a bad time at the party isn't a foregone conclusion unless you decide it will be so. Likewise, predicting you won't be successful in losing weight increases the chances that you won't.

Those who fail at losing weight or keeping it off are vulnerable to fortune-telling because of their past experiences. However, weight management is possible for everyone when they make permanent changes in their food choices and exercise. The National Weight Control Registry (NWCR), established in 1994, has conducted the largest investigation of long-term successful weight loss from then to the present. They have tracked and examined weight-loss strategies of thousands of people. They report that, while there is a wide variety of ways that people lose weight, most succeed in keeping it off by maintaining a low-calorie, low-fat way of eating with high levels of activity.

Maintain hope that the future brings new possibilities and be open to them. Rely on real evidence and facts to anticipate what the future will bring. In the meantime, bring your focus to the here and now, and be open and receptive to your experience without judgment. Remember that if you eat less and exercise more, you will be closer to achieving your healthy lifestyle goals.

Filtering and Disqualifying the Positive

Filtering is a thinking error that involves paying selective attention to information. When thinking through a mental filter, you might focus only on the negative aspects of a situation and filter out all the positive ones. With filtering, you notice only those things that conform to your current beliefs and ignore information that disputes them.

Filtering causes you to miss information you need to more effectively cope and control your behavior. For example, you may notice all your faults—what you did wrong and how you failed—while at the same time filtering out all your good points—what you did right and the successes you have had. Filtering, disqualifying the positive, or discounting success causes you to neglect important information by deciding that anything positive that happened was due to luck or external circumstances. For example, if you lost 2 pounds despite having had an eating indiscretion you might decide, "Oh, the weight loss doesn't really count because I messed up on eating this week."

Many dieters make filtering and discounting interpretation errors. You may be able to recite examples of how you failed and reasons why you don't have what it takes to succeed with weight management, while not paying attention to the many times you made healthy food choices, managed your behavior well, or achieved other small successes. For some reason, when it comes to your eating behavior, giving credit where credit is due just doesn't happen.

To overcome the error of filtering, become aware of bias in your thinking. Stop blocking out important information and start paying attention to evidence of success as well as of shortcomings. By filtering and discounting, you are minimizing your accomplishments and sabotaging your chances of making lifestyle changes.

You also need to understand that weight loss is not linear; it takes a longer time than expected for changes to show up. Don't lose sight of the fact that what counts are not small slips but the overall trend of behavior change. As healthier choices are made more frequently and exercise is increased gradually, adjustments in weight will follow. Weight change follows long-term behavior, not short-term deviations. This is why the focus needs to be on behavior change and not pounds lost. Some people make small changes in their diet and expect instant, big weight loss, but slower, gradual changes bring your weight to the level that is right for your body.

Emotional Reasoning

Emotions are important sources of information. They are usually the first alert system that tells you to bring conscious awareness to bear on something and take necessary action. Emotions, however, are best used in conjunction with rational thinking. When action is the result of all or mainly emotional stimulation, trouble can result. People who use *emotional reasoning* decide things about themselves or situations based exclusively on a feeling, not facts. For example: "I feel sad (*conclusion*: so I must not measure up)." "I feel guilty (*conclusion*: so I must be bad)." These conclusions are based on nothing more than feelings and subsequent thoughts. Sometimes feelings present themselves and we reason backward to explain them, as in the examples just given. Remember that feelings are not facts. Feelings serve an alerting function and are only one tool you have for understanding the world.

"Should" Thinking

When you want things to be different from the way they are, you are engaged in *"should" thinking*. In this thinking, you believe that the way things are is wrongheaded and your way is right. People who engage in "should" reasoning seem to have a little rule book in their heads entitled *The World According to Me*. They operate on assumptions they make about right and wrong. This is because they misjudge or don't want to accept certain realities. As a result, they often feel angry and protest when these assumptions are violated. "Things should be fair." "Should" reasoning is often used by people who need to be right and refuse to entertain a contrary point of view.

Adopting mindfulness—which is an open and receptive attitude that does not include judgments of right and wrong—is an antidote for "should" thinking. It allows you to stay present in the moment and not get sucked into right/wrong thoughts, which often create discomfort or pain and can cause trouble in relationships. Staying mindful allows you to simply notice your beliefs and hold them lightly.

Empathy—understanding the other person's point of view without necessarily agreeing with it—and open mindedness are required to overcome should statements. "Should" thinking provides the perception of control—of knowing "the rules" (at least as you see them) and having standards you go by. People who indulge in "should" thinking try to control events and others by deciding and acting on what they declare to be "right." Such thinking is often inflexible and unproductive. Not getting caught in "should" thinking allows you to take reasonable or realistic steps to change the situation at hand. The challenge is to set aside anger and "should" reasoning and be open to another approach to a difficult situation.

Taking Things Personally

Sometimes you may erroneously interpret people's behavior as being all about you. A woman who was about 20 pounds overweight was having lunch with a large group of people when one person at the table made a comment about another overweight person passing by: "How can people let themselves go like that?" The overweight woman at the table interpreted the unkind remark as meant for her. She had fallen victim to the interpretation error called *personalization*—taking things personally. As a result, she felt bad.

People who take things personally tend to have self-doubts about their own worth. As a result, they expect others to not value them very highly either. Others' remarks and behavior are regarded with suspicion, and they react to perceptions of being devalued with hurt feelings, indignation, and withdrawal. They usually nurture feelings of anger about the perceived slight or insult, not realizing that by being attached to a core belief that they are unworthy, their own negative self-view is the real cause of their emotional upset. (Core beliefs are the subject of discussion later in this chapter.)

If you tend to take things personally, feeling that other people are putting you down or mistreating you on purpose, you should examine your beliefs about yourself. Low self-esteem and self-critical beliefs create the expectation that others are out to hurt you. In most cases, this is not true. The tendency to take things personally also arises from the belief that being loved and respected by everyone is a dire necessity. If you find yourself feeling hurt by others' remarks, consider what beliefs you hold that may be giving rise to these feelings.

Even if an unkind remark or act *is* meant for you, you don't have to take it personally. To preserve your self-esteem, learn how to hear and use criticism but not let it hurt you. Perhaps the person is just being insensitive. Of course, not every personal remark or comment made by another is meant to be hurtful. It could contain some truth worthy of consideration. Consider the often-painful situation of undergoing a job review. You may hear critical things about your work that hurts your feelings. You may feel the comments are unfair or biased. Try to evaluate feedback for what it is—just information. It may or may not be fact. If there is some truth there, use it. If not, discard it. Refer to the Alcoholics Anonymous admonition: "Take what works for you and leave the rest." Sometimes you feel blamed in a situation. It is hard to not take this personally. In such a case, consider if you have any responsibility for what happened. If so, take ownership of it and, if necessary, apologize. But sometimes you don't deserve the blame or, at least, not all of it. Give yourself time to "sit" with the blaming situation. Often you can think more clearly with time and distance from the situation. Don't just react immediately to feeling blamed, which can lead to feeling angry or upset. Notice your feelings and try to correct the other's misperception or just let go of the situation.

Labeling

Another interpretive error is *labeling*. This involves making a judgment about yourself or another person and putting a negative label on the person or yourself such as "jerk," "idiot," "judgmental," "narrow-minded," or "hypersensitive." Making a sweeping conclusion about someone is labeling. Deciding that someone is "defensive all the time" or "hard to get along with" is also labeling and causes you to form an expectation to see them and treat them in a particular way. Once you label, you find evidence to support your conclusion and you overlook any information to the contrary. Often the impetus to label comes from the arousal of an emotion, perhaps anger or a negative interaction with the person being labeled or even disappointment with yourself. Sometimes labeling takes the form of a catty, offhand remark. Even so, labeling biases your thinking about yourself and other people.

Consider the man who made a judgment about a person the first time he met them and then labeled that person as "dumb as a board." This judgment kept him from taking any information seriously that did not confirm his original and probably unfounded opinion. When he moved from an artistic section of a large city to a small academic community, he decided that the people in his new neighborhood were too "linear," and he just couldn't relate to them. He missed his old friends and made few efforts to make new ones. Having labeled the people around him in a negative way, he closed off the opportunity to learn more about them and perhaps come to like them. Feeling isolated and lonely, he ate himself into a weight problem.

Labeling does not recognize the nuances of people's personalities or consider other evidence. Often labeling is used to shift blame to another person or entity and is accompanied by feelings of anger, irritation, or annoyance. To avoid labeling, first notice when you are doing it—it is usually signaled by pejorative words such as "stupid," "selfish," or "idiotic." When you find yourself labeling, ask yourself what it is you are not letting yourself notice and whether, in some way, you are labeling to protect yourself or your feelings.

Helping and Hindering Self-Talk

Identifying your cognitive distortions is one way to begin adopting thinking that can help you manage your weight and adopt a healthy lifestyle. Learning to recognize and promote positive or *helping self-talk* is also a good way to further your weight-management goals. Attaining your goal weight and maintaining it over time remains the biggest challenge for weight management. Some people reach goal weight by simply changing what they eat. Those who do, research shows, eventually also incorporate regular exercise into their lifestyle to help maintain weight loss. Many variables have been investigated in the hope of shedding light on what predicts success. Researchers agree that there are multiple causes of obesity and that obesity is probably not a unitary phenomenon. Increasingly, obesity is being conceptualized as a chronic, prevalent, and refractory (resistant to treatment) disorder. Research suggests that self-talk is one of many factors that play a role in weight management.

Self-talk can fuel emotions, and emotions can, in turn, produce *negative* self-talk—also known as *hindering self-talk*. Research shows that people who are depressed have a hard time thinking anything other than depressing thoughts. What's worse, depressing thoughts lead to more feelings of depression. Likewise, ruminating over angry thoughts can make a person even angrier. (It's not true that "getting anger out" releases the energy; it only rehearses it.) Similarly, thoughts of being alone without social interaction can increase feelings of loneliness. A person with a positive outlook on life generally experiences pleasant thoughts, and their actions tend to reflect those of a happy person or one with a positive attitude. The person who is a pessimist, however, tends to have gloomy thoughts and sees things in the worst possible light.

Some scientists have been able to demonstrate that the ratio of positive to negative thoughts characterizes various mood states and the ability to cope. This doesn't necessarily mean one should try to get rid of negative thoughts and replace them with more positive ones, which is common—but unhelpful—advice. However, recognizing the difference between helping and hindering thoughts can be useful. The idea of negative or positive self-talk suggests that some thoughts *feel* bad while some *feel* good—that is, such thoughts imply emotions. A more useful way to characterize your self-talk is to ask the question: "Does my self-talk help achieve my goal and is it consistent with my guiding principles and values, or does it lead to hindering action, which impedes progress toward my goal?"

For example, research has shown that some kinds of self-talk—*helping* thoughts—characterize those who succeed in managing weight, while other types of self-talk—*hindering* thoughts—typify those who fail. An example of a helping thought would be: "Just stay away from the food table and focus on talking to friends." This helping thought gives you an instruction about what to do. Alternatively, a hindering thought might be: "I might never get a chance to eat this food again." This hindering thought gives you permission to overeat by making an excuse or rationalization.

Self-Talk of Those Who Fail Versus Those Who Succeed. Research has demonstrated that people's self-talk influences their coping ability. When people exhibit more positive self-talk than negative self-talk, they are less prone to depression and are better able to cope.

Some research has shown that there are important differences in helping and hindering self-talk between those who succeed in losing and maintaining weight loss versus those who still struggle to lose weight. This research looked closely at how much helping self-talk versus hindering self-talk characterized those who were successful at losing weight and keeping it off. To watch a YouTube video about self-talk and beliefs that are learned in childhood, search for "Support Yourself with Upbeat Self-Talk" by communication expert Dr. Bill Lampton.

In research, people who are able to maintain weight loss show a relatively healthy ratio of two-thirds helping to one-third hindering self-talk, whereas unsuccessful dieters tend to have lower proportions of helping self-talk and higher proportions of hindering self-talk. However, the exact ratios depended on two factors: (1) *The situation.* For example, socializing with friends can often lead to excuses to overindulge (hindering self-talk) for both those who succeed and those who don't. (2) *How far from their goal weight the dieter was at the time of the study.* Those who had more weight to lose exhibited more hindering self-talk. Those closer to their goal weight but still dieting showed better ratios of self-talk than those further away. Likewise, the longer maintainers had been at their goal weight, the better their ratios were. Early maintainers had slightly less healthy ratios.

Unsuccessful dieters' hindering self-talk takes many forms: excuses and rationalizations, self-blame, blaming others, losing sight of goals and guiding life principles and values, looking for immediate gratification, feelings of deprivation or resentment, deliberately abandoning goals and guiding life values, or simply the cessation of thinking (that is, going blank or spacing out). In contrast, the helping self-talk of those who succeed is characterized by: the use of self-instruction, acknowledgment of personal accomplishments, maintaining an optimistic attitude and positive expectations, keeping sight of and staying mindful of goals and guiding life principles and values, staying mindful of long-term consequences, focusing on immediate rewards for "doing the right thing," and remaining conscious, aware, and mindful. For examples of hindering and helping self-talk, see table 11.2 on pages 260–261.

Many people combine several kinds of hindering thoughts at one time. See table 11.3 on page 262 for examples of combined self-talk

Table 11.2 Comparison of Hindering and Helping Self-Talk

Hindering Self-Talk	Helping Self-Talk
1. Using excuses, rationalizations and justifications. *Examples*: "Just one won't hurt." "I may as well eat it now and get it over with." "I better eat it so it doesn't go bad." "I need to rest today instead of trying to exercise." "I'll start tomorrow." "I can't ask others to change their way of eating because I need to lose weight."	**2. Using self-instruction.** *Examples*: "I'll wait ten minutes before I eat and I'll focus on doing something else for now." "Stay out of the kitchen. Enjoy reading your book." "Stop. Don't go there. Do something else." "Let's get going to the gym now." "Just drink some water and go back to bed."
3. Engaging in excessive self-blame, self-criticism, or self-denigration. *Examples*: "I'm ashamed of myself." "I hate my body." "I'm disgusting." "I'm a failure." "There is something wrong with me." "No one could like anyone as fat as I am."	**4. Providing acknowldgement of personal accomplishments.** *Examples*: "I've worked hard to lose all this weight." "I can stay in control." "I'm pleased that I'm getting stronger." "It's okay to give myself pats-on-the-back for small successes." "I bought a whole box, but I only ate one, then I threw away the rest."
5. Blaming others or external circumstances. *Examples*: "I have to take clients out for lunch almost every day, so I can't control my calories." "They keep bringing food to work." "With my schedule, I just can't fit in time to exercise." "She insisted that I eat. I didn't want to offend her."	**6. Having an optimistic attitude and positive expectations.** *Examples*: "I think I can do it this time." "If she can do it, I can do it." "I feel empowered in a way I have never felt before about managing my weight." "I can handle this." "I'm going to complete a 5K race next month even if I have to walk part of it."
7. Losing sight of goals and guiding life principles. *Examples*: "What's the use?" "Who cares?" "Why bother?" "Why keep trying?" "What's the point?" "It won't matter."	**8. Attending to future consequences of proposed actions and staying in touch with goals and guiding life principles.** *Examples*: "If I eat this, I could lose control." "I want to maintain my success." "I want to be healthy and this won't help." "If I eat a little bit, I'll probably eat more and then I'll feel bad."

Table 11.2 **Comparison of Hindering and Helping Self-Talk** (*continued*)

Hindering Self-Talk	Helping Self-Talk
9. Focusing on immediate gratification. *Examples*: "It would taste so good." "What looks good to eat?" "I'll feel better if I eat." "I love chocolate."	**10. Attending to long-term consequences to avoid doing the "wrong" thing.** *Examples*: "I'll keep gaining weight if I keep binge eating." "If I want to be healthy, I have to stop making excuses to eat inappropriately."
11. Focusing on being deprived and resentful. *Examples*: "Why can't I eat like other people?" "Why me?" "I hate having to change what I eat." "Why can't I eat what I want?" "I wish I didn't have to do this." "I hate exercise." "Low-calorie food doesn't taste good." "Poor me, I have to give up everything I like."	**12. Focusing on immediate rewards of "doing the right thing."** *Examples*: "I'll feel better about myself when I choose something healthy to eat." "Making good food choices makes me feel good." "I feel like I've accomplished something every time I finish my exercise routine."
13. Deliberately abandoning goals and guiding life principles. *Examples*: "I know I should stop, but I don't want to." "I just need something to nibble on so I'm going to eat." "I want something sweet."	**14. Maintaining a single-minded focus on goals and guiding life principles.** *Examples*: "I've worked too hard to blow it now." "I'm taking it one day at a time." "Is this what I really want?" "Does this accord with my values?"
15. Not thinking and just eating. *Examples*: Going blank, numb, or spacing out. Choosing not to think. Going into a trance. Not thinking.	**16. Remaining conscious, aware, and mindful of overriding values and guiding life principles.** *Examples*: "A healthy lifestyle is important to me." "I want to be healthy." "Exercise is what I do." "I make healthy food choices."

statements. It is helpful to tease apart the types of self-talk you use and ascertain your ratio and proportion of helpful versus hindering self-talk. Doing so will help you recognize which thoughts have distressing content or hinder your weight management efforts and which thoughts keep you focused on your goals and values.

Table 11.3 Combining Types of Hindering Self-Talk

❖ "It was Super Bowl weekend (*blaming external circumstances*) and I was bad (*self-blame*)."

❖ "Someone brought doughnuts to the meeting (*blaming others*) and they were just there in front of me (*excuse and rationalization*). Before I knew it, I had eaten several (*abandoning conscious control, going blank*)."

❖ "I decided that it had been a rough day and I deserved a treat (*excuse and rationalization*), so I ate one of the cookies offered (*abandoning conscious control*), and afterward I couldn't stop thinking about how good they were (*focusing on immediate gratification*). I just had to go to the store and buy some more (*excuse and rationalization, deliberately abandoning goals*). Afterward I felt terrible for eating the whole bag (*self-criticism*)."

Assessing your Goal-Related Self-Talk

A good first step in attempting to improve your self-talk is to take the Self-Test 11.1, The Inventory of Goal-Related Self-Talk, on page 263, which was developed and validated as part of a research project on self-talk. This self-test helps you identify the ratio of your helping to hindering types of self-talk. Complete the questionnaire and follow the scoring instructions provided. If your ratio of helping to total self-talk is less than .50, you may be experiencing distressing thoughts, or your self-talk may be undermining your weight-loss efforts. After you complete the self-test, look at table 11.4, The Key to Goal-Related Self-Talk on page 265, which is a key to the types of helping and hindering self-talk each item of the inventory represents. Refer to table 11.2, Comparison of Helping and Hindering Self-Talk, for more examples.

Dimensions of Helping and Hindering Thinking

In the research study mentioned, the sixteen types of self-talk described in the table 11.2 and assessed in Self-Test 11.1 were subjected to a statistical procedure called *factor analysis*. Results suggest that these types of self-talk tap into four important dimensions of helpful versus hindering problem thinking.

Self-Test 11.1 **Inventory of Goal-Related Self-Talk**

Instructions: Put a check mark by each of the statements that is true for you:

_____ 1. I find excuses for eating what I know I shouldn't, or I rationalize that I will start making better food choices later.

_____ 2. I tell myself what to do and how to cope so I can stay, or get back, on track.

_____ 3. I get down on myself and become self-critical because of my weight or my eating.

_____ 4. I periodically remind myself that at times I have been able to do well at managing my weight or my eating.

_____ 5. I think that others or circumstances beyond my control are often the reason for my eating or my weight-management difficulties.

_____ 6. I try to stay optimistic and have positive expectations for succeeding.

_____ 7. When the opportunity to eat presents itself or I want something good to eat, I avoid thinking about future consequences of eating, such as gaining weight or feeling bad later.

_____ 8. I frequently remind myself of why I want to lose weight or maintain weight to stay motivated and avoid overeating.

_____ 9. I get to thinking about how good something will taste, and I forget about everything else.

_____ 10. I focus on how bad I'll feel if I do something unhelpful, such as over-eating or skipping my exercise.

_____ 11. I often feel deprived, tired of doing without, or annoyed by having to manage my eating or my weight.

_____ 12. I usually focus on how good I'll feel for doing the right thing now to manage my eating or my weight

_____ 13. I often don't care about what I "should" do, and I focus more on what I want to do.

_____ 14. I use mindfulness to stay present in the moment.

_____ 15. Sometimes I stop thinking altogether and just eat; only afterward do I think about what I've done.

_____ 16. I want to be healthy and I value regular exercise.

See page 264 for scoring ▶

Self-Test 11.1 Scoring:

❖ Count all the check marks in the even-numbered statements: _____

❖ Divide your total number of checked even-numbered statements by 16: _____

❖ If you have no even-numbered statements checked, use a "1" as the numerator—that is, divide the number 1 by 16 to get your result.

❖ Interpretation: If your result is less than .50, your self-talk is probably hindering your weight-loss efforts.

For five of the hindering self-talk items in table 11.2 (#1, excuses and rationalizations; #3, self-blame; #9, immediate gratification; #13, deliberately abandoning goals and life principles; #15, not thinking, blanking out, going numb), the results suggest that people using these types of thoughts function at the level of *program control.* That is, the behavior of people having these sorts of thoughts is automatic and requires minimal conscious control. These hindering thoughts reflect inadequate self-vigilance, selective or misdirected attention to information, or the intentional neglect of information that could be helpful in attaining a goal.

Two items of hindering thoughts (#5, blaming others or external circumstances; #11, feeling deprived and resentful) and one that is the opposite of a helping thought (#6, optimistic attitude) seem to reflect a kind of *peevishness* dimension. That is, taken together, blaming others or circumstances, focusing on feeling deprived or resentful, not having an optimistic attitude suggesting ill humor, having a querulous temperament, being obstinate, and being difficult to please are attitudes likely to hinder goals.

Peevishness can produce thoughts such as "Why me?" and "No one is going to tell me what I can and can't eat." Many who struggle with a weight problem also struggle with the seeming unfairness of it. "Others seem to have it easy and not have to watch their weight,"

Table 11.4 Key to "Inventory of Goal-Related Self-Talk"

1. I find excuses for eating what I know I shouldn't, or I rationalize that I will start making better food choices later. (*excuses, rationalizations, and justifications*)

2. I tell myself what to do and how to cope so I can stay or get back on track. (*self-instruction*)

3. I get down on myself and become self-critical because of my weight or my eating. (*self-blame*)

4. I periodically remind myself that at times I have been able to do well managing my weight or my eating. (*acknowledgment of accomplishments*)

5. I think that others or circumstances beyond my control are often the reason for my eating or my weight-management difficulties. (*blaming external circumstances*)

6. I try to stay optimistic and have positive expectations for succeeding. (*optimistic attitude and positive expectations*)

7. When the opportunity to eat something presents itself or I want something good to eat, I avoid thinking about future consequences of eating, such as gaining weight or feeling bad later. (*losing sight of goals and values*)

8. I frequently remind myself of why I want to lose weight or maintain my weight to stay motivated and avoid overeating. (*attending to distant consequences, reminding self of goals*)

9. I get to thinking about how good something will taste, and I forget about everything else. (*immediate gratification*)

10. I focus on how bad I'll feel if I do something unhelpful, such as overeating or skipping my exercise. (*attending to distant consequences*)

11. I often feel deprived, tired of doing without, or annoyed by having to manage my eating or my weight. (*deprivation, resentment*)

12. I usually focus on how good I'll feel for doing the right thing now to manage my eating or my weight. (*focus on immediate reward*)

13. I often don't care about what I "should" do, and I focus more on what I want to do. (*deliberate abandonment of guiding life principles*)

14. I try to stay mindful and stay present in the moment. (*maintain single-minded focus on goals and guiding life principles*)

15. Sometimes I stop thinking altogether and just eat; only afterward do I think about what I've done. (*dissociation, not thinking*)

16. I want to be healthy and I value regular exercise. (*aware/conscious of life values*)

they think. Resentment can lead to feelings of entitlement. You may refuse to set limits on yourself regarding food or you may avoid regular exercise, which reminds me of a joke: "When I think of exercising, I have to lie down." These kinds of poor attitudes can produce internal quarrels between that part of you that wants to lose weight or be healthy and the other part that declares, in essence: "I don't care." When the latter sentiment wins, attention narrows to the idea of eating. Making healthy choices is ignored.

The final two types of hindering thoughts (#7, losing sight of goals and guiding principles or values, and the inverse or opposite of #16, not staying in touch with goals for a healthy lifestyle) involve *avoidance* of thinking about one's behavior or the future consequences of one's behavior. These findings are supported by other research, which found that those who are obese frequently reject notions of self-control, avoid placing limitations on themselves, and doubt the possibility of change.

Unsuccessful dieters' struggles appear to be hampered by poor information management in the form of cognitive distortions, fluctuating and poorly defined values, and attention directed at immediate gratification. The hindering self-talk typical of failure shows a bias toward distorting or selectively considering information, blaming external circumstances, avoiding self-discipline, failing to refer to guiding principles, and neglecting to notice the rewards associated with goal-facilitating behavior.

Six of the helping thoughts in table 11.2 (#2, self-instruction; #4, acknowledging accomplishments; #8, attending to future consequences of proposed actions; #10, attending to consequences to avoid hindering behavior; #12, focus on reward for doing the right thing; #14, maintaining a single-minded focus on goals and guiding life principles) reflect thinking that is guided by principles and values. These helping thoughts reflect *principle control*. The person whose thinking is guided by principle control is consciously directing attention to observable elements of the situation as part of cognitive processing and is comparing intended action with beliefs about the healthy way to behave. There is a high level of self-vigilance and consciousness, and cognitive strategies to delay gratification are employed. (For example, such people remind themselves of their goal to be healthy and, when faced with temptation, may delay the decision to eat and instead get involved in another activity.)

Taken together, this research suggests that those who succeed in losing weight and keeping it off tended to stay in conscious control of their behavior and keep sight of their goals and valued life principles, whereas those who struggle with their weight are more likely to operate on automatic, feel resentful about having to engage in weight-management efforts, and often avoid thinking about the consequences of their behavior. Those who are most likely to succeed exhibit principle control thinking, and those who struggle are more likely to be under program control.

Program Control

When you are under *program control*, you lack clarity about or lose sight of your personal life values or guiding life principles. (Recall that *values* are chosen qualities of life and point you toward the direction for action.) In its simplest form, program control means automatic functioning without reference to overriding values. It seeks immediate gratification without regard to long-term goals. Program control means getting caught up in hindering thinking so much that it dominates other useful sources of behavior regulation, like values and principles. When you are under program control, you lose touch with what you want in the long term, and this allows you to indulge or, more specifically, avoid in the present moment.

The combination of hindering self-talk and cognitive distortions can make it hard for people to make positive long-term changes. Recall that the behavior of people experiencing cognitive distortions is often automatic and not under conscious control. Hindering self-talk also tends to be automatic as well as dismissive of goals and values. This mindless kind of thinking is characteristic of program control. You are experiencing program control when hindering self-talk, avoidance (choosing not to think about consequences), and peevishness cause you to lose sight of, or deny, a guiding principle related to health and weight management. When you are under program control, you seek to have only short-term positive, or feel-good, experiences in the here and now, and to avoid negative, or feel-bad, experiences. Experiential avoidance, an ACT concept discussed earlier in the chapter, involves trying to control or alter private events (such as, thoughts, feelings, sensations, or memories) in a way that is harmful to your personal well-being in the long run. Eating can be a way of avoiding the experience of a painful reality and the thoughts it might generate. Giving into eating lets you forget about the need for self-discipline in weight management.

Consider a feel-bad thought like "I don't measure up" or "I'm fat." You could attempt to suppress this thought by thinking of something else. Such experiential avoidance doesn't work very well; usually the thought returns. Then when suppression doesn't work, the thought can lead to a feel-bad emotion, such as anxiety or sadness. In an attempt to escape the unpleasantness that the thought and feeling engender, you might get something to eat or have a few drinks to numb yourself. Unfortunately, trying to control anxiety just evokes more anxiety, and that leads to more attempts to escape. It is better simply to be aware of the unpleasantness and tolerate the feelings until they pass. As one person put it, "I guess I have to learn to be comfortable with being uncomfortable."

Storytelling

Often those under program control are attached to a story that determines their thinking and behavior. Here's one person's story: "I'm so busy at work I sometimes forget to eat lunch. I have an open-door policy and anyone can come in for my assistance. Unfortunately, I often can't get everything done during working hours, so I have to stay late. Sometimes I don't leave work until 8 o'clock. Fortunately, my husband cooks, but I'm so hungry by the time we eat that I often have second or third helpings. After dinner I'm exhausted so I just go right to bed." And another story: "I'm a binge eater. I started eating this way when I was in college and whenever things get really stressful, I binge. I've tried therapy but nothing helps. I am now 50 pounds overweight and I can't stop bingeing."

While everything said in these two stories is probably true, each person is fused or joined with their story and is trying to solve their problems without giving up or acknowledging their story. The problem is that real solutions may not exist for the story—at least not for the story being told in this way. The storytellers have created a conceptualization of themselves that is narrow and cages them in, and inflexible behavioral patterns are the unavoidable result. Many of us are fused to stories that limit our options. Consider, instead, transcending the story you tell about yourself by choosing to define and live life in a meaningful way by clarifying and contacting larger principles and values. These larger principles and values can serve as the chosen standard by which other things and behavior are evaluated.

Let's consider the people in our stories. In the first story, the person defines themselves as being available to anyone at work at any time that they wish to drop in. Setting limits that allow work to get done in a timely fashion so there is time for lunch is not even considered. The person regards themselves as kind and giving. By this definition of self, they have allowed themselves no options and, thus, there is no way out. To find a way out of this story, the person must adopt firmer boundaries. They have to take care of their own needs first.

The second story is about a person who is stuck in the avoidance of pain (stress) by engaging in bingeing and, as a result, does not have the ability to behave effectively. What if they were to accept that stress is an inevitable part of life that everyone must address, and that binge eating is simply their personal means of escaping stress? What if they could make contact with a higher value—wanting life to be about more than food or weight, wanting life to be about healthy living despite the stresses she faces? What if they used other strategies for dealing with stress, like going for a walk to reduce the tension that makes them vulnerable to binge eating?

Changing or abandoning your victim story is the first step in defusing (or reducing the tension from) your story. *Defusing* allows you to step back and observe the story without becoming stuck in it. By taking the point of view of the observer of your thoughts and behavior, you may be able to see other choices. What function does the caretaking in the first story serve? What other options are there? What function does the binge eating serve in the second story? How can the binge eating be overcome? Only when you can see you are telling yourself a story and are willing to let it go can you find a new ending. In so doing, it is necessary for you to confront your underlying core beliefs and reconsider them.

Core Beliefs

Core beliefs are underlying and deeply rooted assumptions. They are called *core beliefs* because they are so central to self-concept—how we see ourselves—and how we see other people, the world, and the future. Such beliefs can be extremely emotionally loaded and can give rise to thoughts that cause emotional distress. For example, a thought like "I am a fraud" or "I can't succeed" emanates from a core belief such as "I'm weak" or "I'm can't make it on my own." A core belief such as "You can't trust people" is one that makes it hard to get along with others.

Your beliefs are usually formed when you are a child. They may reflect your family's—especially your parents'—viewpoints and, eventually, you adopt them as your own. This happens unconsciously. When it is happening, you do not realize you are absorbing others' ideas about yourself and the world. Take the person who has been overweight since childhood and whose sisters and parents constantly picked on them about their eating in their early years. They probably developed a core belief about themselves, their weight, and their eating that may sound something like "I don't measure up." Or the person who as a child was frequently criticized for all manner of things may have the core belief "I'm not lovable." For an example of how core beliefs are formed, watch Dr. Shad Helmstetter's "The Story of Self-Talk" on YouTube.

Beliefs have a powerful impact on many of your attitudes, moods, and behaviors. The person mentioned previously who was picked on as a child for their weight and eating feels pessimistic about ever changing, and today as an adult resents anyone commenting about their eating. The person who was severely criticized as a child is likely to struggle with depression and may use food to escape bad feelings.

People who let others walk all over them, or feel they have to please others to be liked, may have a core belief that they are worthless or undeserving. For these people, taking care of others before themselves is a way to compensate or deflect such feelings. Those with low self-esteem, fear of rejection, and fear of failure may believe "I need others to accept me" or "I can't deal with rejection." Core beliefs that can lead to hindering behavior include:

❖ I don't count.

❖ I'm not lovable.

❖ I'm worthless.

❖ I'm undeserving.

❖ I'm defective.

All people have core beliefs that are not self-hindering. "I'm an intelligent person" is a core belief that usually facilitates good performance in a job. "I get along with other people" is another. Core beliefs can be life enhancing. Some people view themselves as personable, trustworthy, honest, reliable, or good natured. But some deeply held core beliefs reflect fears about the self, such as "I'm different. I don't fit in." "I'm weak and need support from others."

Destructive core beliefs often give rise to automatic thoughts—painful ideas that come into your head without warning. They may seem to materialize for no reason. The obese person may have the automatic thought "I hate myself." Or the person who is trying to manage their weight might have the sudden thought "I just can't do this." Such thoughts often stem from some deeply held, self-hindering, core belief. These thoughts can be so automatic and familiar that they are difficult to pinpoint unless you listen in on your self-talk and keep a record of your thoughts. Once you do that, you may be able to "hear" the thought and identify the underlying core belief. As with thoughts, beliefs are constructions of the mind. They are not facts. When you uncover a hindering core belief, you will recognize it for what it is—a leftover from an earlier time that should not be believed or acted upon anymore. It may be painful to acknowledge your fears about yourself but doing so allows you to rise above them and define the direction you want your life to take now.

Principle Control

Principle control is different from program control. When your behavior is under program control, you are operating "on automatic." When your behavior is under *principle control*, you are consciously in touch with guiding principles and personal values that provide direction for the life you want to live. As a conscious human being, you are mindful and able to stay in touch with the present moment more fully. You are flexible and able to change or persist based on what the situation affords in service to overarching values.

Values

As discussed earlier, values are not ends unto themselves but rather directions without a destination. They are about living in a chosen and meaningful way. Values provide the compass heading for your life. Values guide the process of living but do not end; they usually continue throughout life. A value is not "to lose weight." (That is a goal.) The value is "to have a healthy lifestyle." Values point the way to the behavior.

There are those who have never defined socially acceptable personal values. The values these people embrace may be self-serving in the short run, like personal gain by any means. Some people who were taught good values by their families or their religion consciously forsake them. But most people have just forgotten or lost touch with what is important to them, or they never took the time to think about it. To move forward and address hindering self-talk and core beliefs, it is important that you define your values, stay mindful and present in the moment, accept life's difficulties and suffering, and take action based on your guiding principles.

When you are guided by principle control, you are aware of hindering self-talk without giving into it. You can simply notice a hindering thought without being overwhelmed by it. To do this, you must recognize that thoughts and feelings are transient and need not dictate behavior. With principle control, you can let go of the struggle with the inevitable pain of life and do what is necessary to live according to your stated values. It is not necessary to eliminate hindering self-talk so much as it is important to focus on helping thoughts. You can accomplish this by staying focused on the larger values of your life and listening to the helping self-talk that points the way to your goals.

Hindering self-talk defeats goal achievement and avoids or loses touch with guiding principles and life values. Helping thoughts are those generated with values in mind—thoughts that help you live your life according to chosen principles. Thoughts and feelings are transient; they come and go. An example might be, "This is too hard." If you attach to this idea—that is, fuse with it—you might quit. This is likely just a thought that popped into your head. All you need to do is notice the thought and then turn your attention into an action you can take right now, in this moment. In other words, you need to keep moving toward your goal.

Climbing a high mountain is a good analogy. It isn't easy to climb up over boulders hour after hour and, if you look too far ahead, you might get discouraged by the thought "I have so far to go." On the other hand, if you take it one boulder at a time, in due time you will reach your destination.

The Funnel of Awareness

To succeed in managing food temptations, you need to stay in touch with your values so you can win arguments between the thoughts in your head that advocate for giving up and the thoughts that want you to keep trying. If you can stay in touch with your values, you have a better chance of winning the argument for healthy behavior. You need to avoid being persuaded by thoughts that argue "It's too hard." If you give up, you are likely to lose touch altogether with values and fall into mindless behavior.

Awareness or consciousness can be broad or narrow. When awareness is broad—that is, when you are mindful—values and guiding principles are present and accessible to conscious thought. When awareness is at its most narrow, thinking is at a minimum, if it exists at all. When awareness or attention to eating narrows too much, thinking can actually stop. Instead, there exists just a stimulus and response behavior—food/eat/food/eat—where food is consumed as if the eater is in a trance. This is mindless behavior.

To understand this, imagine a funnel shape that is divided into thirds. "Values" are in the widest part at the top. In the middle, there are "arguments" between inner voices (parts of yourself). And in the smallest bottom third is the "trance," the stimulus/response state where thinking no longer goes on at a conscious level. This concept is illustrated in figure 11.1.

For successful weight management, it is important to keep your awareness in the upper third or widest part of the funnel. This is where abstract and future-oriented thinking goes on. When your awareness is at the top of the funnel, you are in touch with the values and guiding principles that you want to define your life. You are mindful of the here and now. When you slip into the middle of the funnel, your awareness narrows. This is where you get caught up in your own thoughts. Here is where "inner voices" can be heard arguing and engaging in a tug of war to get you to give in to temptation. If you lose the argument and the tug of war, you slip down into the

Figure 11.1 **Funnel of Awareness**

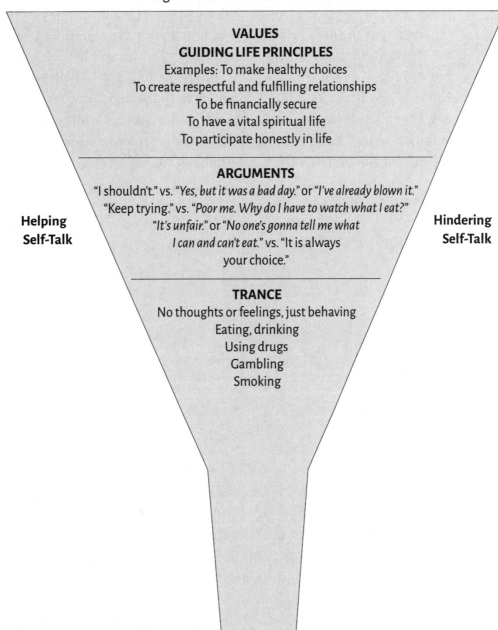

VALUES
GUIDING LIFE PRINCIPLES
Examples: To make healthy choices
To create respectful and fulfilling relationships
To be financially secure
To have a vital spiritual life
To participate honestly in life

Helping Self-Talk

Hindering Self-Talk

ARGUMENTS
"I shouldn't." vs. "Yes, but it was a bad day." or "I've already blown it."
"Keep trying." vs. "Poor me. Why do I have to watch what I eat?"
"It's unfair." or "No one's gonna tell me what
I can and can't eat." vs. "It is always
your choice."

TRANCE
No thoughts or feelings, just behaving
Eating, drinking
Using drugs
Gambling
Smoking

narrowest part of the funnel, the trance state. At this point, thinking stops. This is where overeating and binge eating occur.

The key is to stay mindful and in touch with your goals and values. If you find yourself slipping down the funnel and having arguments with yourself about what to do, be careful not to believe the hindering self-talk. Don't let yourself give in to such thoughts. They are, after all, just part of you—the part that resists conforming to your value of living a healthy lifestyle. The next chapter focuses more on identifying and defying these internal voices.

12

Challenging Your "Inner Voices"

Sophia's mother died when Sophia was only 15. For years before her death, Sophia's mother insisted on weighing Sophia once a week and lecturing her on the perils of getting fat. Between weigh-ins, Sophia's mother constantly watched and commented on what Sophia ate. Now, as an adult, Sophia had a serious rebellious side when it came to food or eating. "I don't want anyone telling me what to eat or what to weigh." Despite the presence of that strong, internal rebel, Sophia wanted to lose the extra 30 pounds she had gained since giving birth to her first child. "I think I would just feel better if I dropped these extra pounds. The problem is, I start losing weight and my rebel pulls success out from under me." Once Sophia recognized that she had an internal Rebel voice—sometimes called a subpersonality—she was able to identify it and also hear the other inner voices that helped her make better choices.

Sophia is not alone in having to face and come to terms with her subpersonalities. An academic journal included this description of a case of emotional eating: a young female college student described an inner voice that often put her down by saying things like "You're not good enough." These thoughts seemed to occur automatically, and they attacked her self-esteem or her ability to do well. She had another voice as well that worried her boyfriend did not find her attractive or that she would do poorly on her exams and not get into graduate school. Such thoughts happened most often after eating so much that she felt uncomfortably full. After overeating, she would feel guilty and worthless and become even more self-critical. Her inner voices included the Critic and the Worrier.

What Is Inner Dialogue?

An article entitled "The Inner Dialogue" by Remez Sasson, an author of several books on positive thinking, advises people how to become mindful of the mind's incessant chatter, which is often negative, and encourages a more positive voice. Check the author's advice on the internet by googling "Remez Sasson" or "Inner Dialogue."

Mr. Sasson notes that most people conduct an automatic inner dialogue—an inner conversation with themselves, which occurs silently in our minds. It is the habit of the mind to keep thinking—to keep conducting internal dialogues or "voices" that sometimes even have arguments with one another. That's normal. Do you sometimes ask yourself, "Should I eat this?" and then start weighing the pros and cons in your mind. Do you sometimes torture yourself about what you did eat or whether you should have gotten more exercise? Just think of all the times you tried to convince yourself to do something or to avoid something. How many times have you commented, analyzed, or reviewed something about your weight or what you ate in your mind? Do you spend a lot of time having negative, destructive thoughts in your head? Continuous conversation goes on in everyone's head. Such thinking is sometimes called the *inner voice dialogue*. It is:

- ❖ The process of asking and answering questions in your head.

- ❖ The process of repeating words and thoughts in the mind.

- ❖ The little voice inside that comments on your life, circumstances, situations, and other people.

Voice Dialogue

A helpful way to understand inner voices is a method called *Voice Dialogue*. Search the internet for "Voice Dialogue," or google Hal Stone, PhD, and Sidra Stone, PhD, to find their books. These two clinical psychologists developed Voice Dialogue as a way of contacting, understanding, and working with the many selves that make up your personality.

The goal behind the Voice Dialogue method is not to try to change thoughts, get rid of them, or help them grow up and be more sensible. Rather, the goal is to allow yourself greater choice in behavior by identifying the parts of your personality with which you are fused and the parts you have disowned—that is, denied, ignored, put aside, or refused to allow to emerge. The Voice Dialogue technique allows you to unhook from those selves that have dominated your behavior and begin to explore and become acquainted with their opposites.

Chapter 11, "Managing Thinking and Self-Talk," introduced the concepts of *the thinking self* and *the observing self*. Recall that the thinking self is the part of the mind that is responsible for all your self-talk, beliefs, memories, judgments, fantasies, and so on. It has a strong influence on behavior and emotions. The observing self is that part of you that is aware and mindful of whatever you are thinking, feeling, or doing at any moment without getting caught up in the content. In Voice Dialogue, the *ego* is the equivalent of the thinking self and the *aware ego* is the same as the observing self. For our purposes here, we will continue to use the terms *thinking self* and *observing self*, rather than the terms used by Voice Dialogue.

Subpersonalities

According to Voice Dialogue, the thinking self (ego) is composed of various parts or subpersonalities, which may also be referred to as *selves* or *inner voices*. One of these parts starts developing at birth. Voice Dialogue calls this part of the thinking mind the Protector/Controller, which is nonverbal in the beginning. This self learns what behaviors are safe and what behaviors bring rewards. It also notices what behaviors bring pain and which are punished. Early on, the Protector/Controller subpersonality figures out the world from a child's perspective and, over time, adopts a code of conduct. Eventually this self matures and, by adulthood, it becomes what Voice Dialogue calls the Operating Ego—the mature version of the Protector/Controller. It still has the job of protecting the individual and trying to control the environment, however, it shares space with other subpersonalities that also develop as we mature.

Voice Dialogue calls these additional subpersonalities *primary selves* because they dictate adult behavior. For example, the authors call one of these voices, or subpersonalities, the Pusher. A Pusher voice may develop to make sure we get done what needs to be done. If it pushes hard enough, we graduate from school or become successful in our career. Another such subpersonality is the Pleaser. A Pleaser subpersonality generally causes us to be polite and behave in socially beneficial ways. The Critic—another Voice Dialogue subpersonality—develops to keep us living according to our own personal code of conduct or our expectations for our behavior. The Rule Maker is that subpersonality that decides how things should be and how people should act. Sophia, from the chapter-opening vignette, has a Rebel voice that refuses to be bound by other people's expectations. This voice is similar to Voice Dialogue's Rule Maker.

Disowned Voices

The subpersonalities that are primary—the primary selves that govern present behavior—have opposite (or disowned) parts, and these are not always conscious. For example, in Voice Dialogue, the Pusher may drive a person to be a workaholic, but the disowned and opposite part of the Pusher is associated with playfulness or relaxation, even laziness.

Voice Dialogue provides this example: Consider the surgeon who refused to take vacations because he had so much work to do. His Pusher wouldn't let him consider taking time off. This was the primary self with which he identified. When he was at home, he spent his time reading medical journals or writing articles for publication. He ignored his family and refused to give himself time off for relaxation. He didn't even realize how his Pusher subpersonality was robbing him of his personal life. He embraced his Pusher and rejected his Relaxer, his disowned self. This man was so fused with his thinking self and not in touch with his observing self that he didn't even realize he had a choice in his behavior.

There are other common examples of opposite selves according to Voice Dialogue. Some people have a Procrastinator inner voice, and they disown their Proactive self. Other people have a Self-Distrusting voice, and they spurn the part that is Self-Confident. Those people who are more rational and intellectual have often lost touch with their Experiencing or Emotional Self.

Conflicting Selves

The observing self can notice and accept both the primary inner voices and the disowned selves on the other side without identifying with either. Your observing self is functioning when you are being mindful. (Remember that mindfulness is a process, not a destination.) The results of becoming more mindful are that you gain access to, and acceptance of, more of who you are. When you are mindful of your inner voices, you realize it is okay if they disagree with one another. When this happens, your thinking self can also feel conflicted. Sophia wanted to lose weight, but she also resisted implementing self-discipline, which she regarded as being demands from others. However, you can decide what to do even though there is bound to be another part of you that prefers an alternative. By embracing more of your inner voices and their often-conflicting needs, you can make more conscious decisions rather than acting out of habit or compulsion. You will experience more self-acceptance and self-understanding, and you will become more accepting and understanding of others as well.

Inner Voices and Behavior Change

A number of voices can chime in when you want to lose weight or are faced with changing a habit or behavior. Let's consider those inner voices now.

Each inner voice or subpersonality has its own type of self-talk. It also has its own set of beliefs and prescribed ways of behaving. A common inner voice is that of the Critic. This voice is self-critical and can precipitate emotions such as guilt or shame. Another commonly heard voice is that of the Worrier. The Worrier frets about real and imagined threats and whether you can cope, which then spirals up anxiety. The voice of the Caretaker (or People Pleaser) advocates anticipating the needs of others and meeting them, often at the sacrifice of your own needs. It advocates assuming responsibility for other people. Some people have a Victim voice that expresses self-pity or complains about unfairness. The Blamer lays the fault at the feet of others and can elicit anger. The Enforcer (also called the "Rule Maker" in Voice Dialogue) talks about the rules and what needs to be done according to your rules, which it holds dear (many of which are not universally held). The Rebel, on the other hand, rejects rules and setting limits. The Perfectionist urges you to set high goals for yourself as a measure of your self-worth, and sometimes your perfectionism is inappropriately applied to others. If others don't meet up to your standards, the Perfectionist can be joined by the Blamer voice and become critical. Alternatively, perfectionism can be driven by believing that others will value you only if you are perfect. The voice of the Pessimist sees things in bleak terms. It engenders expectations of failure.

The Crowd

There are many internal voices. In Voice Dialogue, the multiple inner voices are called the Crowd. In Twelve-Step programs, participants call these multiple voices the Committee. These names ring true since several inner voices talking at once sound like a crowd or committee that can't make decisions or get along. Members of the Crowd (or the Committee) can get into arguments with one another. One voice may express one opinion while another voice disagrees or even argues back. Some of the voices of the Crowd or the Committee may sound quite rational, while others employ emotional arguments: "I feel so stressed. I have to get something to eat." "No, you shouldn't. You'll feel bad if you do."

Some voices collude with each other. The Critic and the Perfectionist often go hand-in-hand, as do the Caretaker and the Victim. In certain situations, the Enforcer can call in the Blamer for help. Similarly, the Blamer and the Victim are often partners.

Voices can form coalitions against other voices in the Crowd. The Victim and the Blamer get together and argue against the good advice of the Healthy voice and the Responsible voice:

VICTIM/BLAMER VOICE: "My boss was really rough on me today. He causes me stress."

HEALTHY/RESPONSIBLE VOICE: "Well, go for a walk to reduce your stress. After all, it's your reaction to your boss that's causing the stress. Give yourself time; the upset will pass."

VICTIM/BLAMER VOICE: "I shouldn't have to put up with his antics."

Is Hearing Voices Bad?

Everyone has a set of inner voices, but some people worry about their meaning. Some people ask, "Aren't crazy people the only ones who hear voices?" Actually, no. Everyone "hears" his or her own thoughts. The difference between those who are seriously mentally ill and other people who "hear" themselves think and act on voices is that the mentally ill don't realize that the voices belong to them, and they find them seriously disruptive and disturbing. They think someone or something outside themselves is telling them what to do, inserting thoughts into their head, or whispering behind their backs.

It may come as a surprise, then, to hear that many people who "hear" voices in their heads experience some of them as positive. Some voices are adaptive in life, contrary to those voices like the Blamer and the Critic that can foster goal-defeating behavior. Some people may understand an inner voice as a dialogue with God or a connection with a higher power. Many people describe inner voices as being a positive influence in their lives, comforting or inspiring them as they go about their daily business. (This voice might be called the Comforter/Inspirer.) Those who are in tune with their healthy voice often hear thoughts about the need to get regular exercise and make healthy choices.

The experience of childhood trauma can give rise to destructive voices, such as the Victim or the Pessimist, while those who have had more positive life experiences and have formed more healthy beliefs about themselves and other people are more likely to develop voices with a helpful perspective. The Self-Confident voice provides self-talk that is assured, positive, and secure: "I'm training to run a 5K race in a few months. I'm excited about it."

Where Voices Come From

Early experiences with family and caregivers contribute to the formation of each person's various selves or inner voices. What people heard said to or about themselves or others in the past gets internalized and integrated into their thinking and inner voices, and is often expressed in their behavior. People learn what to expect from others and what others expect of them by the way they were treated as they grew up. These expectations shape each person's sense of self-worth and self-esteem. Different selves develop, and these selves influence feelings and behavior in the present moment.

Parents and family are important role models for children. If a parent is a worrier, the child is likely to develop an anxious attitude toward life and develop their own worrier voice. If a parent is critical of a child, the child will internalize the parent's criticisms and eventually develop an internal critical voice. The child who is told repeatedly that they are fat and lazy and are treated as if they can't manage themselves come to think they don't measure up and act accordingly. They may develop a pessimistic internal voice or try to compensate by becoming a caretaker for others to increase their self-esteem. Criticism people receive from parents, teachers, coaches, or others is often internalized as true statements. A person who gets negative feedback may try to compensate by becoming a perfectionist. Children who are teased or bullied by peers or siblings are likely to internalize the belief that they are inadequate or unacceptable. They might find themselves saddled with an internal victim voice in adulthood.

Take the example of Sophia, whose mother took her to doctors and enrolled her in programs to lose weight when she was a child and early adolescent. As a result, she developed the idea that she was not okay and, that to be loved, she needed to be thinner. Kids at school teased her about her weight even though she wasn't much overweight. She was chosen last for teams and had few friends. Eating was a way of escaping the pain of being ostracized. As she grew older, when her mother commented that she shouldn't be eating, she became angry and belligerent: "Don't tell me what to do." To escape her mother's criticism, she snuck food into her room. As an adult, she still had a strong rebel internal voice, but she also developed a voice that reflected her feelings of vulnerability. Part of her wanted to be healthy and not eat indiscriminately.

On the other hand, children who are told "You can do it" are more likely to believe in their abilities and to try new challenges. Being praised or acknowledged for good achievements, even if the achievements aren't perfect, contributes to higher self-esteem and greater self-confidence. Children absorb not only what parents say, but also what they do. Parents who are supportive when a child's actions fall short boost the child's self-esteem. Such a child probably has an inner voice that offers messages of self-confidence and promotes a positive, take-charge attitude.

In a similar way, the child who has high-achieving parents may internalize the nonverbal message that it is important to set high expectations and do well even if the parents never actually say so. The father who gets into arguments easily and acts aggressively toward others may influence his son to behave in a similar way. A parent who defers to others and is meek and unassertive teaches a child to be the same. The mother who models taking care of others first and being a people pleaser is likely to raise a child who also becomes a caretaker and a people pleaser.

This is what happened to Gaby, mentioned in the opening vignette in chapter 1. Her mother was a caretaker, and Gaby adopted caretaking behaviors as a teen that continued into adulthood. As such, she took on responsibility for other people's thoughts, feelings, and behaviors. Saying no was difficult for her. Also, like her mother, she rarely let others know when she was upset. Those few times when she expressed her anger, she quickly "took back" her feelings and apologized. After even minor conflicts, she would eat to forget about her negative thoughts. Gaby had a Caretaker voice that lacked assertiveness and needed approval and love from others.

Another woman realized that she regularly confronted anyone she thought did not treat her well. Growing up, her father had demanded she fight back both physically and verbally in such circumstances. She learned to be vigilant for any transgressions people might make. Being always on the alert kept her stirred up. Eating, especially at night, let her relax and provided relief from needing to watch out for people who might offend her. Anger was a prevalent emotion for her, and it was often hard to control. This was her Blaming internal voice.

Some children adopt behavior that is the opposite of one of their parent's and identify instead with the other parent or an admired person, such as a teacher or coach outside the immediate family. One man who had an angry father became a caretaker like his mother, eschewing conflict as she had always done. Another person whose mother was highly critical of others adopted the more forgiving attitude of their father. Another had a friend whose mother was supportive and whom they thought of as a "second mother." This support offset the criticism experienced at home.

In general, the comments and attitudes expressed by parents, caretakers, peers, and significant others eventually become incorporated into a person's inner voices, each of which can be characterized by its own kind of self-talk.

Identifying Your Inner Voices

It is usually possible to name each of your voices according to the things each one says, its perspective, and beliefs. In this section, you will find descriptions of common "voices" that characterize self-talk for many people. At times, some voices are more prominent than others. Each voice reflects a subpersonality or part of your personality. Identifying your most primary and, perhaps, troublesome voices allows you to figure out the disowned voice that is its opposite. In doing so, you will have greater choice in how you behave and will be less likely to fuse with either voice.

It is unlikely that these voices will disappear altogether or change significantly, and that is not the aim. Voice Dialogue, however, suggests that a helpful strategy can be to introduce more healthy self-talk to your Operating Ego. According to Voice Dialogue, your Operating Ego is the more mature part of you that was originally the Protector/Controller self. This self, armed with healthy self-talk, speaks from your internalized understanding of what is best for you. You may choose to give this self/voice a different name, such as Best Friend or

Wise Self. For now, consider which of the following voices give you trouble, and which voices are their healthy opposites.

The Critic

The Critic is judgmental, faultfinding, and self-critical. At times, this voice may sound like a scolding parent, pointing out your faults and commenting on shortcomings. It may discount achievements and is likely to attribute successes to luck, timing, or an accident of fate. You may hear the Critic in your head make "you" statements, as in: "There must be something wrong with you that you're not losing weight." "You are so stupid." Or the Critic may use "I" statements: "I should know better." "I hate my fat thighs." "Compared to her, I'm really fat." "I'll never measure up." "I hate myself for being fat." "I don't deserve to eat anything."

The Critic steals your self-confidence, undermines your self-esteem, and demoralizes you. It promotes shame and guilt. The Critic can prevent you from even making an effort, or ensure that you give up your efforts prematurely by calling upon your Procrastinator voice to join in: "I'll start my diet tomorrow." At its worst, the Critic can create or exacerbate depression by saying: "I'm the problem." "I'm never going to change." "My life is a mess."

The Critic's judgments may extend to others as well, finding faults with their behaviors, ideas, and accomplishments. The Critic can be self-righteous or envious of others: "Why don't people just mind their own business and leave me alone?" "She thinks she's so great because she's skinny." The Critic may join hands with your Perfectionist voice, which holds others to high standards: "She doesn't measure up."

The Critic wants to be "right" in all matters of opinion. To be right, the Critic believes the other person must be wrong. As a result, the Critic can be argumentative and unreasonable. Here is where the Critic joins forces with the Blamer: "She's wrong."

The opposite of the Critic, the disowned self, is that part of you that is accepting and forgiving. It has self-compassion and compassion for others. The disowned self readily feels empathy for others and is kindhearted. Its manner is soft, gentle, and easy. It pardons the self and others when something doesn't go well. A good name for the self that is opposite the Critic is the Compassionate Self.

The Worrier

The Worrier voice whispers thoughts that make you fearful and anxious. It predicts dire events that usually have a low likelihood of happening or that cannot be controlled. The Worrier voice often starts thoughts with "What if . . .": "What if I gain weight?" "What if they don't like me?" "What if I make a mistake?" "What if I say something stupid?" "What if I have a panic attack?" With these catastrophizing thoughts, your Worrier voice makes you feel upset, anxious, fearful, inadequate, and even panic-stricken at times.

Or, the Worrier may have thoughts that start with "Maybe . . .": "Maybe I'll regain the weight I lost." "Maybe they won't like me." "Maybe I'll make a mistake." "Maybe I'll say something stupid." "Maybe I'll have a panic attack."

Other Worrier thoughts take the form of if/then predictions: "If a man were to see my body, then he wouldn't love me." "If I make a mistake, I'll get fired." "If I lose my job, I'll never get another one as good." "If I have a panic attack, then I won't be able to cope."

The Worrier voice ruminates about scary events that haven't happened yet and generally have a low probability of happening. One man worried he would lose his job if he made a single mistake even though his job reviews were consistently good. A college student worried that if she did poorly on a single test she wouldn't be admitted to graduate school. A woman worried that she would regain the weight she had lost if she made a single high-calorie food choice.

Worrying cannot control any of these events. The Worrier engages in a variety of cognitive distortions, such as fortune-telling and all-or-nothing thinking or catastrophizing. (See chapter 11, "Managing Thinking and Self Talk" to learn more about cognitive distortions.)

One person worried that he might have married the wrong person even though he admitted that he was mostly happy in his marriage. Another person worried that she would run out of money even though she lived frugally and had a substantial portfolio. Yet another woman, who was promoted to a high-ranking job, worried that if anyone found out she came from a blue-collar family she would be removed from her position. Such worries are unfounded fears.

Often the Worrier worries about situations that cannot be changed or influenced. One woman worried that her son might never marry even though he was only 31 and had regular dates. Another worried that others would think badly of her even though she had no way of knowing what they were thinking. She engaged in a mind-reading cognitive distortion. As a result, she avoided social situations. With such worrying, anxiety increases and getting something to eat can be a wrong-headed solution used to help reduce anxiety and provide a distraction.

The Worrier is hypersensitive to threat—real or imagined. The Worrier may expect others to be critical and disapproving, and fears being the target of disapproval, criticism, and rejection. The Worrier compares their performance to that of others and worries, "I don't measure up." As a result, the Worrier voice can lead you to avoid situations in which you think someone else will find fault with or criticize you. By trying to anticipate and avoid problems, the Worrier creates actual problems caused by their spiraling out-of-control anxiety. If you are a Worrier, you can get caught up in a swirl of worry thoughts, like so many dry leaves kicked up by the wind. The part of you that is the opposite of the Worrier thinks rationally about the reality of threats and your ability to cope. It is cool-headed and discerns what can be influenced and what cannot and accepts the latter with equanimity and calmness. If anxiety appears, the Equanimity voice is cool and steady. It knows anxiety is just a feeling that comes and goes, and to fight it is to make it worse. Equanimity is self-confident and self-assured. Fears may present, but Equanimity is able to use common sense and maintain the necessary presence of mind to handle situations that can be influenced.

The Caretaker

The Caretaker voice tells you to put the needs of others first. This voice is sometimes known as the People Pleaser. It advocates that you nurture other people or try to make them happy, often at your own expense. The Caretaker hopes that if you are nice to others, they will like you better or overlook the faults you think you have. The Caretaker says things like: "I can't ask my children and my family to change their way of eating for me." "It's not right to make others go without treats and suffer because I need to lose weight." "It's not polite to ask the hostess to change the menu for me. I don't want to hurt her feelings." "I would rather suffer than see someone else suffer."

The Caretaker tells you not to risk hurting or disappointing others, even if that means hurting or disappointing yourself. The Caretaker is afraid to take assertive action in relationships even when assertiveness is called for. It says yes when it really wants to say no. It instructs you to curry the approval of others by being nice, polite, agreeable, and undemanding. The Caretaker reminds you that to be liked and loved, you must defer to others. If you heed all the Caretaker's demands, you are likely to end up feeling unappreciated and resentful, as well as exhausted. Getting something to eat serves as a quick reward and "grazing" on food throughout the day can keep such feelings out of your mind altogether, at least temporarily.

An example of someone whose behavior was governed by her Caretaker voice was the woman who insisted on carrying bundles for others, even when the other person was not overburdened. "But I want to help," she would say when they protested. She felt good when she was helping, and she hoped she would be appreciated. She did everything for her husband, including fetching him a beer when he was watching football on TV. Quietly, however, she resented his apparent helplessness and insensitivity to her needs. She ate to feel better and, over time, she gained 40 pounds.

The opposite of the Care*taker* is the Care*giver*. The Caregiver gives without strings attached—without expecting approval in return. The Caregiver understands that taking care of oneself first enables you to better care for others. The Caregiver self doesn't assume responsibility for others' needs but, rather, offers assistance when necessary. The Caregiver respects others' rights to be responsible for their own thoughts, feelings, and behavior. This self has good boundaries and can say no without guilt.

The Victim

The Victim voice expresses feelings of helplessness and sometimes martyrdom. It may complain: "Poor me, why can't I be normal." "It's not fair that others can eat what they want, and I can't." "I can't help myself." "No one is there for me." "I can't get what I need." "I do so much for others but get nothing in return." Sometimes the Victim voice expresses despair and the expectation of failure: "I've been fat all my life. There's no hope for me." Because such thoughts are based on wrong assumptions, they lead to more bad decisions that are likely to lead to more pain, failure, and discouragement. The Victim voice can keep you from trying to change your lifestyle. It reminds you that you feel bad and eating helps you feel better for a while.

In some cases, the Victim complains of being different and not belonging. The Victim voice tells you to expect to be excluded by others and advocates avoiding situations where this could happen. One man explained: "No one would want to go out with me. No woman is attracted to a bald, fat man." A woman described her predicament: "I'd like to make friends, but I don't know how. I had a friend once, but she stopped calling. Even people at work don't seem to like me." Both people rely on food to distract themselves from bad feelings.

Of course, some people have suffered at the hands of others or have been dealt blows by events in their life. Even if this is so, allowing yourself to feel like a Victim and pitying yourself can become a bad habit that interferes with creating future happiness. Some people even embrace being a Victim because they feel it proclaims to the world how badly they have been treated. They fear that giving up their Victim story would allow others to think the situation couldn't have been so bad after all. One divorced woman said, "If I were to get on with my life and maybe even date again, it would mean I wasn't so hurt by all he did to me."

Allowing your Victim voice to prevail can cause you to feel like you are owed something, that you are entitled to compensation. This can be where the Victim and the Rebel join forces. "If it weren't for my mother harassing me about what I ate as a child, I'd be able to have more self-discipline. Now I feel like I should be able to eat whatever I want, when I want it."

The Victim can also join with the Blamer or the Critic and reveal feelings of anger or bitterness. One man felt betrayed by his own body, and he punished himself repeatedly with angry binges. His voices said things like: "I hate myself." "I can't control my eating." "I'm disgusting." "I have a lousy family and a lousy life." Or the Victim and Blamer may voice complaints together: "Doctors' offices should have bigger chairs without arms. After all, large people have to wait for doctors too." "I'm sick and tired of seeing all those magazines at the checkout stand showing skinny women." "Obesity is a handicap. Airlines should offer larger seats without additional charge for handicapped people like me."

The opposite of the Victim is the voice of Responsibility. This part of you thinks you are responsible for your life and what happens to you. This voice doesn't think you caused your pain and misfortune but, rather, that you must cope with it. It acknowledges that there is pain in life, and no one gets through life without some pain and disappointment. The Responsibility voice promotes self-esteem and confidence. It questions negative thoughts and doesn't become fused with them. When Responsibility joins with Optimism, life goes smoothly.

The Blamer

The Blamer voice shifts responsibility for behavior to others or to external circumstances. The Blamer believes: "It is not my fault." It doesn't let you take responsibility for whatever role you played in the outcome of events. The Blamer constantly is blaming others, the past, or "something unknown" for life being difficult: "It's not my fault I can't lose weight." "Nobody cares." "If it weren't for my (children, stress, schedule, . . .), I'd be able to (exercise, stick to a diet, lose weight, . . .)." Often the blaming and defensiveness is to cover up feelings of defectiveness or failure. The Blamer encourages feelings of helplessness and anger.

Sophia, from the chapter-opening vignette, had a strong Blamer voice as well as a Rebel: "My mother dragged me to weight control programs when I was a kid. That's why I hate dieting." Another woman shifted responsibility for her overeating to her spouse: "He always wants to go out for fast food. He makes it too hard for me to control my weight." When someone else or something else is seen as the source of problem, the Blamer fails to notice his or her own responsibility and, thus, sees little point in trying to change behavior.

Do you tend to find fault with others frequently? Do you think that if only "they" would change, things would be okay? If you do, consider that in almost every situation, there is more than enough responsibility, if not blame, to go around. Consider what part you play in the way things turn out. If you engage in "the blame game," you may eat to express your anger, or you may eat to feel better when something goes wrong.

The opposite of the Blamer is the Accountability voice. This voice enables you to be accountable for the part you play in outcomes or to see things from a more neutral place without placing blame. In essence it asks: "What are the facts? Just give me the facts." Instead of negativity and criticalness, Accountability sees both sides of things: "When he criticized my work, I knew he was under a lot of stress from his boss. I do need to take more care when I send emails." Accountability enables you to be objective and do what you can to improve a situation. It helps you reach your full potential and avoid the pitfalls of blaming: "Losing weight takes self-discipline and I need to do better with this." Search the internet for videos on how to stop blaming behavior and become empowered. Dr. Brian Walsh, author of "Unleashing Your Brilliance," has a video on YouTube that speaks to this situation.

The Enforcer

The Enforcer voice (sometimes called the Rule Maker) has a penchant for orderliness, perfectionism, and rigid control. The Enforcer demands that you pay attention to rules, details, procedures, lists, and schedules at the expense of flexibility, openness, and efficiency. It tries to reduce uncertainty and control circumstances by making and enforcing rules. The Enforcer often requires that you pay extraordinary attention to detail and repeatedly check for possible mistakes: "I have to exercise every day." "I have to be doing something productive." "If I have a dessert, I have to do extra exercise." "I must avoid eating all fat."

The Enforcer feels that rules are necessary to get things done. It wants a rule for every situation. It is uncomfortable when there are no rules and shocked when someone breaks the rules, no matter the justification.

The Enforcer tells you that you "must" do things in a certain way. It tells you to do more, even when you are already doing too much. One person's Enforcer told him that he must guard against making a mistake. If that meant working overtime to get something just right, he did it. As a result, he often felt exhausted from working long hours and fretting about doing things perfectly. For this man, eating provided temporary relief from the expectations of the Enforcer.

The disowned opposite of the Enforcer is more relaxed, flexible, and laid back. This voice might be called the Easy voice. It can go with the flow and adapt to circumstances. It argues that rules should not be followed blindly, and it may allow you to follow the spirit of a rule in lieu of following the rule to the letter. It is aware of and comfortable with guidelines but doesn't need rules to feel safe. Fun is part of this voice, but Easy never takes fun too seriously. It can have a sense of humor: "Whoa, I think I blew that one." Easy is flexible in matters of authority and procedures while still being conscientious: "I really feel like having eggs Benedict, even though it's not one of my usual selections. It's on my 'rarely chosen' list and I don't have this often, so once in a while is okay."

The Rebel

The Rebel voice displays a strong sense of entitlement. It tells you that you should have what you want when you want it, and that self-discipline regarding eating is a bother and an infringement on personal choice. In the guise of self-acceptance, it can relieve you of the responsibility of doing something to curb your eating or your weight. It may even put down those who delay gratification or exercise moderation in their food choices.

Kirstie Alley is an actress who rose to fame on the late 1980s television show *Cheers*. Subsequently, she gained over 100 pounds. Despite admitting she didn't like how she looked, she was quoted as saying, "I haven't worked out for three years. I'm just going for the stuff that looks yummy." She said she tended to eat the most when she was really happy. The actress rebelliously acknowledged a taste for what she called "abundance"—she said she would have "twenty cakes" in a row, if she could.

Another woman, who also had a strong Rebel voice, was often touchy and easily annoyed by others who made suggestions to her about anything. "I told my doctor that I don't want to hear about my weight." Others found her touchiness and her bitter complaining about dieting and weight to be off-putting. Unwillingness to use self-discipline to control her eating urges made it difficult for her to follow a diet for long.

Sophia's Rebel voice conflicted with her Healthy voice. Her Healthy voice kept telling her that she would feel better if she lost some weight. She had a tough time resolving the conflict. Her Healthy voice won her over as it kept reminding her of the life value she held to want to feel better about herself and move around more easily. Even so, her Rebel voice kept up a constant barrage of hindering thoughts. Sophia recognized the hindering voice that didn't want her to exercise self-discipline and she chose to listen to her Healthy voice instead.

The Pessimist

The Pessimist focuses on how bad things are and sees everything in a negative light: "Life is boring." "The job is boring." "Life isn't fair." "Something is bound to go wrong." "Things will never get better." This voice ruminates about what went wrong in the past and uses this as evidence that the future is bound to be bleak. The Pessimist engenders expectations of failure. It is the voice of doom and gloom. Often, listening to the Pessimist voice is a way of fending off disappointment. The Pessimist is demoralizing. It whispers: "I've tried before and failed, so why should things be different now?" "No one else really cares, so why try?" "Bad luck is the story of my life."

If you have a strong internal Pessimist voice, others may think of you as having a negative attitude. The Pessimist in you can keep you from beginning a weight-management effort or cause you to quit prematurely. If you expect to fail, your ability to sustain effort is diminished. When your outlook on life is negative, food and eating may be the only bright spot in your day.

The Optimist is the obvious counterpart to the Pessimist. Research has shown that an optimistic worldview carries certain advantages. Optimists live longer and experience less stress. The Optimist sees hardships as "learning experiences." The Optimist voice tells you to believe in yourself and your abilities, and to expect good things to happen. Negative events are minor setbacks to be easily overcome, while positive events are evidence of more good things to come. The Optimist sees events as short term, changeable, and mostly under their control; the Pessimist sees events as long-lasting, out of their control, and subject to luck or other external forces.

Dr. Martin Seligman, the author of a book entitled *Learned Optimism: How to Change Your Mind and Your Life,* explains why it is best to be an optimist. To hear Dr. Martin Seligman discuss his ideas about optimism, search YouTube for his videos on "learned optimism."

The Excuse Maker

The Excuse Maker finds excuses, provides justifications, and offers spurious rationalizations to make it okay for you to take actions that deviate from healthy behavior. The Excuse-Maker argues "Yes, but . . .": "I'd like to eat better, but with my schedule, it's impossible." "I shouldn't eat dessert, but I deserve a little treat now and then." "I shouldn't eat this extra serving, but no one will see me, so why not?" "I've blown it already today, so why not eat what I want." The Excuse Maker undermines motivation, hinders coping behavior, and defeats efforts to manage eating or weight. It's easy to come up with excuses for letting your impulses get in your way: "I'll have just one."

The Excuse Maker says: "I'll start tomorrow" "I'm not ready yet." It ignores or minimizes facts about the health effects of disordered eating, or it attempts to convince you that it's okay to delay taking action: "Yes, I'm overweight, but my blood pressure and cholesterol are fine." "Just because I weigh 220 pounds doesn't mean I'm not fit." "I'm only 40. I don't have to worry about heart disease yet." Excuse making keeps you stuck wanting change but not doing anything to achieve it. Granted, it helps you avoid the pain of acting, but it keeps you from getting what you say you want.

The opposite voice to the Excuse Maker is the Responsibility voice that reminds you to take personal responsibility for your actions. This voice tells you to remember your values and goals and act accordingly. It calls you out when you make excuses and spurious rationalizations to behave in ways that undermine your health and weight-management effort. The Responsibility voice knows that you are in charge of your behavior and not any person or anything can "make you do it" except yourself. It reminds you that everything is your choice. Taking responsibility for your life is the extra ingredient that makes action a more natural thing. Your Responsibility self reminds you to be proactive, not passive.

Working with Your Inner Voices

The first step in working with your inner voices is to develop a greater awareness of which ones are the most prominent in your thinking and most affect your eating behavior. When you read the descriptions in the previous section, did any of these voices sound familiar to you? If so, these are the voices that most influence you. To start listening in on your self-talk, keep a journal in which you record what you are saying to yourself. Try to capture as best you can what each of your voices typically says. As you record your thoughts, you will notice that certain themes emerge.

You probably don't have all the voices listed in the chapter, and you may have others that are not described here. Some of your voices are likely to be more prominent or troublesome than others. Use your observing self to notice which voices and thoughts run your life.

An interesting video by Mary Lore, author of "Managing Thought: How Do Your Thoughts Rule Your World," talks about watching inner thoughts and observing them rather than acting on them. Search on YouTube to find it.

Helping Your Supportive Voice

After identifying your voices from the preceding section, you need to develop a new voice—your supportive and protecting voice. You can give this voice a new name if you wish—one that means something to you. You might call it your Wise Self, your Best Friend, the voice of the Conscious Self, or the voice of the Coach.

The Coach is a particularly good metaphor for a supportive voice. If you have ever participated in a sport and had the benefit of a good coach, you know that such a coach is always on your side. Even when he or she offers criticism, it is never mean or disparaging. A good coach is willing to show you how to improve, is truthful about your problems, is encouraging when things get rough, and can guide and inspire you.

To help your supportive voice, you need to find thoughts that will counterbalance—that is, oppose or offset—the negative and hindering thoughts expressed by some of your subpersonalities. It is unlikely you will ever entirely rid yourself of all hindering inner voices, but you can moderate their effect on you by creating and rehearsing counterbalancing statements or self-talk. These may sound like the thoughts of the disowned opposite voices that were described in the previous sections. You need to develop counterbalancing thoughts for your "Coach" or "Healthy Self" or whatever you wish to call the voice that will help you achieve your goals.

Creating Counterbalancing Statements

We all need help learning how to pay attention to thoughts that will help us and that will not hinder our efforts at living a lifestyle that is consistent with our guiding principles and values. The following list details some helpful guidelines for constructing counterbalancing self-talk. After the guidelines, you will find examples of hindering thoughts and counterbalancing statements you can use to counter such negative self-talk.

1. If there is some truth to a negative or hindering thought, create a compound sentence in which the first part of the sentence acknowledges that truth. In the second part of the compound sentence, create a thought that opposes or offsets the negative idea with a helpful one. For example: "I sometimes overeat so I need to use portion control." The first part of the sentence, "I sometimes overeat," is the hindering thought, and the second part of the sentence, "I need to use portion control," is a helping self-instruction that offsets the idea that you sometimes overeat.

2. Use the conjunction *and* (not *but*) to connect two sentences, one hindering thought and one counterbalancing thought.

(The conjunction *but* negates the sentence that goes before; instead, to be believable to you, the negative or hindering truth needs to be acknowledged and validated.) Don't say: "I need to lose weight *but* it's hard." Say: "I need to lose weight *and* it's hard." The "and" balances the thought and leaves room for change.

3. If the hindering thought doesn't contain a truth and instead expresses an opinion, attitude, conclusion, worry, or other kind of hindering thought, create an opposing thought that expresses a truth, a preference, or gives a self-instruction. Instead of: "I think losing weight is too hard," substitute: "Even though losing weight is hard, I am going to try by using portion control."

4. Make sure you can believe the counterbalancing thought you create and that it is relevant to you. Take the example in #3: you have to believe portion control is something that works and that you can do it.

5. Remember that all thoughts are short-lived and do not necessarily constitute an objective truth. Encourage your observing self to simply notice hindering self-talk and make note of its opposite voice. You might have the thought: "I can't do this." Remind yourself that this is just a thought, not a truth. It just so happens that this thought appeared, and as long as you don't hold onto it—fuse with it—that thought will soon be replaced by a different thought.

Examples of Hindering and Counterbalancing Thoughts

The following are examples of counterbalancing thoughts created to offset or balance self-defeating or hindering thoughts:

Hindering thought: "Poor me, why can't I eat like other people."

Counterbalancing thought: "Some people do seem to be able to eat what they like, and I can't if I want my weight to be healthy." (This counterbalancing thought acknowledges the truth—some people seem to be able to eat what they want—and it redirects thinking to long-term health goals.)

Hindering thought: "I should do better."

Counterbalancing thought: "I'd prefer to do better, and I need to focus on what I need to do right now." (This counterbalancing thought replaces a "should" thought with a preference thought and links it to a self-instructional thought.)

Hindering thought: "What if they think I'm stupid?"

Counterbalancing thought: "I can't control what people think and worrying about it just makes me anxious." (This counterbalancing thought states the fact that you can't control what people think and refutes the worry thought by reminding you of the consequences of worrying about something that can't be controlled.)

Hindering thought: "I feel fat."

Counterbalancing thought: "I'm my worst critic, and I need to focus on making healthy choices instead of berating myself." (This counterbalancing thought states the fact "I'm my worst critic" and redirects the focus of thinking to managing behavior.)

Hindering thought: "I've blown it. I may as well give up."

Counterbalancing thought: "Okay, I made a poor choice. I need to learn from that mistake and start again right now to get back on track." (The first sentence in this counterbalancing thought states that fact that "I made a poor choice" and gives a self-instruction that tells you what to do instead of giving up.)

Hindering thought: "I can't control my eating."

Counterbalancing thought: "Sometimes I don't control my eating, and there are other times when I do. I need to stay focused on doing the best I can." (This counterbalancing thought shifts the all-or-nothing evaluation that "I never control my eating" to one that reflects a moderate position, "sometimes I lose control," and it then provides an instruction to "focus on doing the best I can" that can motivate appropriate action."

13

Managing Stress

Madison just couldn't say no to others' requests. Madison worked as a personal cook, and she planned all the meals five days a week for the family of her employer. Planning and managing menus were stressful. Occasionally Madison's employer would ask her to do a Saturday party for twenty to thirty people on short notice. Madison was afraid to decline this request for fear of losing her job. She nibbled as she cooked and often ate the leftovers. Her weight kept climbing, and she worried that her employer might begin to object to her appearance. Then she learned to be more assertive. She also learned how to elicit the relaxation response and use deep breathing to relieve stress. As she learned to take better care of herself, her anxiety eased, and her nibbling diminished.

Stress is a physical, mental, or emotional experience that causes bodily or mental tension. Stresses can be external, like going to a party where lots of exciting foods are available, or internal, like worrying about having to deal with food temptations.

Humans experience stress when we perceive a threat and view it as taxing or exceeding our resources for coping. Events or problem situations do not themselves produce stress; rather, the way we understand an event determines our personal reaction to it. As the philosopher Epictetus once said, "Men are disturbed not by things, but by the view they take of them." Echoing this sentiment, Shakespeare wrote, "Nothing is neither good nor bad, but thinking makes it so." When you encounter something that feels threatening and you aren't sure you can handle it, you feel stressed. A different person facing the same event is not as likely to feel stressed if they believe they can handle the situation.

For example, if you are unable to meet a deadline for a project at work and you decide you won't be able to make it, you will be quite upset. You might even put off starting or working further on the project to avoid thinking about it and having to experience the anxiety about the deadline. Someone else might not see the same situation as terrible and would simply negotiate a new deadline with the boss. That person is unlikely to feel as stressed as you, either because they see the situation as less threatening or because they feel they can handle it. How you appraise, or assess, a perceived threat and your ability to cope determines your stress level.

If you would like to find out your perceived stress level, a self-test developed and validated by psychologist Sheldon Cohen and associates is available on the internet. Search for "Perceived Stress Scale." The Perceived Stress Scale (PSS) is the most widely used psychological instrument for measuring the perception of stress. It is a measure of the degree to which situations in one's life are considered stressful.

Appraisal of Stress

Stress appraisal is a two-stage process. In the *primary appraisal stage*, you decide whether a threat is real or imagined and how dangerous you believe it to be. Sometimes it is hard to tell whether the perceived threat is real. In that case, further investigation is needed to determine the accuracy of your perception. It is helpful to consider the probability versus the possibility of the threat being real. (Theoretically anything is possible; the real question is how probable is it?) For instance, it is not very probable that you will become obese from a single overindulgence, and your fear that you will is likely imagined. Of course, repeated indulgences can lead to weight gain.

If you decide the threat is real and probable, you must then decide whether it is significant. How much is it likely to hurt you physically or emotionally? It could be that the threat is real, but you may be overestimating how bad it really is. It may be true that a single indulgence could lead to some weight gain, but it will probably not result in large, sudden weight gain. Sometimes people perceive threats where there are none. For example, you aren't likely to develop diabetes from eating just a little sugar, though eating lots of sugary foods will put you at greater risk for diabetes if such eating leads to obesity.

What if the threat is significant and highly probable—like planning to go to dinner at your grandmother's house where you know she urges you to eat more? Of course, the best thing is to avoid exposure to avoidable threats. If a threat is unavoidable, like having your car break down on a dark highway or visiting your grandmother, you must cope with it as best you can. It may be helpful to have a contingency plan at the ready for coping with a car breakdown, like having a charged cell phone with you at all times. At your grandmother's house, you might try being more assertive.

The *secondary appraisal stage* is about evaluating your options for coping. If you think you can cope with a threat, you are likely to be less stressed though still alert to taking necessary action. If you decide you can't cope regardless of whether or not the threat is actually real and significant, you will feel stressed, and you may try to avoid or escape the thoughts of a perceived stressful situation. Stress results when you perceive a threat to be real and significant or you think you will be unable to cope. Whether or not you experience an event as stressful depends on three factors:

1. The degree to which the event or thought is evaluated by you as potentially harmful, threatening, or challenging: The more harmful, threatening, or challenging the event, the greater the stress. Remember, anything is theoretically possible; what makes a threat significant is the probability (not the possibility) that it is likely to happen. For example, if you think going to a party will provide food temptations, such a threat may be real and probable.

2. The options you have for coping: The more options you have, the less stressed you feel. If you have a plan for coping with food temptations at a party, you are less likely to feel stress (and you'll enjoy the party more).

3. The coping strategies you use to deal with the event: The more adaptive or helpful your strategies are, the more likely stress will be reduced. If you plan in advance to give yourself permission to eat just three food options at the party, knowing your limits will help you.

Stress and Coping

Stress demands coping. That is, it requires some sort of adaptation or response to the demand or set of demands that are perceived as stressful. Research dissects coping strategies into three broad components: (1) the brain and body's response to stress, (2) the mind's cognitive or thinking response to stress, and (3) how you have learned to respond to stress.

The body has its own way of coping with stress. Any threat or challenge that an individual perceives in the environment triggers a chain of neuroendocrine events. One of these is the secretion of *catecholamines*, such as *epinephrine* and *norepinephrine*, which stimulate the "fight or flight" response, which in turn lead to an elevated heart rate and a rise in blood pressure. This is followed by the release of *cortisol*, the stress hormone. Prolonged secretion of cortisol will lead to health problems, such as the breakdown of the cardiovascular system, the digestive system, the musculoskeletal system, and the immune system. When a person cannot recover from ongoing or chronic stress, physical exhaustion results.

The cognitive component of stress is based on how an individual appraises the situation. According to Lazarus and Folkman in their book *Stress, Appraisal and Coping*, a person's appraisal of threat and the unique coping strategies they use determines their level of stress. In chapter 12 of *Maximize Your Body Potential*, we discuss the overestimation of threat, which causes anxiety and stress, and the underestimation of coping ability resulting in catastrophizing.

The learned component of coping with stress includes a wide range of stress-management techniques. These include changing the way you think about a situation (for example, becoming better at appraising threat and your ability to cope) and using techniques like the relaxation response, deep breathing, engaging in meditation, guided imagery, and exercising. There are also failed strategies for stress management and these result in lack of control over stress. One is the phenomenon of *learned helplessness*—giving up without trying hard to survive stress. This phenomenon has also been linked to depression. (The opposite of learned helplessness is *learned optimism*, discussed in chapter 12.)

Both the mind (the cognition and learning components) and the brain/body play a role in stress and coping. Once threat is perceived and coping is initially evaluated cognitively, the body experiences arousal. Cognitive coping is clearly a complex process influenced by both personality characteristics of the person experiencing the stress and even the social and physical characteristics of the setting. A strong-willed person who has good social support is likely to be better at coping with stress. And there is an optimal level of stress that facilitates good performance; some experienced stress stimulates action. But when coping strategies are overwhelmed by demands of the environment, such as not having enough food, experiencing high temperature or noise that irritates, the possibility of injury, or having your coping strategies fail, stress becomes unhealthy.

Consider the example of the person whose home air conditioning failed and her house temperature rose to an uncomfortable level. First, she called a company that fixed air conditioners, but they couldn't come for two days. Next, she changed into cooler clothes, but the heat in the house was starting to overwhelm her. Finally, she knew she had to get out of the house until the temperature cooled down as the sun went down. She opened all the windows, knowing that, by evening, the temperature outside would become more reasonable. Then she took a book, made some iced tea for herself, and went into her backyard where she sat on a lawn chair under a shady tree. Once she sat down to read her book, she was pleased to notice there was a cooling breeze.

In this example, heat in the environment caused stress. She tried several coping strategies before she hit on one that worked. In the meantime, she experienced considerable stress.

Coping Skills

Coping is any cognitive or behavioral effort you make to handle stress. Some of these strategies are more effective than others. Coping skills for managing stress can be either problem-focused or emotion-focused. Let's look at a few.

Problem-Focused Coping

Problem-focused coping involves problem-solving and other active attempts to change a problematic event or stressful situation. The person whose house air conditioning failed had to do problem-focused coping. This type of coping is also helpful for making positive changes in lifestyle. It is best used when a situation or event can be influenced or changed in some way. Many people with an eating or weight problem don't use problem-focused coping. They often believe it is better to avoid a problem than to confront it directly.

They may use eating as a way of distracting their attention from problems or difficulties. Or they may just give up trying to make a change because they don't know how to go about it, or they think their efforts will be in vain.

Suppose you are attempting to incorporate exercise into your life. Two approaches might be to join a gym or to hire a personal trainer to come to your house at times that are convenient for you. One of these solutions might work, but what if you have one or more small children and/or a career to manage, and there appears to be no time in your schedule for exercise? Now the question is: How can you modify the situation to make time for regular exercise given that you have limitations? Engage in problem-solving: perhaps you can exchange time with another parent, work out during your lunch hour at work, or get your spouse to watch the kids while you take time for exercise. It helps if your spouse or employer is willing to work with you to find a solution. The core problem is how to make time for exercise. An associated problem is how to find someone to watch the children while you exercise or how to balance your need to exercise with the demands of your career. When you practice problem-solving coping, you work to address the problems that are stopping you from exercising.

Some people don't use problem-focused coping because they think there is no easy or available solution. Or perhaps they think they have no right to ask someone else to change (if the solution to the problem involves another person). Thoughts such as "I don't want to inconvenience my spouse or coworker" or "What if they get upset?" may prevent the person from taking action. Once the decision is made that the situation cannot be changed, they simply give up and find some other means—usually eating—of forgetting about the problem.

Here's an example: Hannah had a husband who snacked in front of the TV every night. His snacking made it hard for her to resist snacking too. She thought it was not fair of her to ask him to change his behavior just because she wanted to change her eating habits.

This belief kept her from broaching the subject with him until her therapist urged her to bring it up for discussion. To her surprise, he agreed that he too shouldn't eat "junk" food, and they decided to adopt healthier eating together.

In a similar, but more difficult, situation, the wife of a man needing to lose weight did most of the shopping and the cooking. She too was overweight but wasn't motivated to do anything about it. She bought sweets and snack foods for the children and herself, and these were readily available to tempt him. He had to find other ways to cope. Sometimes he could do the cooking, but mostly he had to decide for himself to use portion control at mealtime. When snacks and goodies were available, he had to decide what foods to eat. His value of good health was the guiding principle he used when faced with temptation. This focus helped him ignore the temptations.

Sometimes it is relatively easy to influence a difficult situation with problem-focused coping, but more often it is necessary to find creative solutions to make change. When a difficult situation is not amenable to influence, the problem becomes how to make the best of it. For instance, suppose Hannah's spouse had refused to change his snacking while in front of the TV. Hannah then would be faced with finding another way to solve her problem—perhaps watching TV or reading in another room. It's possible she would also have to manage her hurt feelings or irritation about his lack of cooperation. In that event, she would need to employ effective emotion-focused coping strategies as well.

Emotion-Focused Coping

Emotion is defined as a strong, subjective feeling often accompanied by a physical reaction. The emotional "knowing system" is like the cognitive knowing system and is another, but separate, way of experiencing ourselves and the environment. Emotions alert the mind to evaluate the situation and act.

Effective emotion-focused coping helps mitigate the negative thoughts and feelings that accompany a stressful situation. Such coping is most needed when there is little chance of changing or influencing a difficult situation. Even if the situation can be changed, good emotion-focused coping skills are often needed to manage residual upset or stress.

Take the example just given of Hannah. Before she worked up the courage to ask her husband to change, she worried he would refuse. She was anxious for several days as she considered what she wanted to do. Not knowing how he would react, she put off doing anything. Finally, she worked up her courage and asked him to change. When he agreed, she was relieved.

Emotion-focused coping strategies can be either effective or ineffective. Ineffective emotion-focused strategies include avoiding, distancing, minimizing, or discharging. Examples of *avoidance strategies* include overeating, drinking too much, gambling, overspending, and abusing drugs. These behaviors divert your attention from the problem and its associated thoughts and feelings. *Distancing* is an emotional escape strategy that involves emotional detachment or denial. The person using this strategy stops caring or insists that there really is no problem at all; they know there is a problem but decide to live with it. With *minimizing*, the person acknowledges there is a problem but discounts its importance. For example, "Yes, he drinks, but it's not that much." *Emotional discharge strategies* are verbal or behavioral expressions of unpleasant emotions that serve to reduce tension, especially anger-related tension. Examples of discharge strategies include yelling, cursing, hitting, throwing things, and slamming doors.

These emotion-focused coping strategies may temporarily divert attention from painful feelings or provide the appearance of a solution to a problem, but in the long run they create a worse problem. These strategies do nothing to change the existing stressful situation. Furthermore, reliance on avoidance, distancing, or minimizing interferes with assessing the problem properly and delays the adoption of more effective coping strategies. Unfortunately, people who are prone to stress tend to fall back on ineffective emotion-focused coping because they have not been good problem-solvers in the past. In particular, those with an eating or weight problem tend to rely on ineffective emotion-focused coping strategies.

Effective emotion-focused coping uses the observing self to notice thoughts and feelings that are occurring and, rather than struggling with them or trying to avoid them, the observing self simply notices and does not become embroiled in what the mind and emotions are doing. More on emotion-focused coping is provided later in this chapter.

Improving Problem-Focused Coping

Effective problem-focused coping involves assessing and defining a problem accurately, generating possible solution alternatives, deciding which to try, and evaluating how effective your choices might be in influencing the situation. If none of the solutions work, you have probably not defined the problem accurately; go back to the first step and redefine the problem.

Defining the Problem

Defining a problem correctly is a crucial part of good problem-solving skills. It involves seeking out available and relevant facts, describing these facts clearly, separating facts from assumptions, and identifying obstacles and conflicts. Take the example of the woman who minimized her husband's drinking by telling herself, "He doesn't drink that much." She could consult her doctor or a therapist and discuss how much he drinks to find out if it is a problem. Or she could search the internet for information on problem drinking. Her first step is to face the problem by getting accurate information and then acting.

Some people may have difficulty defining a problem due to their tendency to describe problems in overly vague, general, exaggerated, or negative terms. For example, you may lump several problems into one and feel overwhelmed or unable to find a solution. Feeling overwhelmed should be your first clue that several problems are being lumped together with others; you need to tease apart the problems and tackle each one separately.

Take the example introduced earlier of the man whose overweight wife was not particularly supportive of his weight-management efforts. He had to break the big problem down into more manageable pieces: "How do I handle meals?" "How do I handle tempting goodies?" "What do I do when the wife and kids are snacking in front of the TV?" And so forth.

In defining a problem, it is important to be concrete and focus on behavior. For example, rather than defining the problem as "I need to lose weight," break this into specific component problems that focus on behavior: "I need to reduce calories by cutting back portions," "I need to eliminate sweets," "I need to avoid snacking after dinner," or "I need to schedule time for exercise." Although the objective is to lose weight, the problem definition directs focus to the specific behavior changes that need to be made to achieve your goal rather than focusing on the goal itself.

Self-monitoring can be helpful in defining a problem. This technique was introduced in chapter 7, "Changing Behavior." Self-monitoring is a means of gathering information about behavior patterns by identifying the antecedents and consequences of a particular behavior. One way to self-monitor is to record information about your food habits, such as time of day, food eaten, location, level of hunger, thoughts, feelings/emotions, physical sensations, and how you felt afterward. Once you have this information, decide where you can make changes in your behavior.

Brainstorming Alternative Solutions

Brainstorming involves generating lots of possible solutions without screening or evaluating them. This invites creativity and encourages you to see a problem and be able to think of different ways to cope. After defining your problem and coming up with a list of various solutions via brainstorming, you will want to evaluate each solution for its merits. For example, one person who saw lack of exercise as a problem generated the following list of possible solutions: (1) contact a friend to walk with on a regular basis, (2) hire a personal trainer, (3) join a gym, (4) purchase or rent workout videos to do at home.

Implementing and Evaluating a Solution

Once you have generated a few possible solutions, consider how practical, as well as how effective, each alternative is likely to be. Then choose one or more and try them out. Be sure to give each alternative a fair chance to work.

After you have implemented a solution, evaluate the results. If the solution you tried brings partial success, consider how you might improve on it, or decide if partial success is good enough. Be sure you aren't being unrealistic in your expectations. For example, if you try brushing your teeth to interrupt an urge to eat and it works some of the time but not all of the time, it may still be a good strategy to use. If the solution you try doesn't work at all, try another. If nothing works, consider the possibility that you have not defined the problem accurately; in this case, it is likely there is more than one problem in your initial definition. Go back and start again. Table 13.1 summarizes the steps involved in problem-solving.

Improving Emotion-Focused Coping

Successful emotion-focused coping strategies include eliciting the relaxation response; using mindfulness, deep breathing, imagery, and meditation; learning distress-tolerance and emotion-regulation skills; learning to be assertive; and managing interpersonal conflict effectively.

Stress and the negative emotions that accompany it are often the precursors to overeating. Using relaxation to cope with stress and subsequent urges to eat can be helpful. Learning to be more relaxed in general, not just when the urge to eat is present, helps control anxiety and reduces your vulnerability to stress and episodes of overeating. There are several ways to elicit the relaxation response. One of

Table 13.1 **How to Problem-Solve Effectively**

1. Isolate and identify problems in concrete and specific terms. Define each problem in terms of behavior to be changed.

2. Treat "feeling overwhelmed" as a signal that several problems are being treated as one big one.

3. Brainstorm as many possible solutions to each problem as you can.

4. Choose one or more solutions and try them out.

5. Evaluate the effectiveness of the solutions you tried; be sure you have given them a fair chance of success.

6. Review the results. If one solution didn't help, try another. Return to step 4 and repeat the next steps until you find a solution. If you do not, go to step 7.

7. If none of the solutions you try work, go back and reassess the problem. Look for several problems masquerading as one problem.

the best ways to begin your relaxation training is with progressive deep-muscle relaxation. Search the internet for videos on how to do deep-muscle relaxation. Learning this basic skill will allow you to move on to master the more immediate method of using deep breathing to relax. Focusing on breathing while doing guided imagery is another way to find relaxation. YouTube gives examples of doing guided imagery, or you could google "guided imagery" to find other resources. Meditation is a mind relaxation technique and teaches you to not attach to thoughts as they pop into your head. Again, YouTube provides many examples of how to meditate.

Progressive Deep-Muscle Relaxation

If you do not know how to relax, progressive deep-muscle relaxation is an important place to start. You can purchase audiotapes, videotapes, DVDs, or streaming content that will introduce you to progressive relaxation techniques. Check your local bookstore or use the internet to find suitable material. Google "relaxation recordings" for various options. YouTube videos on the topic are a resource as well.

It is also possible to teach yourself deep-muscle relaxation. The aim of the process is to learn the difference between muscle tension and relaxation in two phases. The first phase involves learning how a tense muscle feels. The second phase involves discovering what tension *release* feels like. With this knowledge, you can tense and relax smaller muscle groups until, ultimately, you can tense and relax the whole body as one. Once you learn the long version—using smaller muscle groups and working up to doing the whole body— you can progress to a shortened version of relaxing your entire body at once to elicit the relaxation response more quickly.

To begin learning progressive deep-muscle relaxation, find a quiet, relaxing place where you will not be disturbed for ten to fifteen minutes. Sit or lie down, remove contact lenses or glasses, and loosen tight clothing. Start with your right hand. Make a fist as if you were having blood taken from your arm. Notice how your fist feels when it is tightened. Your muscles will be taut and strained, maybe even trembling. (Never tense so hard that it hurts.) Hold the tension for a few seconds, and then let go. Relax your fist, and let the tension slip away. Notice the warmth that flows into your hand when you let go and relax. Repeat the tensing and relaxing of your right hand a few times and notice the difference between the two phases. Does your hand throb or feel tight when tensed? Does your hand tingle or feel warm when relaxed?

Now progress to the other muscle groups. Move up the right arm to include the forearm with the hand, then the whole arm. Complete that arm, and then do the same sequence—hand, hand and forearm, whole arm—with the left arm. Next focus on your legs—first the right foot, then the foot and calf together, then the whole leg, followed by the left leg. (Do not include your arms when you are tensing and relaxing your legs.) After each tensing and relaxing a particular muscle group, notice the difference in sensations. Pay attention to these physical sensations.

Continue up your torso, tensing the buttocks, then the abdomen, then the chest, shoulders, and neck. For your head, tense and relax first the jaw only, then your forehead. Then tense all the facial muscles at the same time. Finally, tense and relax your whole body at once, including arms, legs, and torso. Notice the difference between feeling tense and letting go of tension. After you have tensed and relaxed your whole body for several repetitions, allow yourself to enjoy total relaxation for a few minutes before continuing your daily activities. Remember what this feels like, and when you are totally relaxed, remind yourself that you can achieve this state of relaxation whenever you choose just by telling yourself to relax and remembering the state of relaxation you achieved before. The feeling of warmth and relaxation tells you that you have elicited the relaxation response. Do the progressive deep-muscle relaxation exercise several times until you can easily slip into relaxation just by bringing your attention to the idea of relaxing. (Eliciting the relaxation response with progressive relaxation is also good for helping you fall asleep.)

After you are proficient at eliciting the relaxation response with the long procedure, you can do a shortened version that includes just four main muscle groups. The first step is to tense and relax both legs, feet, and buttocks at once. Then move up to the abdomen and chest for the second step. Next do the arms, shoulders, and neck at once. Finally do the face and head.

Deep Breathing

To elicit the relaxation response through deep breathing (also known as *diaphragmatic* or *belly breathing*), inhale slowly and deeply through your nose and allow your lungs to breathe in as much air as possible. Let your abdomen relax and expand, so that you take in more air. Once you have filled your lungs, hold your breath for a few seconds. Then exhale slowly through your mouth until your lungs feel almost empty, focusing on letting go of muscle tension throughout your body as you do so.

You may be able to learn to do this more easily by lying on your back on a firm bed or carpeted floor and placing a small accent pillow on your stomach. You should be able to observe the top of the pillow as it moves up and down with your breathing. Notice that the deeper you breathe, the higher the pillow rises. Recall the sensation of relaxation you had when you did the progressive deep-muscle relaxation exercise. Repeat the deep-breathing cycle several times until you feel more relaxed. Remind yourself that you can attain this state of relaxation again, anytime you choose, just by breathing deeply. And you can do this anywhere—in a meeting, at a movie, sitting with friends—without others really noticing.

Check the internet for stress-reducing apps that help you breathe in slow, measured intervals. Find one that allows you to change settings depending on how long you want to inhale and exhale. And look for an app that gives you simple audio and visual cues for pacing your breath. Several apps are available for free on the internet that will help you pace your breathing. One is the "Awesome Breathing: Pacer Timer." Check out other options by searching "breath pacing." Some apps make the sound of rain that rises and falls in sync with your breathing so you don't have to watch the screen. You can tune out and breathe deeply in response to the sound of rainfall.

Imagery

Imagery can also be used to evoke the relaxation response and improve your mood. *Imagery* involves allowing yourself to "see" in your mind's eye scenes or action, as in a movie. Everyone can call up mental images even if they think they can't. Dreams are one example of unconscious "mental movies." Daydreams are conscious "mental movies" that you direct. When you visualize a scene in your mind, you are consciously directing the imagery process. You can use imagery to evoke the relaxation response by visualizing a pleasant or relaxing scene. The scene can be based on a memory of some place you have actually been, or you can invent a place. The steps for doing imagery are given in table 13.2. Search the internet for apps that provide imagery exercises. You should be able to download free audio tracks for muscle relaxation, deep breathing, and imagery.

Table 13.2   **Using Imagery to Elicit the Relaxation Response**

1. Relax.	It is best to find a private place where you will not be interrupted for a period of time—perhaps ten to fifteen minutes. However, if necessary, you could do this anywhere (for example, on a park bench or on a bus) during whatever time you have available. Get as comfortable as you can. Close your eyes and, using the deep-breathing technique described previously, allow yourself to relax. Turn your focus inward and allow an image to arise without trying to control it. Remember, there is no right or wrong way to do imagery and with practice it becomes easier.
2. Picture a relaxing scene.	Allow a relaxing or pleasant scene to come to mind. Examples of such scenes might include a lovely beach, a sunny lake, a picturesque hiking trail, or the green grass of a quiet meadow. Direct your attention to the sensory details—the sounds, colors, smell, touch, and temperature. Notice the enjoyable aspects of the scene and give yourself permission to become more involved in it and more relaxed.
3. Bring the imagery to a close when you are ready.	Continue until you have enjoyed the mental imagery sufficiently and are feeling relaxed and satisfied. Tell yourself you can return to this place (the enjoyable scene) anytime you wish simply by taking several deep breaths. Without opening your eyes, allow the mental images to fade, then gently bring your consciousness back to the present. Open your eyes, stretch your muscles, and continue your day with an improved perspective.
4. Write out and record your relaxing scene ahead of time.	You may find it easier to do imagery if you write out the details of the scene you want to imagine. Then read aloud what you have written and record it on audiotape or on your phone to play back while you are relaxing. When you are recording your scene, take care to speak slowly and use a relaxing tone of voice.
5. Practice doing imagery.	Do imagery at least once a day, repeating steps 1 and 2 each time, until you feel confident in your ability to improve your mood by using imagery. If you wish, try different kinds of images to alter your mood.

Meditation

Meditation is relaxation for the mind. The aim is to quiet the mind by simply watching thoughts and not holding onto any of them. During meditation, the observing self listens to mind chatter as if from afar and doesn't attach to any thoughts that may come and go. Meditation starts by finding a quiet, comfortable place—you need not sit on the floor in a "lotus" position. It is okay to sit on a chair or on pillows on the floor as long as you are comfortable. Choose a time and place when you will not be interrupted. It helps to have a bell to sound your start, but this is not necessary. It also helps to have a clock to check your time, but don't set an alarm. Check the internet for an app that provides meditative white noise or environmental sounds, such as chimes, crickets, ocean and beach noises, and several different kinds of rain. There is an app that provides the sound of a Tibetan singing bowl and also provides a timer for turning off the sound and ending the meditation session. Search the internet to find an app that includes a timer for turning the sounds off at a specified time or after the number of minutes you want to meditate.

Once you get settled, start meditating by paying attention to your breathing. The practical effort required to focus completely on your breathing takes your mind off the constant chatter in your head. It also allows feelings to settle into a time of calm. At first, plan to do a fifteen-minute meditation session. Just focus on your breathing and allow yourself to relax. When thoughts come into your mind, just gently bring your focus back to your breathing and allow the thoughts to float away. Do the same thing with any sounds that may be intrusive. Gradually, the process of meditation takes on its own energy, resulting in feelings of peace and calm, and helping to open your self to new insights. Search YouTube for videos on how to meditate.

Keeping a Stress Diary

Keeping a diary of stressful events is another helpful tool for managing and improving your emotional coping skills. In the diary, record

stress events as you experience them. Identify and rate your feelings during the event from 0 to 10, least stressful to most stressful.
Write down the fundamental cause of the event, your physical symptoms during the event (for example, flushed face, increased heart
rate, sweating hands), and how well you think you handled it. Use
this diary to problem-solve better ways to handle such events in the
future. A printable stress diary template can be found by searching
the internet for "stress diary."

Managing Stress with Mindfulness

Dr. Marsha Linehan, a professor of psychology at the University
of Washington and a clinician, teaches mindfulness, distress tolerance, and emotion-regulation skills for coping with emotional
distress. Dr. Linehan first teaches her patients mindfulness skills,
which she regards as the basis for balancing rational thinking—the
"rational mind," in her terms—and emotional experiencing—the
"emotional mind." According to Dr. Linehan, the *wise mind* is that
part of you that holds both reason and emotion at the same time
and draws wisdom from both. Mindfulness skills can help you
better tolerate emotional distress and cope more successfully with
painful feelings.

Mindfulness lies at the core of Buddhist meditative practices, and
it has a much broader application as well. It is universal in that it has
to do with the ability to pay attention to the here and now, to sustain
penetrative awareness, and to achieve insight that is not available
from simply thinking. The definition of *mindfulness* is "an open and
nonjudgmental attitude." Mindfulness allows the person using it to
see thoughts as thoughts and events as events independent of their
content and their emotional "charge." That is, thoughts and feelings
come and go; they are transient. Using their observing self, a mindful
person can experience emotionally charged thoughts without trying
to change them, replace them, or "fix" them. Rather, thoughts, feelings, and events are simply observed with relative calm or serenity. In this way, it is possible to achieve greater self-knowledge and

self-acceptance.

In their book *Mindfulness-Based Cognitive Therapy for Depression*, Zindel Segal, Mark Williams, and John Teasdale say, "mindfulness is not a technique or method, although there are many different methods and techniques for its cultivation. Rather, it is more aptly described as a way of being, or a way of seeing, one that involves 'coming to one's senses' in every meaning of that phrase." Another way of describing *mindfulness* is systematic self-observation that involves suspending the impulse to judge, characterize, or evaluate experiences. Mindfulness focuses on awareness of inner sensations, perceptions, impulses, emotions, thoughts, and the process of thinking itself, as well as outer manifestations, such as speech, actions, habits, and behaviors. Mindfulness helps you focus your attention, which aids coping with difficult emotions more effectively.

Mindfulness involves learning to observe, describe, and participate with awareness. It also involves taking a nonjudgmental attitude, focusing on one thing at a time, and acting at that moment in a way that is in alignment with your values and guiding life principles. When you actively observe, you attend to events, emotions, and other behavioral responses even if they are distressing, without trying to avoid them or escape. To do this, part of your consciousness must step back from the event itself and act as an observer to whatever is happening. This "observer" part of you is alert and watching what is going on without getting caught up in the experience or reacting to it. When you participate with awareness, you let yourself experience events and feelings without judgment or trying to escape by thinking of something else.

Dr. Linehan describes three "What to Do" and three "How to Do It" skills for achieving mindfulness. Practice these six mindfulness skills (adapted in table 13.3) at every opportunity, not just when things get stressful. Begin with the simple technique of "just noticing" the pressure of your foot on the floor or the pressure of your back against the chair. If you are walking, "just notice" that you are walking and what it feels like to walk without judging whether you

Table 13.3 **Mindfulness Skills**

"What to Do" Skills for Achieving Mindfulness	
1. Observe your experience.	Just notice your experience or what is happening without getting caught up in it. Step aside from yourself and observe, but don't attach your attention to anything. Become a self-observer. Use your observing self to notice your thinking self and its mind chatter. So, for example, notice that you are reading while you read this page. When you are eating, focus on the experience of eating.
2. Describe what is happening.	Put words to the experience. Acknowledge and describe to yourself what you are feeling or what you are doing. Objectively describe the facts. When a feeling or thought arises, or an action occurs, simply acknowledge it and describe it to yourself. For example, the observing self might say, "I am reading this book" or "I am eating."
3. Participate in the experience.	Let yourself experience the feelings or event in the moment, while acting in each situation as needed. Let go of ruminating and stay in the moment. If you find yourself thinking of other things from the past or in the future, bring your attention back to the present. For example, if your mind wanders while reading this page, just gently bring your attention back to reading. Let your observing self notice that your thinking mind wandered away. If you find your mind wandering away from reading, just bring yourself back to the page.
"How to Do It" Skills for Achieving Mindfulness	
1. Be nonjudgmental.	Separate your opinions from the facts. Stay away from notions of "fair" or "unfair," "right" or "wrong," "should" or "shouldn't." When you do find yourself judging, simply release your judgments and return to observing the facts. Your observing self does not make judgments. When you are walking, notice that you are moving.
2. Stay in the moment.	Focus your attention on the present moment. Don't escape by letting your mind think of things in the past or the future. Do one thing at a time. Let go of distractions, again, and again, and again. When you are eating a meal, stay focused on the act of consuming food.
3. Focus on what works at that moment.	Do what needs to be done in the moment. Meet the needs of the situation you are in, not the one you wish you were in, not the one that is more comfortable, not the one that allows you to ignore your feelings in the present situation. Let go of vengeance, useless anger, self-pity, and righteousness. Stay in touch with your values and guiding principles. As you participate in exercise, focus on doing the exercise.

are "doing it right." When you are eating, be aware of the sensations of eating and "just notice" without judging the thoughts, feelings, and experience associated with eating at that time. These small steps are the beginning of becoming mindful. Eventually, you will be able to adopt the observing-self position even when you are in a stress-producing situation.

Mindfulness and Awareness

Mindfulness is an important stress-management tool that can easily be used by a wide range of people. Practitioners of mindfulness report that they enjoy the cultivation of greater awareness and self-knowledge. They say this even though it is sometimes painful because it does not allow them to avoid unpleasantness. However, when unpleasantness is there, they do not struggle with it or try to push it away. Mindfulness is a way of dealing skillfully with both inner experience and external events. It provides a way of "being with" a problem and letting go of the need for an instant solution. Becoming aware of a difficulty and holding it in awareness can provide a time-out from the mind, which can get caught up in old mental routines and ineffective habits. Mindfulness paves the way for "doing what works" in the moment.

Distress-Tolerance Skills

According to Dr. Linehan, who has done years of research on how to manage negative emotions, mindfulness forms a foundation for coping with painful feelings. In addition to becoming mindful, it is also necessary to learn distress-tolerance and emotion-regulation skills.

The ability to tolerate and deal effectively and appropriately with distress is necessary for good mental health. Stress and pain are parts of life and cannot be altogether avoided or removed. Personal growth and change inevitably result in some discomfort, at least in the short term. Distress tolerance involves being able to accept both yourself and your current situation in a nonjudgmental fashion. It is the ability to perceive your environment without demanding that it be different, to experience emotions without attempting to escape, and to observe your current thoughts and actions without attempting to stop or control them. However, acceptance need not lead to complacency. The idea is to accept your present circumstances and work toward changing them if they need to be changed, and if they cannot be changed, then to make the best of the situation. If, for example, you have the thought, "I'm fat" and you feel bad, just notice the thought without getting drawn into it. Don't fight the thought; let it be and focus on eating in a healthy way.

There are many things you can do to help yourself tolerate painful events, thoughts, and emotions. Soothe yourself by engaging one or more of your senses—sight, touch, taste, smell, or hearing. Buy yourself some flowers. Light a scented candle. Apply perfume or lotion. Drink a cup of fragrant herbal tea. Take a bubble bath. Go to an art museum. Listen to music. Engage in healthy activities such as gardening, hiking, or biking. Check the internet for groups and activities that you might participate in. Choose activities that provide opportunities to experience positive emotions—joy, happiness, and satisfaction. Call a friend and ask them to join you. Do something nice for someone else: volunteer your services to a charity. Pay attention to your new activity.

Emotion-Regulation Skills

The ability to manage overall emotional health requires the application of mindfulness skills. It is most important that you remain nonjudgmental when you observe and describe your current emotions. By stepping back from, and becoming more mindful of, your emotional experience, you are less at the mercy of your emotions. Dr. Linehan describes several specific emotion-regulation steps, which are listed in table 13.4.

Table 13.4 Emotion-Regulation Steps

1. Identify and label emotions.	The first step in emotion regulation is to identify and label your emotions. Many people with eating problems have never learned to differentiate one emotion from another; they often lump all negative emotions together into an undifferentiated mass they call "feeling bad." They are like artists who have only one or two colors to work with instead of an entire palette. Having a whole palette of emotions is necessary for good mental health. Being able to identify and label a range of emotions and emotional responses is important. You can more easily identify an emotion if you observe and describe the events that prompt the feeling, understand the meaning or interpretation you assign to the event, and notice where in the body you experience the feeling.
2. Identify obstacles to emotion management.	Emotions work. Generally, emotions function to stimulate your rational mind to take action, but rational thought is not needed for all action. For example, you don't have to decide to jump out of the way of an oncoming bus; you just do it. Emotions also communicate information about you to others. When you show anger, others may become quiet. Emotions motivate your behavior. Feeling anxious can make you want to eat—or may ruin your appetite. Emotions can be used to influence or control the behavior of others, and they validate your own perceptions and interpretations of events. When there is a "payoff" for an emotion—for example, getting others to feel sorry for you or to take care of you—the payoff becomes an obstacle to emotion management. If you stop suffering, you must give up the attention you get for having problems. Suffering is a way of communicating that you have been hurt. To give up suffering is like saying, "It wasn't so bad after all." Likewise, because emotions often trigger a knee-jerk reaction, you may need to catch the emotion earlier in the process to interrupt the automatic reaction. The first step in doing this is to become an observer of your own experience.

Table 13.4   Emotion-Regulation Steps (*continued*)

3. Reduce vulnerability to stress.	Stressful situations, thoughts, or memories make most people emotionally reactive. People with eating problems are hyper-sensitive to threat and very reactive to stressors. If you become a better problem-solver, you are more likely to keep stress under control. Take care of yourself physically—eat properly and get adequate exercise and sleep—to increase your tolerance for stress. Vulnerability to stress is increased when you are tired, hungry, in pain, or otherwise physically compromised. Restrictive dieting or not getting enough exercise also increases your vulnerability to stress.
4.. Change your circumstances or change your attitude.	When you are in a bad situation, take action to get out of it. For example, if you are in an abusive relationship, decide what you need to do to change it or leave it. Perhaps marital counseling will help. If not, consider the possibility of leaving, particularly if children in the relationship are also targets of abuse. (Remember that abuse can be verbal, physical, sexual, or emotional.) If you cannot change a situation—for example, if you feel you must take care of your ill and aging parent—make the best of it. Change your attitude from one of suffering to acceptance. Remember that it may take time for some circumstances to change. And it is sadly true that no one is happy all the time.
5.. Increase positive emotional experiences.	Take action to get involved in experiences that produce good or happy emotions. People usually feel bad for good reason. They are unhappy about their circumstances and they dwell on how awful it is. To compensate for painful emotions, you too need to increase positive experiences and to notice and take advantage of any when they do occur. Find activities that help you to feel better and, if necessary, do what you can to change your situation.

continues ▶

Table 13.4 Emotion-Regulation Steps (*continued*)

6. Increase mindfulness of current emotions.	To increase mindfulness of your current emotions, you must be willing to experience distressing emotions in the moment without judging them, trying to inhibit them, blocking them, or seeking distraction from them. If you feel angry but think you shouldn't be, you are likely to feel guilty as well as angry. This makes distress more intense and tolerance more difficult. It is better to just notice, put into words, and experience your anger and the distressing situation without judging yourself for feeling angry, trying to distract yourself from your anger, or losing sight of what is the most effective course of action to take at that moment. So, if someone remarks on your eating, notice if anger rises in you and consider how to best deal with the situation.
7. Take opposite action.	One way to change or moderate an emotion or mood is to act in a way that is inconsistent with that emotion or mood. Do something that seems contrary to how you feel. For example, you might listen to soothing music or watch a funny TV show—that is, find something to do that is the opposite of how you feel when you are upset. This would be doing what works in the moment. If you feel unhappy, go to the zoo or the gym. One person felt depressed because several people in their family and circle of friends were ill or suffering from various misfortunes, so they started training to run a marathon. Having a goal and training for the race elevated their mood and helped them overcome depression, even though the plight of some of their friends and family members had not changed.
8. Apply distress-tolerance techniques.	It is important to be able to tolerate painful emotions without trying to avoid or escape them. Earlier in this chapter, several techniques were given for tolerating distress. These included self-soothing, engaging in healthy activities that promote positive emotions, accepting present circumstances without fighting the emotions they bring, and taking the best action in the moment to cope. By using these, you will discover that the intensity and duration of your emotions fade sooner than you may expect. When a distressful event happens, acceptance is the only way out. Avoid judging things as good or bad; it is best to acknowledge and accept that which cannot be changed. Make a commitment to accept reality as it is and work with it.

Assertiveness

Styles of Interpersonal Behavior

Assertiveness, *aggressiveness*, *passive/aggressiveness*, and *passiveness* are four styles of interpersonal behavior. Most people use a mix of styles but have one preferred or most frequently used style.

If you behave *assertively*, you express how you feel and assert your rights while still respecting the rights of others. When communicating assertively, you express your wants, ideas, opinions, and feelings directly and honestly, without having to make excuses or apologizing. Doing so allows you to feel self-confident and good about yourself because you increase the likelihood of being heard and getting what you need. Other people are likely to feel that you respect them and are more likely to respect you in return.

Some people confuse assertiveness with *aggressiveness*. In fact, an aggressive interpersonal style is used to overpower, intimidate, or manipulate another for the purpose of achieving a desired end. Aggressive behavior disregards the other person's rights in a situation. Aggressive verbal communication is the outright expression of anger—yelling, cursing, name calling, making sarcastic comments, criticizing, and blaming. Examples of aggressive, nonverbal behavior would include slamming doors, giving "dirty" looks, stomping, or retreating into silence. Aggressive physical behavior includes pushing, shoving, hitting, or blocking another's way. The person who is treated aggressively feels hurt, afraid, angry, intimidated, belittled, or humiliated. Targets of abuse may come to believe they do not deserve better treatment, or they may retaliate with passive/aggressive behavior.

Passive/aggressive behavior is used to express dissent while trying to avoid outright conflict. Since the behavior is subtle, the perpetrator can deny their intentions if the target of the passive/aggressive behavior reacts negatively. Passive/aggressive behavior is intended to look innocent while it is, in fact, covertly aggressive. It can involve little acts of sabotage, such as "forgetting" something important, withholding something of value, making sarcastic comments under the guise of joking, or doing mildly annoying things, such as not being ready on time. At times, overeating can be a passive/aggressive behavior used to irritate others or show defiance. In other cases, overeating is an outright aggressive behavior aimed at punishing oneself.

Passiveness is another style of interpersonal behavior that one can adopt to avoid conflict with others. The passive person does not assert their rights and, by not doing so, they hope to preserve the peace and avoid making waves. Passive behavior says, "You count; I don't." All too often, passiveness characterizes those who don't know what they want or feel, or what their rights are in an interpersonal situation. Sometimes the overweight person who takes a more passive role is looking for a "hidden bargain"—hoping if they are nice to others, they will be liked despite the shortcomings they think they have. Unfortunately, this hoped-for benefit is not always forthcoming, and the passivist pays a significant personal price for it with the decline of their health and self-respect.

Search the internet for tests of assertiveness. You may find some good information about yourself.

Assertiveness and Weight Management

Lack of assertiveness is a problem for many who are overweight. On the other hand, some people who are overweight or obese feel vulnerable and may resort to an aggressive style of communication as a defense against criticism. Some defend their size, claiming that obesity is not a health problem, but dieting is. (Refer to chapter 1 for the answer to "Can you be healthy at any weight?")

More often, those who are obese feel they are not entitled to speak up, and they act passively. This passivity shows up when the overweight person puts others' needs first, becomes the caretaker of others, or when they act the part of "doormat" and let others walk all over them. Although they may be assertive in some circumstances, such as at work or with strangers, they may fail to be assertive with their significant others. To avoid conflict, they do not stand up for their rights in the hope that others will not bring attention to their weight. They tend to accommodate others excessively or keep quiet about feeling hurt. They may fear displeasing others, hurting another's feelings, or losing the relationship. Often, they ignore their own anger or upset. If emotions do surface, they may minimize or rationalize the actions of others that contributed to the hurt feelings. Likely they don't know their personal rights. They then turn to food to avoid or suppress painful feelings. Table 13.5 provides a list of some of the basic rights that every person has.

Becoming More Assertive

Even though you may have one preferred interpersonal style (assertive, aggressive, passive/aggressive, or passive), there are times when another style is called for. It is unreasonable to expect that you will

Table 13.5 Everyone's Personal Rights

You have the right to:

❖ Be treated with respect and dignity.

❖ Have your own values and standards.

❖ Make your own choices and decisions.

❖ Make mistakes and not be perfect.

❖ Have and express feelings appropriately.

❖ Ask questions and seek clarification.

❖ Negotiate for change.

❖ Say no and refuse requests.

❖ Make a request.

❖ Change your mind.

❖ Have your own personal space.

❖ Refuse to take responsibility for someone else's thoughts, feelings, or behaviors.

❖ Refuse to live in a verbally or physically abusive environment.

never communicate in an aggressive or a passive fashion, even if your preferred style is assertive. If a robber holds you at gunpoint, it is better to cooperate passively than to react in either an aggressive or an assertive fashion. Occasionally meeting another's aggressive communication with your own aggressive responses may be appropriate if you think the person is trying to bluff you, but more often it is better to step away, if possible, and say nothing in the moment. When someone is overly emotional, it is better to wait for things to cool down before asserting yourself. Likewise, you need to choose the right level of assertiveness. For example, "Please don't do that" is a low level of assertiveness, "Don't do that" is an intermediate level, and "Stop" is a high level of assertiveness.

To be properly assertive, you need confidence that you have the ability to handle the situation. You need to be clear—the message should be clear and easy to understand. And finally, you need to deliver the information you want to convey in a calm and controlled manner. Check the internet for more information on how to be properly assertive.

Improving Your Weight-Management Assertiveness

To be successful in weight management, you must be able to say no and stick to it. But first, you must believe that you have the right to refuse. Instead of just saying "No" or "No, thank you," it is tempting to add on an excuse or justification for refusing. People often invent or embellish an excuse so that the refusal will be more easily accepted or because you feel you should provide an explanation. Sometimes you do it to soften the "blow" of saying no to another person or so you appear to be a "nice" person. Or you may make an excuse to take yourself "off the hook." Unfortunately, you can get so wrapped up in inventing an excuse to go along with the refusal that you feel even more awkward, or you make yourself vulnerable to the other person's counter to your refusal. Table 13.6 gives guidelines for making an effective refusal.

Table 13.6 Guidelines for Making an Effective Refusal

1. Be direct and avoid making excuses.	An example of a refusal with an excuse is, "No, thanks. I'm trying to cut down on my sugar intake, and I don't think it is a good idea to have any cookies." Then the other person may say, "Oh, come on, one won't hurt you. Here, share one with me." A refusal without explanation would be less likely to invite counterarguments. If the other person continues with a counterargument, you need to increase your level of assertiveness: "No. I don't want one."
2. Acknowledge the other person's good intentions.	For example, "I know you made the cookies yourself, and I'm sure they are excellent, but no, thanks."
3. If necessary, offer a compromise.	"I see you have gone to a lot of trouble to make this lovely dessert. I'll have a bite of my partner's portion, but don't give me my own serving, please."
4. Avoid people who won't take no for an answer.	If every time you go to lunch with a friend, they order a dessert and insist you share it, avoid going to lunch with them. Suggest the two of you take a walk instead.
5. When necessary, increase your level of assertiveness.	There are levels of assertiveness ranging from politeness or being warm to firmness. It is best to try politeness first, but if the other person is insistent, you may have to become firm. In that case, you must go from "thanks, anyway" to a strong "no."

Using "I" Statements

Assertive communication means using "I" statements instead of "you" statements. A "you" statement is usually a blaming statement, such as "You make me mad when you leave dirty dishes in the sink all day." An assertive "I" statement communicates from your perspective and your experience. By using an "I" statement, you take responsibility for your feelings and don't assign responsibility to someone else. Such statements objectively describe the facts of the situation and ask for a change in behavior. For example,

I've noticed several evenings now that, when I come home, dirty dishes are still in the sink. I thought we agreed that each of us would take care of our own dishes promptly. After I've spent a long day at the office, I'd like to come home to a neat kitchen. What do you think we could do to make this situation work better? It would sure make my day nicer if the kitchen were neater, and I think we'd get along better too.

Notice that in the assertive "I" statement, the first thing the speaker does is describe the situation objectively, including the speaker's understanding of the "dishes" agreement. (If there is no agreement about the dishes, the first step is to negotiate one.) Be careful that your tone of voice does not convey anger or annoyance with the situation. Next the speaker describes their desires and suggests that both parties participate in finding a solution. Finally, the speaker spells out the benefits of addressing the problem constructively. The use of assertive "I" statements is less likely to result in conflict. Of course, there are times when even reasonable assertive communication leads to interpersonal conflict.

Managing Interpersonal Conflict

An important part of assertiveness is being able to respond appropriately to another's anger or criticism. Conflict arises for a variety of reasons—values differ, assumptions are made, expectations don't match, or someone takes offense. Actions that are perceived as unfair, wrong, or insensitive can produce conflict. A difference of opinion or perspective is at the bottom of virtually all situations that engender conflict or bad feelings. Some people get prickly if they feel guilty about failing to do something or when attention is called to an insensitive remark they made. Even the best relationships can encounter situations that bring up conflict.

Communicating assertively may bring you into conflict with others, especially if they have been used to getting their own way and now you seem to be changing the rules—that is, you are becoming more assertive. At such times, you may encounter another person's anger because they prefer that you continue to be passive. If this happens, there are ways to make confrontation easier and to facilitate a better outcome. Many of these are listed in table 13.7.

Depression and Weight

A cluster of depression, overeating, and body-image distress is frequently seen in those with obesity and disordered eating. One study found that 74 percent of women seeking treatment for bulimia and 48 percent of those seeking help for binge-eating disorder had lifetime prevalence rates for major depressive disorder. Another study found that clinical samples of obese binge eaters had prevalence rates of 65 percent for major depressive disorder or chronic low-level depression.

Atypical depression is marked by overeating and oversleeping. Research shows that obese individuals consume significantly more calories than people of normal weight. Eating can be a way of medicating feelings of depression, but it may be that eating certain foods also contributes to depression in addition to creating negative emotions and more depression following overeating.

Overcoming Depression

Medications are available that can help alleviate both severe and chronic, low-level depression. However, antidepressant medication alone does not generally cure depression. Therapy alone or in combination with antidepressant medication has been shown to produce the best results for overcoming moderate to severe depression. Research has shown that several therapy approaches are effective in treating these disorders. Cognitive-behavior therapy (CBT) and its newest iteration acceptance-based therapy (ACT) focus on

Table 13.7 Guidelines for Managing Interpersonal Conflict

1. Don't let yourself get hooked into someone else's anger.	Maintain your "cool" by using supportive self-talk (see chapter 11) and distress-tolerance skills covered in the current chapter. Avoid taking things personally. Stay relaxed. Be careful not to let your "buttons" get pushed; if you lose your temper as well, the argument is likely to escalate.
2. If someone is angry, don't try to reason with them at that moment.	Let things cool off and discuss the situation at a later time—a day later perhaps. Listen attentively and let the person know you understand their concerns. You can acknowledge you know they are feeling upset, but you do not need to agree that anger is justified if it isn't. Suggest that you table the discussion until later. Set a time to revisit the problem and be sure to get back to the issue when tempers have cooled, usually the next day.
3. Make conciliatory gestures to defuse another's anger.	You may be able to defuse the situation by finding something to agree with—without agreeing to everything. For example, in response to the accusation that you never put away the dishes, you might say, "It is true that I sometimes wait to put away the dishes." Or see if you can agree in principle. For example, "If you believe that I never put away the dishes, I can imagine why you feel upset." Watch for words such as *always* and *never* in arguments. When you hear these words, you can usually find a chance to agree in part or to agree in principle thereby defusing anger.

problematic thought patterns and beliefs that contribute to depression and promote mindfulness and active acceptance of troubling thoughts and feelings. CBT and ACT seek to identify hindering self-talk, cognitive distortions, and core beliefs. An important step is to disengage from such thoughts and beliefs and see them, instead,

Table 13.7 Guidelines for Managing Interpersonal Conflict (*continued*)

4. Handle verbal abuse carefully.	Try not to take it personally. Remember that verbal abuse is the angry person's attempt to gain control or to intimidate you. One way to handle verbal abuse is to state assertively: "Please don't talk to me that way." Then raise the level of assertiveness if you have to: "If you don't stop cursing and yelling, I am going to leave." If this does not stop the verbal abuse, go to another room or get out of the house. If verbal abuse looks like it might escalate to physical abuse, or if the verbal abuse continues and you are afraid in the situation, don't hesitate to call 9-1-1.
5. Ask for a time-out.	When emotions escalate, ask for a time-out. A time-out is a break to cool down and collect your thoughts. Be careful that you don't use a time-out to ruminate over anger-engendering thoughts. A time-out should provide a chance for emotions to cool down and for logical thinking to prevail. You need to have an agreement beforehand with your partner that either of you can call a time-out. During the time-out, consider what you may have done or failed to do that contributed to the original issue.
6. Resolve residual stress.	Once a conflict situation passes, remember that you are likely to have residual arousal. Be prepared to take care of yourself by finding a way to let go of tension. Use relaxation techniques, like progressive relaxation and deep breathing. Take a hot shower or go for a brisk walk around the block.

as an observer on the shore watching waves wash in and wash out might. It is not necessary to act on a particular thought or feeling. Defusing from your thoughts and feelings can help defeat depression. Likewise, engaging more in behaviors that are rewarding is helpful in overcoming depression.

Exercise

Exercise is as good as antidepressant medication for decreasing depressive symptoms. Research has shown that those who become and remain fit are less likely to suffer from clinical depression. Once depression has developed, exercise can reverse it. Starting to exercise does not mean having to become a "jock" or engaging only in aerobic exercise. Weight training can work, and even simply increasing your regular activities of daily living—walking the dog, gardening, doing chores around the house—by as little as thirty more minutes a day has important therapeutic benefits.

Sleep

Getting eight hours of restful sleep a night is recommended for good physical and mental health. Lack of good sleep hygiene is a contributor to depression. Staying up late and sleeping in may be fun at times, but it is important to keep a regular sleep schedule to maintain or improve good mental health. Check the internet for information on sleep hygiene.

Eat a Healthy Diet

Some people with depression don't feel like eating, while others overeat. To help with depression, eat regularly throughout the day— three meals and planned snacks as necessary. Avoid or minimize simple sugars. Follow the rule of thumb that if it is white, replace it with a healthier alternative. Replace white potatoes with sweet potatoes. Substitute whole grain bread for white bread. Use brown rice or wild rice in place of white rice. Avoid products made of unrefined, white flour, such as cookies, cakes, pastries, pasta, and many types of bread. Try to have some protein at every meal. Satisfy your sweet tooth with fruit. Include lots of vegetables in your diet. Choose fish over red meat often. Have a meatless meal once or twice a week. Most of all, avoid junk food and fast food.

Minimize or Eliminate Alcohol

If you are depressed, alcohol should be minimized, if not eliminated altogether. Alcohol is a central nervous system depressant. Although it may seem to relax you at first and help you forget about your problems, there is a good possibility of a depressive rebound, especially if you drink more than one or two drinks a day. Drinking too much interrupts the body's ability to have a good night's sleep, which leads to fatigue, overeating to feel better, and so on. And, of course, drinking alcohol is an easy way to take in lots of calories. Even if your alcohol intake does fall within socially acceptable limits and health recommendations, having a mood disorder such as depression makes you more sensitive to the effects of alcohol. Even a small amount of alcohol in the midst of depression can cause early morning awakenings and disrupted sleep.

Plan Positive Activities

Some theories hold that depression results from a lack of rewarding experiences. It is easy to get bogged down with boring or tedious chores and forget to include fun activities. Such activities can be as simple as setting aside time to read a book, taking a walk with a friend, or arranging to have someone watch the kids while you go to an exercise class. Consider what things you did in the past that gave you pleasure. Or what would you like to do now or soon that would be satisfying? Think of ways to replenish yourself emotionally by balancing everyday routines with fun activities. Develop a plan for acting on them. When you get moving in a positive direction, you are less likely to feel depressed and less likely to eat as a quick way to feel momentarily better.

Seek Social Support

Social support is helpful in coping with depression. The tendency of many depressed people is to withdraw from social activities. They may watch television (and eat) to distract themselves from feeling down rather than reach out to other people. Some depressed people become more dependent on the internet as a means of distraction—a substitute for "real" relationships. The comfort of family and friends is a great antidote to depression.

If you're not comfortable sharing your feelings of depression with family and friends, consider finding a support group. It often helps to know that others are struggling with similar problems, and the opportunity exists for making new friends that provide mutual support. Group therapy that provides a CBT or mindfulness approach for overcoming chronic depression might be a good choice. Also, some churches offer self-help groups for depression. Online depression support can be found by doing a search on "support groups for depression," but be careful of people who masquerade online as "therapists." Check credentials before you take the advice of an online therapist and be sure they are legitimate.

Fight Back Against Your "Inner Bully"

Stop blaming, criticizing, and attacking yourself. Don't compare yourself to others or to the excessively high standards you or someone else might have imposed on you only to find yourself lacking. Be more compassionate with yourself. What you say to yourself silently matters. Review chapter 11 on managing thinking and self-talk.

14

Stopping the Binge-Eating Cycle

Rachel confessed she was a secret binge eater. When she left work in the evenings, she stopped and ate a complete dinner at a restaurant, and then went home and dined again with her family. Rachel also picked her face and got upset with herself afterward, just like she did when she binged. Rachel felt completely helpless to stop either the binge eating or the skin picking. Finally, she sought the help of a therapist with experience in dealing with compulsions.

When most people think of binge eating, they think of *bulimia nervosa*, an eating disorder that involves binge eating followed by attempts to compensate for the calories consumed by vomiting, misusing laxatives or diuretics, restricting calories, or exercising to excess. Those with bulimia are typically within the normal weight range, although some may be slightly overweight. Bulimics have concerns about weight and shape that cause great distress. Bulimia is uncommon among those who are obese.

Binge-Eating Disorder

Binge eating is also the central feature in a more recently recognized eating disorder—binge-eating disorder (BED). The person with BED also engages in binge eating but does not regularly use the compensatory behaviors that the person with bulimia uses. Those with BED may diet periodically or even vomit occasionally after an eating binge, but these behaviors do not occur on a regular or frequent basis. Individuals with BED are usually moderately overweight or obese. Those with BED who also overvalue their shape and weight tend to suffer more psychological distress—depression, anxiety, eating pathology—than do binge eaters who don't have significant concern about their weight or shape. This is true regardless of actual weight.

Binge eating is often the paradoxical consequence of attempts to restrict calories to lose weight or maintain weight loss. Unable to cope with feelings of hunger or deprivation or other unpleasant feelings, the binge eater eventually succumbs to an overwhelming urge to eat. Those with BED gain weight because their bouts of excessive eating provide more calories than they expend, whereas those with bulimia or anorexia compensate for excess calories consumed. Between 25 and 50 percent of obese people suffer from BED. The more severely overweight a person is, the more likely it is that binge eating will be a problem.

Understanding Binge Eating

Some binges are triggered by hunger precipitated by strict dieting. Those who skip meals hoping to cut back on calories are particularly susceptible to hunger-induced overeating. Feeling bad is another trigger for eating binges. Self-criticism or criticism from others about weight or shape results in lowering self-esteem and can set the stage for a binge. Habit or simple pleasure-seeking can also contribute to binge eating. In some cases, obsessing or ruminating about a desired food can trigger a binge.

Emotional reasons—the desire to be comforted, avoidance of upsetting situations, painful emotions, or distraction from boredom or loneliness—are frequent triggers for binge eating. In such cases, the binge serves to escape unpleasantness or forget difficulties. Some people are unable to identify specific triggers for binges but report feelings of persistent tension and anxiety that are relieved by binge eating.

What Keeps Binge Eating Going?

Most people continue to binge because it "works." The binge is an effective means of escaping upsetting thoughts and painful emotions—anxiety, anger, depression, loneliness, and boredom—or pain or fatigue. A binge can temporarily shut out self-criticism and hindering self-talk. In some cases, a binge provides a certain amount of satisfaction because it is a way to express anger or to rebel against rules. In other cases, it affords a much-needed relief from tension. In some cases, the binge eater doesn't even enjoy the act of eating, yet they keep eating as if in a trance; their behavior is mindless.

The events that follow a binge serve to reinforce it. Escaping thoughts and painful emotions by bingeing is reinforcing because it helps avoid pain. Because binge eating works, it continues to happen. For example, eating a cookie that tastes good makes you want another cookie. The good flavor in your mouth leads to wanting and, probably, eating more cookies. If the cookie didn't taste good, you might not have another one unless you are just eating mindlessly. The consequences that follow a behavior make it more or less likely to happen again. This kind of cue and reward can devolve into mindless eating.

Furthermore, immediate consequences carry more influence on behavior than do distant ones. The good taste of a cookie now is more important than worries about deviating from a healthy way of eating or gaining weight later. The desire to escape stress and tension by binge eating is compelling, especially if the binge eater has no other way to cope. Good consequences now usually win out over future negative consequences.

Of course, a binge has its downsides. Eating excess calories produces weight gain. After a binge, most binge eaters feel disgusted, guilty, and ashamed of their behavior. Or they are just numb—they feel nothing. Yet the relatively distant consequences often do not stop the binge behavior from happening again and again. The fact that a binge provides immediate relief from stress or hunger outweighs most of the eventual negative consequences.

Identifying the Binge Pattern

If you are a person who binges, to stop the binge cycle you must identify the behavior pattern that triggers the binge, the thoughts and beliefs that accompany it, and the reinforcers that perpetuate the behavior. Deconstructing the behavior pattern using the ABC model introduced in chapter 7, "Changing Behavior," helps you decide how to change your behavior in the future. The ABC model is a way of understanding a behavior pattern. As discussed in that chapter, the antecedents, or As, are events that precede and elicit or trigger behaviors and thinking, Bs are often the beliefs we hold and the

Table 14.1 Criteria for Diagnosing Binge-Eating Disorder

1. Eating in a discrete period of time (for instance, any two-hour period) a large amount of food and experiencing a lack of control overeating.

2. Three or more of the following:

   a. Eating much more rapidly than normal

   b. Eating until feeling uncomfortably full

   c. Eating despite not feeling hungry

   d. Eating alone

   e. Feeling disgusted with oneself, depressed, or very guilty afterward

3. Marked distress afterward.

4. Engaging in a binge, on average, at least once a week for three months.

thoughts we have about an A event. Bs are the behaviors—thoughts or actions—that are cued or triggered by the A. Consequences, the Cs, follow and reinforce the behavior and influence whether it happens again in the same context. Once you identify the antecedents or triggers, the thinking or behaviors, and the consequences or rewards that reinforce a binge, you are better able to influence the pattern. For example, one person felt bad about being severely overweight. When someone at the supermarket remarked about the ice cream in their basket at checkout, they felt ashamed and went home and had an eating binge. Afterward, they felt overly full and distressed about their behavior. They resolved never to lose control like that again.

Revisit chapter 7 and review the information on self-monitoring of behavior patterns. Then begin monitoring your binge patterns. Record the date and time, what you ate (not necessarily the calories), what kind of binge it was (stress binge, opportunity binge, and so on), and what you thought and felt before, during, and afterward. Study your notes on each binge and write out a plan for coping with them in the future.

Characteristics of the BED Binge

According to the American Psychiatric Association, a *binge* is characterized by a perceived lack of control over eating (for instance, feeling that one cannot stop or control what or how much one eats) and eating within a discrete period of time, typically two hours, an amount of food that is definitely larger than most people would eat in a similar time period under similar circumstances. However, this description of a binge better fits the type of binge experienced by those who are bulimic or anorexic rather than the binge of those with binge-eating disorder.

For the "person on the street," a binge means losing control, whether eating or drinking too much or spending too much money. A loss or suspension of control, or inability to stop eating once it has begun, are hallmarks of eating binges. The amount or type of food eaten and the number of calories consumed can vary. Some BED binges may involve eating large amounts of food in one sitting; in other cases, the binge can have a stop-and-start pattern. A BED binge can last for days at a time rather than a couple of hours. Some binges may involve continuous snacking throughout the day that blends into mealtimes. This type of eating is called *grazing*.

A BED binge eater may keep large stores of candy bars or chips in their desk drawer to snack on throughout the day. Sometimes grazing begins in the late afternoon and continues until bedtime. Such binges are often associated with watching TV or using the computer. Most binges end when a person goes to sleep, but some people get up at night to eat again.

A binge may involve eating a meal before arriving home only to eat another meal that was prepared by a spouse (like Rachel did in the chapter-opening vignette). Or a binge may begin by eating just one tasty item and then going to the store to purchase a larger quantity and consuming it all. Binge eating is often followed by self-criticism, which is painful, and can lead to more binge eating later.

When a binge involves large quantities eaten quickly, it usually involves eating when not physically hungry, eating until uncomfortably full, and eating in secret. It is usually accompanied or followed by feelings of disgust with oneself, depression, shame, anger, or guilt. Low self-esteem and dissatisfaction with appearance accompany binge-eating disorder.

The type of food eaten during a binge varies, but it typically includes sweet, high-calorie foods, such as ice cream, cookies, cake, pastries, or candy. Starches are also preferred binge foods for many—especially bread, cereal, bagels, and the like. For others, chips, nuts, and other salty snacks are preferred. Some people get hooked on red meat because of its high-fat content. If an eating episode violates a self-imposed rule about "good" eating, it can trigger a binge.

BED binges are often triggered by negative emotions. Eating serves to block out thoughts and feelings, at least temporarily. Binge eaters are usually distressed about their inability to control their eating and about their weight. In some cases, the person with BED was once anorexic or bulimic. Most have a long history of dieting. Some continue to try diets, whereas others have given up all efforts because of repeated failures. Increasingly, bariatric surgery (surgery that reduces the size of the stomach or alters the gastrointestinal tract to reduce the number of calories consumed or absorbed) for the obese is considered necessary when dieting and exercise efforts fail, though even surgery may not eliminate binge eating.

The BED person does not seek to be thin; generally, they would be happy just to be average, or even somewhat above average, weight. Binge eaters are often sedentary and may have obesity-related physical problems that interfere with exercising, such as foot or knee problems. Because of their considerable dissatisfaction and shame about their bodies, they may avoid sexual relations. Many obese binge eaters are in marriages that have been asexual for many years. They may believe that their spouses look at them with disgust; in fact, their own body dissatisfaction is a contributing factor to the lack of sex in their relationships. The American Psychological Association provides information on BED and its treatment. To learn more about binge eating, search the internet. The American Psychological Association provides a good deal of information on the topic and is an excellent resource.

Types of Binges

Depending on the cause or the triggers, binges come in a variety of forms. These include the hunger binge, the deprivation binge, the stress (or emotional) binge, the opportunity binge, the vengeful binge, the pleasure binge, and the habit binge. Let's look at each.

The Hunger Binge

The *hunger binge* is triggered by physical deprivation. To most people, dieting means limiting calories. Dieting can also involve eliminating certain foods or food groups, eating fewer times per day, or following an extensive set of rules about what, when, and how much to eat. Studies on starvation show that fasting and severe caloric restriction produce changes in the body and the brain. Hunger that persists leads to symptoms similar to those of starvation. These include preoccupation with food, eating, and excessive thinking about meals one has had or hopes to have. Mood swings are common with starvation and hunger. Dips in blood sugar can trigger dizziness, hand tremors, and headaches. Irritability is also not uncommon with hunger-inducing, restrictive dieting.

To thwart a hunger binge, it is important to eat regularly and adequately throughout the day. This means eating at least three regular meals with planned snacks as necessary or eating more frequent but smaller meals. Those who think they are saving calories by skipping a meal—usually breakfast or lunch—are setting themselves up for a hunger binge.

Some people claim they *can't* eat three regular meals. They don't eat breakfast because they aren't hungry and can't "face" food that early in the day. Sometimes this is because they have eaten so late the night before that they still feel full. Others don't leave time to eat breakfast as they hurry off to work, preferring to grab a donut or a muffin on the way, or they get something from the vending machine at work. Still others fear that once they start eating, they won't be able to stop, so they delay eating for as long as possible. When they do allow themselves to eat, usually sometime late in the afternoon, they are too hungry to stay in control, or they feel they "deserve" to eat whatever they want after having not eaten all day. That's when the hunger binge evolves into a deprivation binge.

The Deprivation Binge

The *deprivation binge* results from psychological restriction. Making foods forbidden or off limits ultimately leads to feelings of deprivation. The irritability that results from attempts to resist desired foods and to eat low-calorie foods that are unappetizing often means a deprivation binge is not far behind. Foods that are forbidden become more irresistible and compelling, especially if you continually think about eating them. Dieters reach a tipping point that often involves having "just one" or committing a small indiscretion, and the binge begins.

One way to curtail deprivation binges is to eat all foods in moderation. However, sometimes it is necessary to stay away from certain problem or "dangerous" foods (foods that trigger binges) until you feel more confident about maintaining healthier eating habits. Then you can try reintroducing such foods in moderation. If you still cannot eat certain trouble foods without triggering an eating binge, you may need to change your thinking about which foods you choose to include in your eating style.

Consider the approach taken by Alcoholics Anonymous (AA). AA has helped more people overcome alcoholism than any other organization. They promote a policy of total abstinence from alcohol. One of their sayings is "one drink—a drunk." If you experience "one bite—a binge," you may have to decide whether you can learn to live without the food that triggers the binge. Just as it is possible to live without drinking alcohol, it is possible to live without a problem food. This requires a change in self-concept—that is, how you think of yourself. Rather than saying, "I can't eat sweets," you need to focus on saying, "I don't eat sweets" (or whatever your specific danger food is). Be careful, however, not to make large categories of food forbidden.

This author's former binge food was Almond Roca. I could eat other candies without caving into overeating, but with Almond Roca, I could not eat just one. For many years I was okay not eating Almond Roca (and didn't binge), and, in fact, I had no desire for it. I had decided I could live without Almond Roca. One holiday, a gift appeared at my door; it was a tin of Almond Roca. "After all these years [twenty], I can surely eat just one," I thought. Instead, I polished off the whole tin in one sitting. As a result, I concluded I still cannot manage to eat Almond Roca in moderation. Doesn't this constitute making Almond Roca a forbidden food, and isn't that a bad idea? Banning highly desirable foods can lead to feelings of deprivation and is generally not advised. But, in my case, for undetermined reasons, the taste of Almond Roca was more compelling than other desires. I rededicated myself to the decision that I was someone who did not eat Almond Roca. By deciding it was not part of my way of eating, it did not lead to feelings of deprivation.

To change your self-concept means to revise your beliefs and assumptions about yourself. Take the example of the person who achieves sobriety through AA. They change one of their beliefs about themselves from "I'm trying not to drink" to "I'm a recovering alcoholic. I don't drink." Notice that the latter statement is focused on the present moment, not the future. A future-focused statement would be "I'll never drink again." While never drinking again may be a goal, in the words of AA, it is necessary to take it "one day at a time." A person in recovery doesn't necessarily have to change all their beliefs in order not to drink. For example, they might say, "I wish I could drink. I liked the high. I miss drinking." But the bottom line is, "I don't drink." For my Almond Roca binges, I didn't wish I could eat the candy; I defined my eating pattern as not including Almond Roca. It was a danger food for me.

When choosing to adopt a healthy eating pattern, consider the following. There are people who define themselves as vegetarians because they don't eat any kind of meat. As vegetarians, or non-meat eaters, they don't pine for meat. Their values—how they think of themselves—guide their eating. Perhaps they chose these values for health reasons, moral reasons, or other convictions. They may reveal that in the past they were not vegetarians, but at this time, they think of themselves differently. Defining some aspect of self-concept today—whether it is related to drinking alcohol, eating meat, or eating certain types of sweets—becomes the guide for current behavior. (Of course, it is possible to change again, as some do, and start drinking or eating meat again.) The point is, you can avoid a deprivation binge by defining yourself as having a particular healthy eating pattern.

The Stress Binge

As stated in chapter 13, "Managing Stress," a person experiences stress when resources for coping are taxed or exceeded in the face of perceived threat and well-being is endangered. Common sources of stress include having unrealistic expectations, as well as being unable to be appropriately assertive or manage interpersonal conflicts, process losses, failures, unsatisfactory relationships, and disappointments. Even some occasions that are normally associated with happiness or celebration, such as weddings, retirement, vacations, or the birth of a child, can bring stress as well as joy. Anxiety, anger, depression, boredom, sadness, loneliness—these emotions and others can result from stressors, and even thoughts about stressful situations, and are at the heart of the *stress binge*.

When stress or emotional conflicts become too intense or overwhelming, a state of dissociation can occur. *Dissociation* involves the breakdown of the usual ability to integrate cognition and behavior. Consciousness, memory, perceptions, and behavior become compartmentalized or split off from one another. Those experiencing dissociation may feel temporally detached from their bodies or from their mental processes. Dissociation can occur when a person is subjected to traumatic circumstances, including severe physical, sexual, or emotional abuse. Eating can, at times, become a state of dissociation because it can temporarily numb feelings and provide distance from difficulties or troubling thoughts. During a binge, some report they aren't thinking at all; it is as if they are in a trance.

When a person is under chronic stress, eating can serve as a coping mechanism and a means of day-to-day survival. If eating is limited due to dieting, anxiety and tension are likely to increase. The stress of trying to diet eventually brings a return to eating as a means of coping and may initiate a binge. The stress binge is an attempt to escape painful self-awareness and to avoid feeling bad.

To overcome stress eating, it can be helpful to identify your problem thinking, challenge your assumptions and underlying beliefs, use more helping self-talk, and learn new coping skills for managing stress and emotions. Cognition and problem thinking were addressed in chapter 11, "Managing Thinking and Self-Talk," where cognitive distortions, self-talk, and core beliefs are discussed. Remember that thoughts and feelings rise and fall away, like waves washing in and out on a beach. You do not have to act on them. Chapter 13 covers both problem-focused coping and emotion-focused coping. Refer to that chapter for suggestions on managing stress eating.

The Opportunity Binge

The *opportunity binge* most often occurs when there is easy access to tempting food and high access to privacy. In some cases, the opportunity binge occurs due to a combination of boredom and unstructured time. The likelihood of such a binge happening is increased if the person dwells on thoughts of eating highly preferred high-calorie foods. The incentive of "getting away with something" is an added factor. Simply realizing that there will be an opportunity to be alone and binge can trigger thoughts about food choices. Expecting an opportunity to binge together with mentally planning what to eat can set the opportunity binge in motion.

Other good times for an opportunity binge involve socially sanctioned eating events such as vacations, holidays, and celebrations. Any feel-good gathering can provide an opportunity to overeat. Ironically, some people in weight-loss programs who lose weight between sessions leave their meeting and celebrate by getting something to eat.

Of course, overeating on occasion is not the real problem for weight management. Most people overdo now and then. It is when overeating occurs frequently—usually occasioned by using some excuse or rationale to permit it—that weight is impacted. Rachel from the chapter-opening vignette admitted that she found lots of excuses to eat at any opportunity: "When I'm out with my friends I want to eat like they do." "Why should I have to set limits on myself?" "It's been a tough day." "I need something to feel better." "I might never get to try this again."

Transitions from one task to another provide opportunities to eat. Getting home from work and transitioning to family time can prompt getting something to eat. This is often the "glass or two of wine plus cheese and crackers" beginning of an opportunity binge. Any change in routine—for example, wrapping up a project, finishing painting the living room, driving home after a meeting—can incite an impulse to get something to eat or drink. Completing a task is often associated with good feelings. Eating serves as a tension reliever and signals it is time to relax. Such transition times can pose a problem if getting something to eat turns into overeating. When eating results in the thought, "Well, I've blown it now, so why not go all the way?" a small incident of overeating can trigger a full-blown binge.

The best remedy for opportunity bingeing is to bring all the cognitive and behavioral tools you have learned in the preceding chapters to bear. These include managing the environment and planning how to cope. For example, decide in advance how to minimize or cope with unstructured time, holidays, and special occasions, and plan to use self-rewards to encourage better behavior. The core principles for overcoming all types of binges include normalizing eating (discussed in detail later in this chapter) and allowing yourself to eat most foods in moderation. Also, learn to direct thinking away from the immediate rewards of eating and focus on your long-term goals. Preventing a small lapse from turning into a major relapse is addressed in chapter 15, "Dealing with Backsliding."

The Vengeful Binge

Fueled by anger, the *vengeful binge* is a way to vent hostility. The target is often the binge eater themselves, sometimes another person, and sometimes the situation. Your body may become a target because it "let me down and became obese." Perceived failure can invite self-punishment. A nagging parent can be the source of vengeful eating. Having a tough time at work can trigger a vengeful binge. Overeating is one way of venting frustration and anger when a situation seems out of control.

Vengeful binge eaters are sometimes people who have been injured emotionally. These binge eaters perceive themselves as wronged, slighted, or, in some way, hurt by others. They usually don't see how their own actions may have contributed. Or perhaps they were, indeed, hurt through no fault of their own and feel they have no way to alleviate their anger. Binge eating is one outlet. A binge can be a way to suppress angry feelings. Unfortunately, the vengeful binge eater must bear a double burden—the original injury plus the hurt, anger, and disillusionment that seem to have no place to go afterward.

Sometimes the vengeful binge is instigated by an inner "Rebel" voice or subpersonality, which resents and rejects the authority of good eating habits and takes delight in flaunting poor food choices. The Rebel eschews self-discipline and undermines dieting attempts. The Rebel is often angry about being "different"—having to eat differently from others or having to cope with obesity. Obsession with this unfairness and the wish for revenge prompts the vengeful binge—a symbolic "No!" that arises when there is no obvious resolution available. Review chapter 12, "Challenging Your Inner 'Voices'" for more on dealing with the voice of your inner Rebel.

To overcome vengeful binge eating, the underlying anger must be addressed so that forgiveness can proceed. In his book *Forgive for Good*, Dr. Frederic Luskin states that forgiveness involves transforming anger into acceptance. Another way of thinking about forgiveness is "giving up the wish that the past was different from what it was" and learning to accept what is and move on. According to Dr. Luskin, forgiveness is not the same as forgetting, pardoning, reconciliation, condoning, justifying, or even understanding. Of course, in some cases, forgiveness may lead to reconciliation, but this is not a necessary outcome. It may be advisable not to allow the offending person back in your life. The goal is to move on with your life and find happiness by staying in touch with your values and overarching principles and acting accordingly.

In their book *Helping Clients Forgive*, Drs. Robert Enright and Richard Fitzgibbons add that attaining retribution for, compensation for, or acknowledgement of the wrong by the perpetrator is not part of forgiveness. Neither is forgiveness achieved by passively letting time heal the wound, nor by simply saying, "I forgive you." Some people want to know if they should confront the person who hurt them. Usually, doing so only leads to more hurt because the other party may likely see things differently or is defensive. Writing a letter to the offender expressing what you feel but not sending it can be cathartic. Doing so allows you to work through the experience by expressing on paper your feelings and opinions. If after writing and rewriting such a letter, you can communicate your opinion and feelings assertively and respectfully in person, then do so. But remember, the other person may still dispute your experience. There are times, however, when standing up for your rights is necessary and appropriate. (Refer to chapter 13 regarding assertiveness skills.)

Dr. Luskin describes preconditions for forgiving. It is important to look closely at the facts about what happened. In what way did your actions or inaction play a part in the outcome of the situation? How did each person involved contribute to the problem? What assumptions did you jump to about the situation? Did you check out your judgments? Looking back on the event and trying to understand the part you played may help you see the situation differently. If you find that something you did, said, or didn't do contributed to how the situation turned out, own up to your part. That can open the door to reconciliation and/or forgiveness.

To heal, Dr. Luskin advises telling your story to a couple of trusted people, but without practicing a victim or grievance story. Remind yourself that clinging to a victim story only reinforces "poor me" and keeps you stuck in the past. After acknowledging what has happened and validating your feelings, it is better to put your energy into looking for a way to get your needs and goals met in the present rather than rehashing past hurtful experiences. When you seek out

Table 14.2 How to Forgive

1. Acknowledge what happened to you, and examine your grievance and anger about it.

2. Write out a description of what happened and your feelings. Don't communicate this to the offending person; the goal is for you to let go of hurt. Writing about the incident will help clarify what happened.

3. Consider what role you played (with your actions or inactions) that contributed to bringing the event about.

4. Tell your story to a few trusted people but don't cling to a victim story.

5. Do not expect or necessarily seek reconciliation.

6. Allow yourself to feel the pain or hurt of the incident without fighting your feelings.

7. Put your energy into looking for new ways to get your needs and goals met in the present.

8. Focus on staying true to your values and getting on with your life.

new ways to get what you want instead of mentally replaying your pain, you will no longer need the vengeful binge. Table 14.2, How to Forgive, summarizes the steps for reaching forgiveness. Remember, the person you most need to forgive may be yourself.

The Pleasure Binge

The *pleasure binge* is triggered by the desire for stimulation and entertainment. Obese binge eaters are vulnerable to this type of binge when they have few other sources of pleasure or satisfaction in their lives beyond food. Eating provides a reliable source of reward. Those who succumb to the pleasure binge describe feeling excited by the idea of eating and sometimes spend a great deal of time thinking and fantasizing about what they will eat next. They enjoy eating food, but later may regret their behavior and its health implications.

For all people, eating should be a pleasure that does not induce guilt or harm health. In every culture, eating and sharing food with others is a central focus of social celebrations and social interchange. The ceremony of "breaking bread" is an acknowledgement of friendship. In ancient historical times, overindulging in a feast was accepted. More recently, Christian tradition has labeled overeating or eating to excess as the "Sin of Gluttony." In modern Westernized society, eating healthy food in moderation was recommended by health experts, which stands in stark contrast to our present-day environment that invites unhealthy eating and overindulging.

One way to avoid the pleasure binge is to exercise portion control. It is also helpful to eat slowly. Eating should not be the only, or even the main, source of pleasure or satisfaction in a day. Redefining self-concept so that healthy eating and regular exercise become parts of self-identity is also necessary for overcoming pleasure binge eating. Think of yourself as someone who chooses to eat healthy foods and engages in regular exercise. The person who defines herself as a vegetarian doesn't wish they could eat meat. Similarly, the runner doesn't wish they didn't have to run; they worry or feel bad when they can't. It's a matter of self-perception. The vegetarian and the runner have a self-concept that defines their behavior.

The Habit Binge

The *habit binge* is the one on automatic pilot—no one seems to be at the controls. This sort of eating involves a basic stimulus–response pattern and is basically mindless eating. The stimulus is readily available food, and the response is eating without much thinking—and often not much pleasure. For example, one person who had a wonderful dinner out, returned to his hotel and kept grabbing handfuls of peanuts from a dish in the lobby, eating them without thinking. Unlike the pleasure binger, the habit binge eater does not especially focus on the taste or pleasantness of food. Another name for the habit binge might be the *grazing binge*—continuous, more or less nonstop eating with little conscious effort to control it and no immediate inclination to feel upset about it. Only later, when body weight increases or obesity is obvious, do negative reactions set in.

The habit binge eater is likely to benefit from self-monitoring. Self-monitoring involves keeping daily records of food eaten and the circumstances, including external events, thoughts, and feelings related to these events. Keeping a record of eating behavior is the first step in identifying problem patterns. It also makes the behavior more available to conscious control and, therefore, more readily changed. The habit binge eater needs to beware of small dishes of snacks that are set out for the taking, for instance, a dish of peanuts on a coffee table. Limiting food consumption to prescheduled meals and planned snacks is important for overcoming all types of binge eating.

Interrupting the Binge-Eating Cycle

Binges commonly have six stages that repeat over and over. The first is the *tension-building* stage when stress is taxing your ability to cope. During this stage, your thoughts and interpretation of situations may cause you to feel stress. At the second stage, the *tipping point*, stress and tension become so seemingly intolerable that you make a decision to binge. The third stage is the *binge itself*, where little thinking occurs. At some point, the binge terminates and is followed by the fourth stage, *self-recrimination and guilt*. If you had a sugar binge, there may also be a period of *fatigue and exhaustion*, the fifth stage. This is eventually followed by the sixth stage—the point at which you *resolve* not to let it happen again. And then stage one, the tension-building stage, begins again. Figure 14.1, The Binge Cycle, is a schematic of what the stages of a binge look like.

The best stage to intervene in a binge-eating cycle is during the first stage, when tension is building but before you reach your tipping point. The tension-building stage may consist of obsessive thoughts about food or eating. Some people admit they plan to binge. Sources of stress and tension—including stress-inducing thinking—need to be identified and reduced before tension becomes overwhelming. Although it is possible to avert a binge before it begins, it is more difficult to do so if the tension has built to a high level. This is especially true if a thought like "Well, I've blown it, so who cares?" occurs.

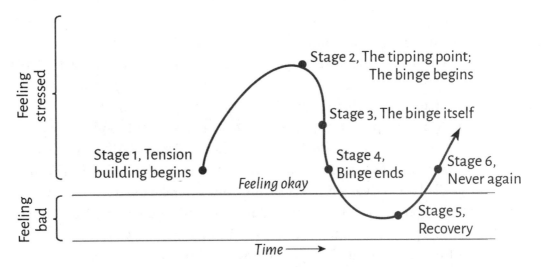

Figure 14.1 **The Binge Cycle**

Once the binge has begun, it is difficult to stop it from proceeding, mainly because there has been an abdication of conscious control.

Success is more likely if you identify the behavior pattern, including the triggers that elicit the binge, the thoughts and beliefs that occur, and the reinforcers that immediately follow it (for instance, avoidance of feeling, temporary relief, or even satisfaction from eating all you want). Effective stress management will reduce tension buildup and decrease the likelihood of a binge. Avoiding the triggers that set off a binge reduces the likelihood of one occurring. Likewise, learning to cope more effectively with tension helps eliminate these cues and prevents the binge cycle from continuing to its conclusion. Identifying self-hindering self-talk and focusing on self-helping self-talk (see chapter 11) is important. Instituting rewards for *not* bingeing is also helpful.

Triggers

The occurrence of one or more events can trigger or elicit a binge. Self-hindering self-talk and how you understand external events can be triggers. It is important to determine which triggers are most likely to set off a binge for you. An event can be external—perhaps an argument with someone or a painful remark made by them. An event can also be internal—a thought, a feeling, a physical state such as fatigue or hunger, a decision, or a reaction to an external circumstance, such as being left alone with an opportunity to overeat. A particularly potent trigger involves obsessing about food.

Self-Test 14.1, Rate Your Triggers for Binge Eating, lists some events that can trigger binges. Identify the thinking or self-talk that is likely to trigger a binge for you. After you take the test, think about how you can use the coping skills covered in chapter 13 to reduce the impact of the ones you rate on the high end—a 4 or a 5. Consider pleasurable or satisfying activities you can use to reduce the likelihood of having a binge because of negative emotions.

Obsessing About Food

Some people are troubled by intrusive and persistent thoughts of food and eating. As they ruminate more and more about a particular food, they reach a point where they can no longer resist eating. Their focus of attention has become so narrow, they can think of nothing else but eating that food. Eating serves to reduce the tension built up by obsessing about it. In some cases, thoughts that turn to eating follow thoughts about a troubling situation. "Wishing it wasn't so" or worrying about the future prompts feelings of anxiety or even anger. Both anxiety and anger are emotions that push the thinker to "do something." A vulnerable person's thoughts may turn to eating when it appears there is nothing that can be done about a troubling situation, thus diverting attention from the problem. The more attention that is focused on eating and thoughts of food, the more compelling eating becomes. Finally, the tipping point is reached, and the binge occurs. It provides temporary relief from worries and troubles only to be followed by self-recrimination and guilt, and a return of worrisome thoughts.

The best way to avoid the binges triggered by obsessive thinking about food and eating is to use the problem-focused and

Self-Test 14.1 Rate Your Triggers for Binge Eating

Instructions: Rate each of the following from 1, not at all likely, to 5, highly likely to trigger a binge for you. Those you rate a 4 or 5 need your special attention.

Rate	Binge Triggers
_____	1. Experiencing hunger from restrictive eating
_____	2. Experiencing anxiety or tension
_____	3. Experiencing cravings
_____	4. Obsessing about food or eating
_____	5. Eating anything
_____	6. Eating something sweet
_____	7. Breaking a dietary rule or breaking your diet
_____	8. Experiencing interpersonal conflict
_____	9. Feeling judged, criticized, blamed, rejected, unappreciated, taken advantage of, or unacknowledged
_____	10. Engaging in irrational thinking, cognitive distortions, self-critical thinking, or self-hindering self-talk
_____	11. Failing to perform up to your own expectations
_____	12. Having unstructured time
_____	13. Having access to privacy and food
_____	14. Participating in social situations.
_____	15. Needing to or feeling like rebelling
_____	16. Worrying about money, sex, family, etc.
_____	17. Feeling overwhelmed
_____	18. Suffering work-related distress
_____	19. Having marital problems
_____	20. Thinking about sex
_____	21. Suffering pain, fatigue, illness, or debilitating physical symptoms
_____	22. Suffering from premenstrual tension
_____	23. Drinking alcohol or using certain drugs
_____	24. Other: _____

emotion-focused coping skills detailed in the chapter 13. If you continually find yourself obsessing about eating, learn to shift your attention to something else. Take a walk. Brush your teeth. Drink a few big glasses of water. Call a friend. If the thought continues to intrude, try telling yourself, "That's just my binge thought," simply noticing and acknowledging it is there. Don't grab onto the thought; just let it pass through your mind as you say to yourself, "Okay, it's just a thought. I don't have to act on it." Keep reminding yourself of this, and shift your attention to something else you need to do now. You may need to repeat this process many times, and it may not always work. Keep trying. (If you have intrusive and unsettling thoughts, such as washing your hands or checking the stove, you may have obsessive-compulsive disorder and should consult a qualified therapist to relieve your anxieties.)

Coping with Cravings

About 50 percent of obese binge eaters report having cravings for certain foods, especially sweet foods. Both hunger and unpleasant emotions such as boredom can set off food cravings. We crave because we seek pleasure and hope to escape pain. For some, a thought about a particular food occurs, and that thought becomes the only thing they can think of. The best thing to do is recognize you are having a craving, remind yourself you don't have to follow through with it, and enlist the Five Ds:

❖ Delay at least ten minutes before deciding to act on the craving.

❖ Distract yourself by doing something else that requires your attention.

❖ Distance yourself from the food or temptation.

❖ Determine if giving into the craving is in alignment with your lifestyle values.

❖ Decide in that moment whether to eat what you crave or to do something else that serves you better.

Use Rewards

In chapter 7, you learned how to use reward to change behavior patterns. You can use the calendar-and-stickers method introduced there and give yourself a reward sticker for each day you don't binge. By using a month-at-a-glance calendar, you will track your progress and see your improvements. Be sure to give yourself a mental pat on the back as well for each day without a binge.

Normalize Your Eating Pattern

To break the binge-eating cycle, you must normalize your eating pattern. To succeed, it is necessary to learn to eat in a way that is naturally healthy. Natural and healthy eating is regulated by feelings of hunger and satiety. Those with an eating disorder such as BED no longer tune in to these signals, or they confuse them with other feelings. For example, anxiety may be misinterpreted as hunger. Those who are grazers never let themselves feel hunger, and those who skip meals usually become overly hungry.

Eating regularly—having three meals and optional, planned snacks each day—is the basis for long-term weight management. If you want to cut calories, eating on a regular basis—perhaps four or six planned meals—throughout the day may initially seem counterintuitive. However, binge eating will be less likely if you learn to eat regularly; when you eat regular meals, you are not stressing your body or your psyche, you are less susceptible to negative moods, and you are less likely to overeat or binge. Regular eating is also a far more satisfying, healthy, and effective way to manage weight over the long haul.

Normalizing your eating pattern must be done in small incremental steps. The first step is to decide on the times of day you want to eat your three meals and two or three planned snacks. You can decide each day what your times will be, and the times may vary from day to day. Or you can plan several days or a week in advance. You can adjust your eating times to accommodate your commitments as long as *no more than three to five hours elapse between eating times.*

Once you establish eating times, eat only during those times. Allow yourself only enough time in your schedule to eat your meal or snack. Breakfast or lunch should take no more than fifteen to twenty minutes to eat. Dinner ordinarily should take no longer than thirty minutes, and a snack no more than ten or fifteen minutes. Focus on eating slowly; remember that binge eaters tend to gulp their food. Eat at the planned times even if you don't feel hungry and use portion control. Don't skip meals or planned snacks; try not to eat at other times. If you do slip and eat at an unplanned time, or you binge, just get back on track as soon as possible.

If you have been on many diets in the past, usually with poor results, the thought of imposing self-discipline, or even just restricting meals and snacks to certain times of the day, may feel overwhelming to you. Some so-called experts advise only eating when you feel hungry. Most overeaters have lost touch with their physical signals and don't know when they are hungry. In fact, they often don't let themselves feel hunger—they snack or eat to prevent hunger, so it is important to plan your mealtimes.

If you have never had much success with setting limits on your eating in the past, perhaps you doubt that you can. By normalizing eating with planned eating, you demonstrate to yourself that you can exercise control even if it is only by limiting eating to certain times of the day. And you will overcome your fear of hunger. Once you find you have more control than you thought, the next step is to make gradual changes in what you eat to move you closer to a healthy diet and a healthier weight. Table 14.3 sets out a plan for making positive changes to your eating habits.

Once you are eating on a regular schedule, begin to make changes to what you eat. Start with small changes you feel are easily accomplished. For example, you might change from whole milk to low-fat milk and, eventually, to nonfat milk. Try eliminating butter on bread, then reduce the amount of bread or change to a whole-wheat bread. Switch from sugary soft drinks to sparkling water with a twist

Table 14.3 Steps to Normalizing Your Eating Pattern

1. Establish set times for eating three meals a day.

2. Eat planned snacks as appropriate.

3. Use the three-to-five hour rule. You should allow three to five hours between eating episodes.

4. Don't skip meals.

5. If you have an eating slip, get back on track as soon as possible.

6. In the beginning, focus more on when you eat and not on what you eat so you can use the three-to-five rule described in #3.

7. Focus on overcoming binge eating before worrying about losing weight.

8. Avoid restrictive eating.

of citrus or tea. Reduce the size of your portions. Remove tempting foods from your refrigerator and kitchen; if you don't have it in the house, you are less likely to eat it. Implement some of the changes suggested in chapter 7.

Succeeding with Planned Eating

When it comes to normalizing your eating pattern, success is achieved gradually. It is not necessary—or possible—to go from never setting limits on eating to being perfect at doing so. Take it one day at a time, one meal at a time. Just tell yourself you'll do the best you can. Each time you succeed at a small goal—for example, limiting one evening's snacking to a predefined time—count that as a success and pat yourself on the back. Analyze what helped you succeed that time and do more of what works. Keep your eye on the big picture, and don't get distracted by small slips. Remember that the road to success is always under construction.

How to *Prevent* a Binge

The best strategy is to prevent a binge from occurring in the first place. Normalizing your eating patterns, as we discussed, as well as implementing the following steps, will decrease the likelihood of a binge:

1. **Start with a healthy breakfast and don't skip meals.**
   Choose foods that are rich in fiber, such as fruit and whole-grain cereal or old-fashioned oatmeal. Fiber is important for keeping the gut healthy and preventing or relieving constipation. Forget "white bread" breakfasts that cause a blood sugar spike and then a premature blood sugar drop. Include a healthy, high-protein food, especially those from plant sources, such as tofu or veggie sausage, at breakfast and other meals.

2. **Eat enough when you eat.**
   That doesn't mean stuff yourself. But don't skip meals or eat tiny diet-sized portions and expect to keep hunger at bay for hours. Include high-fiber items such as beans, vegetables, fruits, and grains.

3. **Know your minimum number of calories per day.**
   Multiply your desired healthy body weight by ten to determine a target minimum. Remember, this minimum doesn't take age or exercise and physical activity into account.

4. **Get exercise and enough rest.**
   Even if you don't go to a gym, you will benefit from incorporating more movement into your usual daily activities, such as taking the stairs, parking in a far corner of the lot, doing yard work, or walking the dog. Regular physical activity helps you sleep better. Beware of caffeine and alcohol, both of which can disrupt sleep. Have a glass of milk before bed or some other food that promotes serotonin, such as a piece of whole-grain toast.

5. **Improve your coping skills for managing stress.**
   Use problem-focused and emotion-focused coping. Remember that thoughts that are upsetting are just thoughts and need

not be acted on. Likewise for emotions. Learn to change that which can be changed and accept that which cannot. See chapter 13 for more stress-management tools.

6. **Stay in touch with your values and guiding principles.**
Remember your health and weight are excellent reasons for preventing or intervening in the binge cycle. What matters are the benefits you have identified for developing a healthy lifestyle that is in alignment with your values. See chapter 6, "Getting and Staying Motivated," for more information about motivation and values.

7. **Meditate.**
Having a meditation practice will also help relieve tension and manage emotions.

How to Binge-Proof Your House

Be sure to binge-proof your home as much as possible. Stock up on healthy foods and don't buy binge foods. For the obese binge eater, having lots of good food around may provide a sense of security and comfort. The idea of keeping tempting foods that can trigger a binge out of the house may cause anxiety. When food and eating have functioned as your primary or only way of coping, not having food available to eat can make you feel vulnerable. This is where emotion-focused coping is needed. Chapter 13 discusses emotion-focused coping. Find other ways to deal with anxiety. Tell yourself, "Not having my comfort food readily available is difficult and focusing on this worry just makes me anxious. I need to remember that feelings are like waves: they build, crest, and pass. I just need to accept my feelings and allow them to pass and, in the meantime, focus on doing something else."

Coping with "Danger" Foods

Even as you binge-proof your house, try not to make any foods forbidden or completely off limits. Instead, categorize foods as "Frequently

Chosen," "Sometimes Chosen," and "Rarely Chosen." As mentioned in chapter 7 on changing behavior, you may need to add a special category for one or two items that are your favorite binge foods. This last category would be your "Danger" foods. You may need to avoid them for a while, but eventually you can try to reintroduce them into your diet. If you find that certain foods are proven to always set off a binge, consider that you can probably live without them. As noted previously in this chapter, binge foods you are not able to eat successfully in moderation are better defined out of your eating style, just as this author did with Almond Roca.

Medical Management of BED

Several medications have been found to be helpful in reducing the symptoms of binge-eating disorder. It appears such medications can reduce the frequency of episodes and hopefully help with weight loss. However, drug research for BED is still in its early stages and more studies are needed.

Antidepressants known as *selective serotonin reuptake inhibitors* (SSRIs) appear to help reduce binge eating by increasing the availability of the neurotransmitter *serotonin* in the brain, which helps improve mood. (Recall that *neurotransmitters* are the chemicals in the brain that control communication among brain cells.) Examples of SSRIs include fluoxetine (Prozac) and sertraline (Zoloft). Take note that once these medications are discontinued, binge eating can reappear. Furthermore, some people experience weight gain with some of these medications.

Developed for controlling seizures, topiramate, or Topamax, has also been found to reduce binge-eating episodes. However, it can cause serious side effects, including fatigue, dizziness, problems in focusing, and burning or tingling sensations.

No medications alone will help you lose weight and keep it off. To do that, you must adopt a healthy lifestyle that includes regular exercise.

15

Dealing with Backsliding

Ethan made good progress on his weight-management effort until he went out with his friends for the evening. He told himself he'd just have one beer and no snacks. After the second beer and some peanuts, Ethan forgot about his weight-management progress and threw caution to the winds. "Who really cares?" he thought to himself. "After all, I've already blown it, and besides, I deserve a little fun once in a while." Then he had a cheeseburger with fries, and, together with the beers, the calories really added up. In short, Ethan backslid—suffered recidivism— when he went drinking with friends. Eventually, he had to face a difficult question: Could he keep associating with his drinking (and eating) buddies and maintain healthy habits? Ethan had to recognize that going out with his buddies was a "high-risk situation," and he needed better coping skills for managing such events or he might have to give up his boys' night out. Ethan also had to decide if alcohol was a problem for him. He went on the internet to get more information about weight-management relapse prevention and to investigate whether he had a problem with alcohol. After his research, he decided he would eat before joining his buddies and then follow one beer with soda water. If that didn't work, he resolved, he would have to take a hard look at his situation and decide if he had to stay away from his drinking buddies or reevaluate his drinking.

Backsliding is a process that leads to a return to old habits. It is a significant problem for weight management. People typically begin to backslide after a period of doing well. Often there is a single small lapse, which may be followed by more lapses. If lapses keep multiplying over time, backsliding has begun, and a complete relapse can occur.

Of course, occasional lapses are common in any behavior-change effort and are to be expected. When you slip, the important thing is to recover and recommit to value-driven behavior and the lifestyle change you say you want. It is important to treat a slip as a learning experience rather than a prediction of imminent failure. Having a small slip invites you to understand what caused the lapse.

Causes of Lapses

In terms of succumbing to a lapse, the biggest hazard is your hindering voice telling you that you can have "just one" or that you can bend the rules "just this time." Such thoughts usually occur in the context of a *high-risk situation*—a situation fraught with temptation. When these small lapses increase in frequency and motivation wanes, backsliding has begun. A series of little lapses, intended or unplanned, accompanied by increasing ambivalence about your ability to maintain success, can result in a precipitous return to bad habits. Most total relapses occur within the first ninety days after altering a behavior, but they can occur later if adverse circumstances and hindering thoughts prevail.

A single lapse usually results from the desire for *short-term gratification*—wanting something now—and losing sight of your core, overarching values and principles. Often because of the single slip, all-or-nothing thinking occurs: "Now I've blown it. I'm a failure." If you see the infraction as evidence of your inability to succeed, you may decide to quit trying. You may feel guilty and remorseful about the lapse, unless you are able to rationalize it away.

To justify having committed one small infraction, you may defend your action and continue to make more unhealthy choices. Perhaps you decide you don't want limits set on your behavior, which weakens your motivation. This eventually leads from a single slip into backsliding. If, on the other hand, you are willing to view deviations from your commitment from which to learn how to be in better charge of your behavior, you can open the way to renewed commitment. A single lapse need not lead to total relapse.

Developing awareness of the process of backsliding and learning how to prevent or recover from a single lapse is key to preventing total relapse.

Emotional Hazards of Lapses

Deciding that a single slip is terrible, or that you are bad and incapable of succeeding because you made an unhealthy choice, moves you closer to backsliding and, eventually, total relapse. Backsliding that leads to full-scale relapse, or sometimes even small lapses, can produce emotional upset and lower your self-esteem.

How upset you get depends on several things. If you feel that the lapse wasn't your fault or that you really did not try your hardest, you might not feel too bad knowing you can fix that behavior. If, on the other hand, you engage in self-criticism and blame rather than problem-solving, you will feel worse. The more effort you have put into changing or the more you feel pressure to succeed, the more upsetting lapses are likely to be. Backsliding after you have maintained a new behavior pattern for a long time is likely to be very upsetting. Likewise, regaining a significant amount of weight can be emotionally devastating. If someone you care about is angry or disapproving because of your backsliding, you will probably be upset too. Feeling that you are losing, or have lost, control produces more negative emotions and may result in abandoning further effort. The more important the thwarted goal is to you, the more upset you will feel.

Backsliding affects not only how you feel but how you think. You may start to wonder if the goal you are striving for is worth the effort. You may begin to focus on the nonmotivation boxes of the cost-benefit analysis (see chapter 6, "Getting and Staying Motivated"). You may try to rationalize the actions that led to backsliding so you can stop feeling guilty about violating your commitment to change. To find a good excuse, you may distort or deny the facts. If you unjustly blame someone else for the backsliding, you may create problems in your relationship with that person or end up resenting or even lying to them. If you place all the blame on someone else, or fail to acknowledge your own accountability, you are less likely to learn from the experience and to reverse the backsliding. Or, conversely, you may completely, and unreasonably, blame yourself for backsliding, with the result that your self-esteem declines and your self-image suffers. Your confidence in your ability to cope takes a nosedive, and you develop an expectation of future failure.

Many things can contribute to backsliding, including high-risk situations, errors in thinking, an unsupportive context, lack of self-management skills, and an unbalanced lifestyle.

High-Risk Situations

Lapses and backsliding start in the context of a particular event or situation—usually a high-risk situation. Such situations may catch you unawares, although sometimes you can anticipate a circumstance, like an office party, that will strain your ability to cope with food temptations. Whether or not you are prepared to cope and how you mentally react to a triggering situation can determine if you will have a lapse and begin to backslide. The real problem is not the high-risk situation per se; it is the failure to anticipate it and to have a coping strategy.

G. Alan Marlatt, the psychologist who first discussed the role high-risk situations play in relapse of alcoholics, has identified two general groups of high-risk situations: those that occur due to intrapersonal determinants and those that are brought about by interpersonal determinants.

Intrapersonal Determinants. *Intrapersonal determinants* are the thoughts you have and the emotions you feel in response to an external situation like a slip or an accident. They include:

* ❖ *Negative emotions, moods, or feelings*: frustration, anger, fear, anxiety, tension, depression, loneliness, sadness, boredom, worry, apprehension, grief, or loss; or stressful feelings that arise in response to situations such as undergoing an examination, responding to a promotion, engaging in public speaking, having employment or financial difficulties, or suffering a personal misfortune or accident.

* ❖ *Negative physical states*: unpleasant physical experiences, such as pain, illness, injury, excessive hunger, or fatigue; reactions associated with drugs or with withdrawal from an addictive substance; or hormonal or chemical imbalances such as those associated with diabetes, hypoglycemia, or premenstrual syndrome (PMS).

* ❖ *Private positive emotions*: desires for, or actions intended to produce, feelings of "getting high," prolonging pleasure, feeling relaxed, satisfactorily finishing a task; or positive feelings of being secure, loved, accepted, or nurtured.

* ❖ *Tests of personal control*: thoughts that rationalize actions on the basis of having "just one"; thoughts focused on testing willpower; or overconfidence in one's capacity for moderate use.

❖ *Urges or temptations*: responses to both sudden inclinations and to enduring desires to give up or return to old habits.

Interpersonal Determinants. *Interpersonal determinants* are influenced by your relationships with other people. They include:

❖ *Interpersonal conflict situations*: such as those you experience in marriage, friendship, family, employer/employee relations, or any other situations involving people that produce frustration, annoyance, anger, arguments, disagreements, fights, jealousy, discord, hassles, anxiety, fear, tension, hurt, apprehension, or guilt.

❖ *Social influences*: situations in which either an individual or a group pressures, coerces, tempts, coaxes, prepares, condones, or makes a gift that influences you to backslide, or situations in which such a return to old habits is prompted merely by observing an individual or group engaging in unhealthy behaviors.

❖ *Interpersonal positive emotions*: social situations that generate feelings of pleasure, celebration, sexual excitement, freedom, and the like.

Typical Triggers for Backsliding

Nearly 75 percent of all backsliding related to behavioral addictions is triggered by just three determinants: negative emotions, interpersonal conflict, and social influences.

Similarly, research has identified three clusters of typical high-risk situations for weight control. The first and most common of these, *social mealtime situations*, usually involve friends or family. In these situations, spirits are high and negative emotions tend to be absent. A second cluster of high-risk situations involves *emotional upset situations*, especially anger, but also situations associated with anxiety, sadness, or depression. Most such emotional upset situations occur when the dieter is alone, although sometimes other people are present. The third cluster of high-risk situations, *low-arousal situations*, is characterized by eating when alone. Dieters report feeling no particular emotions at such times, though occasionally they feel tired or bored. These low-arousal situations involve relaxing, waiting, or being between other activities, called *transition times* (when one task has been put aside or finished and another has yet to begin). These are the times when dieters often find themselves getting something to eat. In these situations, food is present or readily available, and the person often reports feeling "hungry." The *feeling* of hunger may actually be another emotion erroneously interpreted as hunger, perhaps boredom or happiness about finishing a task.

Clearly there are many high-risk situations that can lead to relapse in weight management. You need to determine your own. The best way to do that is to use self-monitoring. Another way is to deconstruct a lapse: determine what led up to it, what beliefs or self-talk were involved, and what you did afterward. From this analysis, you should be able to identify the high-risk situation that led to your lapse and how it can be avoided in the future.

Recognizing High-Risk Situations

Sometimes people don't recognize that they have just encountered, or are about to encounter, a high-risk situation that puts them in danger of having a lapse. We easily recognize that attractive and available foods present a temptation, but other high-risk situations are not so obvious. For example, many people find that feeling good is a high-risk situation, and they not only indulge but also use food to prolong the positive emotions.

Getting bored with a weight-loss program is also a high-risk situation. At the beginning of a diet there is excitement, but, over time, diets can be wearing. Other high-risk situations can arise from having to tolerate a slow rate of weight loss, having to make decisions about what to eat, or getting injured (thus being unable to exercise). That is another reason why diets don't always work—they can lead to boredom.

To substantially reduce the risk of backsliding, it is important to learn to identify and cope with high-risk or crisis situations that can prompt overeating. Success is ensured by developing skills for coping with emotions (including positive ones), dealing effectively with interpersonal conflict, and managing social influences and situations. It is also important to know how to recover from a small lapse and not let repeated slips lead to a full-blown relapse.

Rather than following a diet, adopting a healthy eating pattern helps avoid or manage high-risk situations. Making small changes permanent, and then continuing to strive for a new self-definition that is signified by a new way of eating, leaves room for small deviations. The healthy eating pattern is less likely to founder on the rocks than a diet.

How to Cope with High-Risk Situations

To overcome backsliding triggered by a high-risk situation, you can do several things:

1. **Learn to identify the high-risk situations that may cause you difficulty.** Figure out what causes your eating problems. Once you have identified your personal list, take steps to avoid those situations that can be avoided. For those that cannot be avoided, try to anticipate problems and plan in advance how to effectively cope.

2. **Be prepared with a coping response.** Know what to do. Mentally remind yourself of your values, your commitment, and why you made it. Review the motivation boxes in the cost-benefit analysis you completed in chapter 6. Tell yourself what to do to cope, then take positive action. A coping response should involve both thoughts and actions. If you start to slip into excuses and rationalizations, bring in helping thoughts. Remember, you don't have to act on your hindering self-talk. Be willing to take drastic action if necessary, such as tossing candy or chips in the disposal (instead of rationalizing that you'll save it for the kids or company).

3. **Mentally rehearse.** If you know you will have to deal with a high-risk situation, mentally rehearse to prepare for it. Never let yourself encounter an anticipated high-risk situation without preparation. To rehearse, imagine yourself in the situation before you encounter it. Then imagine effectively handling the situation and feeling good about it. Determine in advance what you will order in a restaurant, at a wedding, or at a party. Plan how you will say no nicely but firmly.

4. **Employ specific skills or techniques for coping.** To avoid backsliding, be prepared to use helping self-talk, exercise, meditation, relaxation, assertive communication, and any other skill or technique that will help you cope more effectively. Review earlier chapters that discuss how to implement such strategies. There is also helpful advice and specific strategies provided later in this chapter in the section that discusses Implementation Intervention Plans.

5. **Avoid "tunnel vision."** When you have "tunnel vision," your thoughts seem to focus only on the temptations—eating, drinking—to the exclusion of other influences, such as your health, your weight resolve, sticking to your commitment, your values, and so forth. Tunnel vision often leads to rationalizations about why you should give up your efforts and is a precursor to falling into a trancelike state in the bottom of the Funnel of Awareness (see figure 11.1 in chapter 11, "Managing Thinking and Self-Talk").

   One trick for avoiding tunnel vision is to keep your cost-benefit analysis from chapter 6 on hand and refer to it when you expect to encounter a high-risk situation or when motivation starts to wane. Be careful not to get caught up in your hindering self-talk; remember that just because you have a thought, doesn't mean you have to act on it. Talk back to your rationalizations and excuses. Think about your life values and guiding principles. Talk yourself out of giving up; reread the motivation boxes (#1 and #4) of your cost-benefit analysis.

Remind yourself why you made this commitment, and recognize and honor the hard work you have already put in.

6. **Learn to recover from a first slip.** Learning to recover from a first slip is a crucial coping strategy. If possible, avoid a first slip, but if you do slip, having coping skills will keep you from backsliding. Most people do not stop at "just one," and recovering from a small slip can be problematic. If you do manage to handle "just one" the first time, you may become overconfident and think you can always handle "just one." But a succession of "just ones" can lead to full-blown backsliding.

   Succumbing to a first slip, however, does not have to signal a full slide backward. Instead of getting down on yourself, focus on what you can learn from the experience so that it is less likely to happen again. Usually, this involves discovering which situations presented temptation and making sure you have coping strategies at hand to deal with similar events in the future.

7. **Use reminder cards.** Another helpful tool for preventing or recovering from a first slip is to carry a reminder card. Like the seat-back pocket card the airlines use to tell you what to do in an emergency, a reminder card tells you what to do in case of a threatened or actual slip. On an index card, write a brief reminder of why you made the commitment to change and also note your values related to health. List what actions you should take to either avoid or recover from a slip if it happens. It's a good idea to include the name and phone number of a friend or weight-loss buddy you can call for support and advice. Carry the card with you. If you ever need it, use it!

Translating Intention into Action

Specific *Implementation Intervention Plans* (IIPs) promote goal achievement by translating intentions into specific, context-linked plans. That is, by writing out what you plan to do regarding a specific category of food, for instance sweets, you are more likely to carry out your intention. An IIP might list when and where you plan to eat a food that is high in calories. Thus, if you plan to allow yourself to choose a pastry on Sunday when you go out for coffee, you would write this on your menu planning form (an example of an IIP is shown in figure 15.1). On the other days of the week, you might not choose a sweet, so you would write down your plan to order only coffee or coffee and fruit—an alternative strategy for handling sweets.

Planning how to translate intention into action within specific contexts promotes goal achievement and weight loss. Planning when, where, and what to eat will help you translate your intentions into actions and prevent backsliding. Likewise, planning when and where you will exercise and what exercises you will engage in helps motivation. Planning how you will cope with risky or tempting situations increases your likelihood of success in high-risk situations.

These food categories and plans for physical activity are listed on the menu planning form because the behavior-change targets in this sample form are: reducing consumption of sweets and processed foods; increasing vegetables and fruit intake; choosing wisely when it comes to bread, meats and protein, and whole-grain foods; and planning exercise. The contents of this form are a suggestion; feel free to customize your weekly menu planning form to suit you.

In addition to completing a menu planning form each week, you need an IIP to help you anticipate difficult situations you might encounter with regard to eating or exercise. Figure 15.2 is a sample completed Plan for Coping with Difficult Situations form. Figure 15.3 is a blank form. After reviewing the sample, complete the blank form, giving as many answers to each statement as you can. Be specific: What thoughts or actions would you take in each situation? Once you have completed the sentence statements, make a list of situations that are specific to you. Write out what the situation is and what you plan to do to cope. For example, what would you do if someone offered you your favorite unhealthy food at a party? How would you avoid eating it? How do you plan to maintain a healthy

Figure 15.1 Menu Planning Form

MENU PLANNING: Week of _____ to _____

Planning when, where, and what to eat as well as when, where, and what exercises to perform has been found to help people translate their intentions into action. Using this form, make an **exact plan** of when, where, and what you will eat, and when, where, and how you will exercise in the next seven days.

Describe:	Monday	Tuesday	Wed.	Thurs.	Friday	Sat.	Sunday
Sweets, Fats, Alcohol *time, where, what*							
Bread *time, where, what, type of bread*							
Snacks *time, where, what*							
Vegetables *time, where, what*							
Fruits *time, where, what*							
Meat/protein *time, where, what*							
Whole-Grain Products, Cereal, Rice, Pasta *time, where, what*							
Exercise, Physical activity *time, where, what*							

Figure 15.2   Plan for Coping with Difficult Situations (Completed Sample)

1. **When I am hungry for something high in calories, instead of eating something unhealthy, I plan to:**

   Remember my guiding principles; know that although temptation is strong, I can take time to make a healthy choice; make a healthy choice that also tastes good; have healthy choices available; be pleased with myself for doing this.

2. **If I have a slip, instead of giving up, I plan to:**

   Think about what led up to the slip; make healthy choices at my next meal because each moment is a new moment to make a healthy choice; resolve to return to my healthy eating pattern.

3. **When I go out to eat, I plan to:**

   Think beforehand about what choices will be healthiest; imagine myself taking no or one piece of whole-grain bread before dinner; review the menu for healthy choices; eat slowly to enjoy my food and realize when I am full enough (not overly full or stuffed).

4. **When I'm out socializing and having a good time with friends, instead of giving myself permission to eat anything that seems appealing, I plan to:**

   Remember my guiding principles; know that the only person I have to answer to regarding my eating is me; be prepared for possible hunger before going out by eating a healthy snack; make healthy choices just as I would try to do if I wasn't out.

5. **When someone brings food into work, I plan to:**

   Remember my guiding principles so I can make good choices; have my own healthy snacks available so I don't feel deprived.

6. **When I'm feeling mad about having to cut calories or exercise, I plan to:**

   Allow myself to feel my emotions but know I don't have to let them take over; be wary of eating out of resentment, anger, or rebellion; take a walk or do something interesting to take care of myself at that moment.

7. **When I'm tempted to do something else besides exercise, I plan to:**

   Think about how good exercise feels afterward; consider doing a different type of exercise (perhaps a class instead of using the elliptical machine); when I start thinking of other things to do, I'll remember that those are just thoughts and I don't have to act on them; remember, I just need to exercise.

8. **When I am tired and don't feel like exercising, I plan to:**

   See #7 comments; remember that when I exercise, I sleep better; give myself permission to exercise for less time while still getting my heart rate up.

Continues ▶

Figure 15.2 Plan for Coping with Difficult Situations (*continued*)

9. When I am feeling overwhelmed and stressed out, I plan to:

Talk to my spouse; go for a walk; meditate; schedule a massage; remind myself that stress will pass, and I'll be okay.

10. When I start getting down on myself, I plan to:

Think about my guiding principles and goals; think about the great things in my life, like my friends and family, my spouse, and my job; find something else to do, like reading a book, going for a walk, or planning meals.

11. When I am bored, I plan to:

Stay away from the fridge; find something to do, like go to a movie, read, go for a walk, plan a fun healthy meal to cook, buy a magazine, go to the library, clean up around the house, surf the net.

12. When I have a binge, I plan to:

Tell myself that slips can happen, and I must not be too hard on myself; try to understand what kind of stress preceded the binge so I can stop another such binge in the future.

13. Describe your own difficult situations and how you plan to cope with them?

My difficult situations are boredom, losing motivation, giving up, resentment, rebellion. When these occur, I plan to cope by using all the ways I mentioned above. I have to remember that I am an adult and I am in control of my actions. I must answer to myself for my heart health, my waistline, and my emotions. My actions are under my control. I'll remember the support systems that I have in my spouse and friends, and I'll talk to them when needed. I'll stay in touch with the values and guiding principles that give direction to my life.

eating pattern? What if family or friends are coming over for dinner? What if you are tempted to forgo your exercise session? How do you plan to expend calories in your ordinary, day-to-day activities?

Cognitive Distortions and Backsliding

Cognitive distortions, or misinterpretation biases, were discussed in chapter 11. You may want to go back and review these now. Cognitive distortions are almost always a factor when backsliding happens, and they contribute to ineffective coping in high-risk situations. Everyone misinterprets now and then and doing so

Figure 15.3 Plan for Coping with Difficult Situations

Instructions: On a sheet of paper, complete the following sentences by writing down as many ways to cope as you can conceive for each situation. Use additional paper as necessary. Be specific: what *thoughts* or *actions* would you take in each situation?

1. When I am hungry for something high in calories, instead of eating something unhealthy, I plan to: _____

2. If I have a slip, instead of giving up, I plan to: _____

3. When I go out to eat, I plan to: _____

4. When I'm out socializing and having a good time with friends, instead of giving myself permission to eat anything, I plan to: _____

5. When someone brings tempting food into work for all to share, I plan to: _____

6. When I'm feeling mad about having to cut calories or exercise, I plan to: _____

7. When I'm tempted to do something else besides exercise, I plan to: _____

8. When I am tired and don't feel like exercising, I plan to: _____

9. When I am feeling overwhelmed and stressed out, I plan to: _____

10. When I start getting down on myself, I plan to: _____

11. When I am bored, I plan to: _____

12. If I have a binge, I plan to: _____

13. Describe your own difficult situations and how you plan to cope with them?

    _____

—

is not cause for self-condemnation. Rather, learning to recognize when you make such errors in thinking and taking steps to reconcile them are important. Cognitive distortions can lead to faulty decision-making.

Faulty Decision-Making

Part of the thinking process involves making decisions about what something means or what to do. Sometimes the quality of decision-making is poor, further compounding the problem.

A faulty decision-making strategy known as *defensive avoidance* involves ignoring or denying the existence of a problem. A person who is using defensive avoidance may procrastinate and delay taking appropriate action. A defensive avoider tends to blame others for the problem, to construct wishful rationalizations that make it acceptable to choose a less difficult alternative, and to minimize probable consequences. The person who rationalizes having "just one" with the thought, "I might never have this again" is an example of faulty decision-making. Buying into such a thought leads directly to making poor choices.

Engaging in defensive avoidance often allows the problem to get worse until it can no longer be ignored, at which point panic may lead to yet another faulty decision-making strategy called *hypervigilance.* This strategy is characterized by searching frantically for a way out of a dilemma and impulsively seizing on whatever solution seems to promise immediate relief. An example of hypervigilance would be seeking a quick weight-loss diet when weight gain has become alarming.

A better approach to making decisions is to be sure you are in touch with what's really happening. Be on guard against tendencies to deny or distort feedback. Armed with a realistic view of things, you can decide, first, if there is a problem and then, second, what to do about it. Avoid trying to make big changes when you feel upset with your weight. Decide to make many small changes over time that will eventually lead you to adopt a healthy eating pattern.

A *vigilant* decision-maker takes care to obtain relevant and accurate information before making a decision, is careful not to distort the facts, and considers various alternatives before making a choice. This person is probably in either the Contemplation or Preparation stage of change mentioned in chapter 6. An example of vigilant decision-making is taking time to learn about gradual changes that will help you adopt a healthy eating pattern and deciding to make the changes as a result.

Change What Can Be Changed

Acceptance means changing, or trying to influence, what you can change, and accepting and working with that which cannot be changed. If you can't put it on a to-do list, you can't do anything effective to change a situation now. If you are having worry thoughts ("what if . . ."), this is a substitute for acting. If there is no effective action that can be taken, worry is not productive.

Consider the example of a woman who had lost 60 pounds the previous year, but now was having trouble maintaining her weight loss. She and her husband had started a new business, and money was tight. He was often upset, and he took out his irritation on his wife, blaming her for a variety of problems and criticizing her excessively. As if this weren't enough stress, their teenage son got involved with drugs and was having problems at school.

The constant stress of this woman's life was making it difficult for her to maintain her new eating behaviors. She was keeping up her exercise, which helped relieve tension and gave her a good excuse to get away from the issues at home, but once home, she would fall back into her old strategy for coping with stress—snacking. The context of her life was not supporting the maintenance of a healthy eating pattern and, indeed, was actively contributing to her return to old habits. An unsupportive context is a special kind of high-risk situation because it is ongoing.

What this woman had the power to do was to continue to exercise and accept that, right now, life was stressful. She needed to stop fighting her feelings. She didn't have to snack when she felt stressed; instead, it would have been better for her to spend ten minutes a day meditating to cope with the stress. Things were tough for her, and she needed to stay focused on her health values.

The Context of Your Life

A variety of things contribute to the context in which change and the maintenance of change take place. Other people in your life make up an important part of the context. The nature and quality of your interactions with them will influence your thinking, your emotions, and your behavior. Your economic situation is another part of the context that influences your ability to maintain change, as is the degree to which you must cope with personal or physical limitations, including addiction, biochemical dependence, genetics, physical handicaps, or the necessity of taking certain medications. Finally, your ability to produce the results you want and to avoid results you don't want is integral to the context of your life.

The context of your life can either contribute to backsliding or help ensure success. When the people in your life are supportive, when your relationships are nurturing (or at least not destructive), when you enjoy an adequate level of economic security, when you are not constrained by outside forces, and when you have abilities commensurate with your needs and goals, you are likely to have a context that supports change and the maintenance of change. Conversely, when the context of your life is not helping you maintain new behavior patterns, you need to take whatever steps you can to create a context that works to support and encourage the maintenance of change.

Creating a Context That Works

Influencing the context of your life so that it works may seem like a monumental task. Remember the woman mentioned previously who, together with her husband, had started a new business and was barely holding herself and her family together day-to-day. Even in this apparently dire situation, there were things she did that, over time, influenced and changed the context of her life. The following strategies can be used to change the context of your life:

1. **Learn to be more interpersonally effective.** To be more effective in interpersonal relationships, it is important to learn how to communicate assertively. It is also important to learn not to take things personally, especially other people's barbs and nastiness. For some people, it is helpful to enroll in programs specifically aimed at helping you to be more assertive or better able to manage conflict. Another good option is to seek therapy, either individual or couples counseling.

2. **Take action to change your environment.** One way to handle a difficult situation is to get out of it. When this is not a realistic option, it is important to identify the resources available to make the situation less noxious. One possibility is to seek the help of a therapist or a local crisis center. Your county mental health department and similar agencies—perhaps even your church—may be able to help. Often, churches can provide pastoral counseling. Once you begin asking for help, you are likely to find assistance sources you didn't know existed. If you think you might be in an abusive relationship, check the internet to learn what you need to do.

3. **Don't automatically buy into your limitations.** While it is important to consider your actual limitations, it is also important not to sell yourself short. It is probably unrealistic to think you will one day compete in the Olympics if you are older or severely overweight, but don't use being over 35 and severely overweight as an excuse for never being able to do something special, such as run a marathon.

   Challenge your preconceived limitations. You may not be as limited as you think; your "limitations" may be completely imaginary. Real limitations are part of your life's context; the limitations in your head come from thinking errors. Richard Bach wrote in his book *Illusions*, "Argue for your limitations, and sure enough they're yours." Take real limitations into account in your planning, but don't let them (or imagined limitations) keep you stuck in a problem.

4. **Use a problem-solving approach.** Occasionally, you may make a valiant effort and still not get the results you want. Perhaps you get no results at all, or you get results you hadn't expected. You might undertake the effort to adopt a healthy eating pattern only to discover that you are not losing weight right away. When something like this happens, give yourself time to learn to adopt healthy eating. Some people make small changes and expect big rewards. Your goal is to overhaul your present eating pattern to make it healthier at a pace you can maintain.

   Instead of throwing up your hands and giving up all efforts, take a problem-solving approach. Ask yourself, "What is the real problem here? Is it a failure on my part, or is it just taking longer than I expected?" Try to determine how your context may be working against you instead of assuming that the problem lies entirely with you. If necessary, get professional advice. Use a vigilant decision-making strategy to decide what to do next.

   Problem-solving involves identifying a problem and finding various solutions. You need only find the solution that is best for you. After gathering the facts, generate a number of possible solutions. Initially, don't try to decide which is "best." Only after you have identified several possible solutions, should you choose one to try. Try one solution and give it a chance to work. Then, if necessary, try another one, and another one, until you get the results you desire, or until you must go back to the beginning and reanalyze the problem.

5. **When necessary, make the best of a bad situation.** Some situations are bad and not amenable to change. One woman with three children and no job skills was married to a man who was alcoholic. With no family support, she did her best to protect the children from his drunken moods and give them as safe an environment as possible. She was able to get support by going to Al-Anon and enlisting the help of her pastor.

6. **Seek spiritual support.** Many people find support for coping with a difficult situation through a spiritual path. This may involve going to a church, synagogue, or mosque, or it may mean using meditation on a regular basis. Prayer is known to help people cope. Some people find spiritual succor from hiking in the wilderness.

Restoring Balance to Your Lifestyle

Your lifestyle can be another major cause of backsliding. A healthy lifestyle is one that has a relative degree of balance between the things you must do (that are potential sources of stress) and the things you want to do (that make life pleasant). An unbalanced lifestyle is characterized by too many "shoulds" and not enough "wants." When there is more work than play, and more obligations than rewards, energy is directed outward, leaving little time or energy for activities that give personal pleasure, satisfaction, or an inner sense of fulfillment.

If you have an unbalanced lifestyle, you may be attempting to cope with the attendant stress by engaging in one or more negative addictions—abusing alcohol, smoking cigarettes, drinking excessive amounts of caffeine, or overeating. Engaging in such behaviors is an attempt to restore balance and to nurture yourself, as well as an attempt to reduce the physical overstimulation that accompanies stress. When your lifestyle is unbalanced, you are likely to feel deprived, possibly with a periodic need for self-indulgence. The probability of backsliding is high unless you bring more balance into

Table 15.1 Negative Addictions

❖ Eating inappropriately—snacking, skipping meals, eating the wrong foods, overeating.

❖ Obsessing about food.

❖ Smoking tobacco and/or marijuana to relieve stress or obtain pleasure.

❖ Using alcohol to excess to cope with stress, tension, or unpleasant emotions.

❖ Using nonprescription drugs or abusing prescribed drugs to deal with stress.

❖ Sleeping too much—napping or dozing without need.

❖ Overcharging credit cards or otherwise spending beyond your means.

❖ Gambling, betting, playing cards, playing games such as Solitaire or Bingo to excess.

❖ Watching TV to excess.

❖ Playing computer games or surfing the internet to excess.

❖ Spending too much time on the computer at the cost of other activities.

your lifestyle by reducing obligations and/or increasing opportunities for reward and nurturing.

Stress in life can come from major life events, such as divorce, illness, loss of employment, the death of a loved one, or from ongoing daily hassles. Although large, traumatic life events can be the source of considerable stress, in terms of health—and long-term success in weight management—the ability to handle day-to-day stress is more important.

Replacing Negative Addictions with Positive Behaviors

To restore balance to an unbalanced lifestyle, begin with an assessment of your current ways of coping. What strategies do you use to cope with the hassles of daily life? Examine the negative addictions

Table 15.2 **Positive Behaviors**

❖ Eating a healthier diet.

❖ Engaging regularly in a well-rounded exercise program.

❖ Getting adequate relaxation and personal satisfaction by engaging in sufficient "want to" activities.

❖ Enjoying satisfying social contacts and engaging in interpersonal activities that provide a sense of acceptance and connectedness.

❖ Getting adequate satisfaction from your job or career.

❖ Having a life philosophy or spiritual grounding that provides guidance for life decisions.

❖ Engaging in a meditation practice.

❖ Having some friends or family you can talk to for comfort and pleasure.

listed in table 15.1 and identify which of these inappropriate ways of coping with stress apply to you.

Having identified your negative coping styles, decide how you will tackle and change them. Where will you begin? What kind of assistance will you need? What positive coping styles do you need to integrate into your life? A balanced lifestyle is characterized by positive behaviors such as those listed in table 15.2 and by having appropriate coping strategies.

Resources

American College of Cardiology. (2018). "Cover Story: Obesity and Cardiovascular Disease Risk. *Cardiology Magazine.* Published online July 23, 2018.

American College of Sports Medicine. (2010). *ACSM Guidelines for Exercise Testing and Prescription*, 7th ed., Philadelphia, PA: Lippincott, Williams, and Wilkins.

Apple, Robin. F., James Lock, and Rebecka Peebles. (2006). *Is Weight Loss Surgery Right for You?* New York: Oxford University Press.

Bach, Richard. (1977). *Illusions: The Adventures of a Reluctant Messiah.* New York: Delacorte Press.

Barnard, Neal. (2003). *Breaking the Food Seduction.* New York: St. Martin's Press.

Beck, Aaron T., John Rush, Brian F. Shaw, and Gary Emery. (1987). *Cognitive Therapy for Depression.* New York: The Guilford Press.

Beydoun, May A., Hind Beydoun, and Youfa Wang. (2008). Obesity and Central Obesity as Risk Factors for Incident Dementia and Its Subtypes: A Systematic Review." *Obesity Reviews* 9 (3): 201–18.

Boyle, Caitlin. (2010). *Operation Beautiful: Transforming Yourself One Post-It Note at a Time.* New York: Gotham.

Burns, David. (1999). *The Feeling Good Handbook.* New York: Plume.

Canning, Karissa L., Ruth E. Brown, Sean Wharton, Arya M. Sharma, and Jennifer L. Kuk. (2015). Edmonton Obesity Staging System Prevalence and Association with Weight Loss in a Publicly Funded Referral-Based Obesity Clinic. *Journal of Obesity.* Published online April 28, 2015, https://doi.org/10.1155/2015/619734.

Centers for Disease Control and Prevention. "Overweight and Obesity," accessed February 3, 2021, https://www.cdc.gov /obesity/index.html.

Deci, Edward. L., and Richard M. Ryan. (1985). *Intrinsic Motivation and Self-Determination in Human Behavior.* New York: Plenum.

DesMaisons, Kathleen. (2008). *Potatoes Not Prozac: Solutions for Sugar Sensitivity.* New York: Simon & Schuster.

Enright, Robert. D., and Richard P. Fitzgibbons. (2000). *Helping Clients Forgive: An Empirical Guide for Resolving Anger and Restoring Hope.* Washington, DC: American Psychological Association.

Filipovic, Jill. (2013). "The Way America Eats Is Killing Us." *The Guardian*, September 26, 2013.

Flegal, Katherine M., Deanna Kruszon-Moran, Margaret D. Carroll, Cheryl D. Fryar, and Cynthia L. Ogden. (2016). "Trends in Obesity Among Adults in the United States, 2005 to 2014." *The Journal of the American Medical Association* 315 (21): 2284–91.

Forsyth, John P., and Georg H. Eifert. (2007). *The Mindfulness and Acceptance Workbook for Anxiety.* Oakland, CA: New Harbinger.

Fradkin, Andrea J., Tsharni R. Zazryn, and James M. Smoliga. (2010). "Effects of Warming-Up on Physical Performance: A

Systematic Review with Meta-Analysis." *Journal of Strength and Conditioning Research* 24 (1): 140–48.

Fryar, Cheryl D., Margaret D. Carroll, and Cynthia L. Ogden. (2016). "Prevalence of Overweight, Obesity, and Extreme Obesity Among Adults Aged 20 and Over: United States, 1960–1962 Through 2011–2014." National Center for Health Statistics Data, Health E-Stats, accessed February 1, 2021, https://www.cdc.gov /nchs/data/hestat/obesity_adult_13_14/obesity_adult_13_14.htm

Gordon, Tavia, Marian Fisher, Nancy Ernst, and Basil M. Rifkind. (1982). "Relation of Diet to LDL Cholesterol, VLDL Cholesterol, and Plasma Total Cholesterol and Triglycerides in White Adults: The Lipid Research Clinics Prevalence Study." *Atherosclerosis* 2 (6): 502–12.

Gross, Stanley J. (2004). *Pathways to Lasting Self-Esteem.* Bloomington, IN: Author House.

Han, Thang S., and Mike E. J. Lean. (2016). "A Clinical Perspective of Obesity, Metabolic Syndrome and Cardiovascular Disease." *JRSM Cardiovascular Disease.* First published online March 3, 2016, https://doi.org/10.1177/2048004016633371.

Hayes, Steven C., Dirk D. Strosahl, and Kelly G. Wilson. (1999). *Acceptance and Commitment Therapy: An Experiential Approach to Behavior Change.* New York: Guilford.

Hill, James O., John C. Peters, and Bonnie T. Jortberg. (2004). *The Step Diet Book: Count Steps, Not Calories, to Lose Weight and Keep It Off Forever.* New York: Workman.

Hyoung-Kil, Park, Min-Kyung Jung, E. Park, C. Lee, Yongseok Jee, Denny Eun, Jun-Youl Cha, and Jaehyun Yoo. (2018). "The Effect of Warm-Ups with Stretching on the Isokinetic Moments of Collegiate Men." *Journal of Exercise Rehabilitation* 14 (1): 78–82.

Kabat-Zinn, Jon. (1990). *Full Catastrophe Living.* New York: Bantam Books.

Kearns, Karen, Anne Dee, Anthony P. Fitzgerald, Edel Doherty, and Ivan J. Perry. (2014). "Chronic Disease Burden Associated with Overweight and Obesity in Ireland: The Effects of a Small BMI Reduction at Population Level." *BMC Public Health* 14: 143. Published online February 10, 2014, https://doi .org/10.1186/1471-2458-14-143.

Khazan, Olga. (2015). "The Second Assault." *The Atlantic*, December 15, https://www.theatlantic.com/health/archive/2015 /12/sexual-abuse-victims-obesity/420186/.

Lazarus, Richard S., and Susan Folkman. (1984). *Stress, Appraisal, and Coping.* New York: Springer.

LeVitus, Bob. (2010). *Incredible iPhone Apps for Dummies.* Hoboken, NJ: Wiley.

Locke, Edwin A., and Gary P. Latham. (1990). *A Theory of Goal Setting and Task Performance.* Englewood Cliffs, NJ: Prentice Hall.

Lee, Jane J., Alison Pedley, Udo Hoffmann, Joseph M. Massaro, and Caroline S. Fox. (2016). "Association of Changes in Abdominal Fat Quality and Quantity with Incident Cardiovascular Disease Risk Factors." *Journal of the American College of Cardiology* 68 (14): 1509–21.

Leech, Joe. (2017). "Good Fiber, Bad Fiber—How the Different Types Affect You." *Healthline.* https://www.healthline.com /nutrition/different-types-of-fiber.

Linehan, Marsha. (1993). *Skills Training Manual for Treating Borderline Personality Disorder.* New York: The Guilford Press.

Lore, Mary. (2008). *Managing Thought: How Do Your Thoughts Rule Your World?* Northville, MI: Ferne Press.

Luoma, Jason B., Steven C. Hayes, and Robyn D. Walser. (2017). *Learning ACT: An Acceptance and Commitment Therapy Skills Training Manual for Therapists.* Oakland, CA: New Harbinger.

Luskin, Frederic. (2002). *Forgive for Good: A Proven Prescription for Health and Happiness.* New York: HarperSanFrancisco.

Marlatt, G. Alan, and Dennis M. Donovan. (2005). *Relapse Prevention*, 2nd ed. New York: The Guilford Press.

Mayo Clinic Staff. (2019). "Nutrition and Healthy Eating." *Mayo Clinic Foundation for Medical Education and Research.* MayoClinic.org.

MedlinePlus. "Cholesterol Levels, What You Need to Know." *National Heart, Lung and Blood Institute*, https://medlineplus.gov /cholesterollevelswhatyouneedtoknow.html.

McCarthy, William J., and Tony Kuo. (2009). "Support for Benefit of Physical Activity on Satiety, Weight Control, and Diabetes Risk." *Archives of Internal Medicine* 169 (6): 635.

Monterio, Rosário, and Isabel Azevedo. (2010). "Chronic Inflammation in Obesity and the Metabolic Syndrome." *Mediators of Inflammation.* Published online July 14, 2010, https://doi.org/10.1155/2010/289645.

National Center for Health Statistics. 2017. "National Health and Nutrition Examination Survey (2014–2015)," https://www.cdc .gov/nchs/data/factsheets/factsheet_nhanes.htm.

Nash, Joyce D. (1993). *Self-Talk of Dieters and Maintainers: States of Mind, Stimulus Situations, Binge Eating, Weight Cycling, and Severity of Weight Problem.* PhD diss., Palo Alto University.

Nash, Joyce D. (1999). *Binge No More: Your Guide to Overcoming Disordered Eating.* Oakland, CA: New Harbinger.

Padwal, Raj S., Nicholas M. Pajewski, David B. Allison, and Arya M. Sharma. (2011). "Using the Edmonton Obesity Staging System to Predict Mortality in a Population-Representative Cohort of People with Overweight and Obesity. *Canadian Medical Association Journal* 183 (14): e1059–66.

Paeratakul, S., Jennifer Lovejoy, Donna H. Ryan, and George Bray. (2002). "The Relation of Gender, Race and Socioeconomic

Status to Obesity and Obesity Comorbidities in a Sample of US Adults." *International Journal of Obesity and Related Metabolic Disorders* 26 (9): 1205–10

Palmer, Sharon. (2010). "Normal Weight but Obese." *Environmental Nutrition* 33 (9): 2.

Peeke, Pamela. (2005). *Body-for-LIFE for Women: A Woman's Plan for Physical and Mental Transformation.* Emmaus, PA: Rodale.

Peterson, Christopher, Steven F. Maier, and Martin E. P. Seligman. (1993). *Learned Helplessness: A Theory for the Age of Personal Control.* New York: Oxford University Press.

Roemer, Lizbeth, and Susan M. Orsillo. (2009). *Mindfulness- and Acceptance-Based Behavioral Therapies in Practice.* New York: Guilford.

Segal, Zindel, Mark Williams, and John Teasdale. (2013) *Mindfulness-Based Cognitive Therapy for Depression.* NY: Guilford.

Sasson, Remez. "The Inner Dialogue." Success Conciousness, www.successconsciousness.com/index_00002b.htm.

Seligman, Martin E. P. (2006). *Learned Optimism: How to Change Your Mind and Your Life.* New York: Vintage Books.

Sharma, Arya M. (2009). "Edmonton Obesity Staging System." *Dr. Sharma's Obesity Notes*, blog dated February 11.

Shiel Jr., William C. (2018) "Medical Definition of Trans Fat." MedicineNet. https://www.medicinenet.com/script/main/art.asp?articlekey=11091.

Sparks, Dana. (May 24, 2018). Trans Fat Is Double Trouble for Your Heart. *Mayo Clinic.* https://newsnetwork.mayoclinic.org/discussion/transfat-is-double-trouble-for-your-heart-health/.

Stone, Hal, and Sidra L. Stone. (1989). *Embracing Ourselves: The Voice Dialogue Manual.* Novato, CA: New World Library.

Trouwborst, Inez, Suzanne M. Browser, Gijs H. Goossens, and Ellen E. Blaak. (2018). "Ectopic Fat Accumulation in Distinct Insulin Resistant Phenotypes; Targets for Personalized Nutritional Interventions." *Frontiers in Nutrition* 5 (77).

US Department of Health and Human Services. "Dietary Guidelines for Americans, 2015–2020," accessed February 3, 2021, https:// health.gov/our-work/food-nutrition/previous-dietary -guidelines/2015.

Willett, Walter C. (2001). *Eat, Drink, and Be Healthy: The Harvard Medical School Guide to Healthy Eating.* New York: Simon & Schuster.

Zitek, Emily, Alexander H. Jordan, Benoît Monin, and Frederick R. Leach. (2010). "Victim Entitlement to Behave Selfishly." *Journal of Personality and Social Psychology* 98: 245–55.

Index

Note: Page numbers followed by *f* or *t* indicate a figure or table on
the designated page